Pocket Guide to
Diagnostic
Tests

third edition

Diana Nicoll, MD, PhD, MPA
Clinical Professor and Vice Chair
Department of Laboratory Medicine
University of California, San Francisco
Associate Dean
University of California, San Francisco
Chief of Staff and Chief, Laboratory Medicine Service
Veterans Affairs Medical Center, San Francisco

Stephen J. McPhee, MD
Professor of Medicine
Division of General Internal Medicine
University of California, San Francisco

Michael Pignone, MD, MPH
Assistant Professor of Medicine
University of North Carolina, Chapel Hill

William M. Detmer, MD, MS
Assistant Clinical Professor of Medicine
Department of Health Evaluation Sciences
University of Virginia, Charlottesville

Tony M. Chou, MD
Assistant Clinical Professor of Medicine
University of California, San Francisco

With Associate Authors

Lange Medical Books/McGraw-Hill
Medical Publishing Division

New York St. Louis San Francisco Auckland Bogotá Caracas
Lisbon London Madrid Mexico City Milan Montreal New Delhi
San Juan Singapore Sydney Tokyo Toronto

McGraw-Hill

A Division of The McGraw·Hill Companies

Pocket Guide to Diagnostic Tests, Third Edition

1 2 3 4 5 6 7 8 9 0   DOC/DOC   0 9 8 7 6 5 4 3 2 1 0

ISBN: 0-8385-8135-8 (domestic)
ISSN:1061-3463

Notice

Medicine is an ever-changing science. As new research and clinical experience broaden our knowledge, changes in treatment and drug therapy are required. The authors and the publisher of this work have checked with sources believed to be reliable in their efforts to provide information that is complete and generally in accord with the standards accepted at the time of publication. However, in view of the possibility of human error or changes in medical sciences, neither the authors nor the publisher nor any other party who has been involved in the preparation or publication of this work warrants that the information contained herein is in every respect accurate or complete, and they disclaim all responsibility for any errors or omissions or for the results obtained from use of the information contained in this work. Readers are encouraged to confirm the information contained herein with other sources. For example and in particular, readers are advised to check the product information sheet included in the package of each drug they plan to administer to be certain that the information contained in this work is accurate and that changes have not been made in the recommended dose or in the contraindications for administration. This recommendation is of particular importance in connection with new or infrequently used drugs.

This book was set in Times Roman by Circle Graphics.
The editors were Shelley Reinhardt, Isabel Nogueira, and Curt Berkowitz.
The production supervisor was Minal Bopaiah.
The cover designer was Mary Skudlarek.
The art manager was Charissa Baker.
R. R. Donnelley & Sons was the printer and binder.

This book was printed on acid-free paper.

Contents

Associate Authors

G. Thomas Evans, Jr., MD
Associate Clinical Professor of Medicine
University of California, San Francisco
Director of Electrocardiography
Moffit-Long Hospitals, San Francisco
Basic Electrocardiography

Sean Perini, MD
Clinical Fellow
Section of Interventional Radiology
Department of Radiology
University of California, San Francisco
Diagnostic Testing: Algorithms, Nomograms, and Tables

Susan D. Wall, MD
Professor of Radiology and Assistant Chief
Department of Radiology
Veterans Affairs Medical Center, San Francisco
Associate Dean, Graduate Medical Education
University of California, San Francisco
Diagnostic Imaging: Test Selection and Interpretation

Mary K. York, PhD
Clinical Professor of Laboratory Medicine
University of California, San Francisco
Microbiology: Test Selection

Preface

Purpose

Pocket Guide to Diagnostic Tests is intended to serve as a pocket reference manual for medical and other health professional students, house officers, and practicing physicians. It is a quick reference guide to the selection and interpretation of commonly used diagnostic tests, including laboratory procedures in the clinical setting, laboratory tests (chemistry, hematology, and immunology), microbiology tests (bacteriology, virology, and serology), diagnostic imaging tests (plain radiography, CT, MRI, and ultrasonography), and electrocardiography.

This book will enable readers to understand commonly used diagnostic tests and diagnostic approaches to common disease states.

Outstanding Features

- Over 350 tests are presented in a concise, consistent, and readable format.
- Fields covered include internal medicine, pediatrics, general surgery, neurology, and gynecology.
- Costs and risks of various procedures and tests are emphasized.
- Literature references are included for most diagnostic tests.
- An index for quick reference is included on the back cover.

Organization

This pocket reference manual is not intended to include all diagnostic tests or disease states. Rather, the authors have selected those tests and diseases that are most common and relevant to the general practice of medicine.

The *Guide* is divided into eight sections:

1. Basic Principles of Diagnostic Test Use and Interpretation
2. Laboratory Procedures in the Clinical Setting
3. Common Laboratory Tests: Selection and Interpretation
4. Therapeutic Drug Monitoring: Principles and Test Interpretation
5. Microbiology: Test Selection
6. Diagnostic Imaging: Test Selection and Interpretation
7. Basic Electrocardiography
8. Diagnostic Testing: Algorithms, Nomograms, and Tables

Intended Audience

In this era of rapidly changing medical technology, many new diagnostic tests are being introduced every year and are replacing older tests as they are shown to be more sensitive, specific, or cost-effective.

In this environment, students, house officers, and practicing physicians are looking for a pocket reference on diagnostic tests.

Medical students will find the concise summary of diagnostic laboratory, microbiologic, and imaging studies, and of electrocardiography in this pocket-sized book of great help during clinical ward rotations.

Busy house officers will find the clear organization and citations to the current literature useful in devising proper patient management.

Practitioners (internists, family physicians, pediatricians, surgeons, and other specialists who provide generalist care) may use the *Guide* as a refresher manual to update their understanding of laboratory tests and diagnostic approaches.

Nurses and other health practitioners will find the format and scope of the *Guide* valuable for understanding the use of laboratory tests in patient management.

In 1998, the contents of this book were integrated with the contents of *Pocket Guide to Commonly Prescribed Drugs,* 2nd ed., by Glenn N. Levine, MD, in a new CD-ROM, *Current Medical Diagnosis & Treatment 1998 on CD-ROM.* An updated version of the CD-ROM, including this book, will be published in 2000.

Acknowledgments

We wish to thank our associate authors for their contributions to this book. In addition, we are grateful to the many physicians, residents, and students who contributed useful suggestions and to Jim Ransom for his careful editing of the manuscript.

We welcome comments and recommendations from our readers for future editions.

Diana Nicoll, MD, PhD, MPA
Stephen J. McPhee, MD
Michael Pignone, MD, MPH
William M. Detmer, MD, MS
Tony M. Chou, MD

San Francisco
September 2000

1

Basic Principles of Diagnostic Test Use and Interpretation[*]

Diana Nicoll, MD, PhD, and Michael Pignone, MD, MPH

The clinician's main task is to make reasoned decisions about patient care despite incomplete clinical information and uncertainty about clinical outcomes. While data elicited from the history and physical examination are often sufficient for making a diagnosis or for guiding therapy, more information may be required. In these situations, clinicians often turn to diagnostic tests for help.

BENEFITS; COSTS, AND RISKS

When used appropriately, diagnostic tests can be of great assistance to the clinician. Tests can be helpful for **screening,** ie, to identify risk factors for disease and to detect occult disease in asymptomatic persons. Identification of risk factors may allow early intervention to prevent disease occurrence, and early detection of occult disease may reduce

---

[*]Chapter modified, with permission, from Tierney LM Jr, McPhee SJ, Papadakis MA (editors): *Current Medical Diagnosis & Treatment 2000.* McGraw-Hill, 2000.

disease morbidity and mortality through early treatment. Optimal screening tests meet the criteria listed in Table 1–1.

Tests can also be helpful for **diagnosis,** ie, to help establish or exclude the presence of disease in symptomatic persons. Some tests assist in early diagnosis after onset of symptoms and signs; others assist in differential diagnosis of various possible diseases; others help determine the stage or activity of disease.

Finally, tests can be helpful in **patient management.** Tests can help (1) evaluate the severity of disease, (2) estimate prognosis, (3) monitor the course of disease (progression, stability, or resolution), (4) detect disease recurrence, and (5) select drugs and adjust therapy.

When ordering diagnostic tests, clinicians should weigh the potential benefits against the potential costs and disadvantages:

(1) Some tests carry a risk of morbidity or mortality—eg, cerebral angiogram leads to stroke in 1% of cases.

(2) The discomfort associated with tests such as sigmoidoscopy or barium enema will deter some patients from completing a diagnostic work-up.

(3) The result of a diagnostic test often has implications for further care in that a test result may mandate further testing or frequent follow-up. This means that a patient with a positive fecal occult blood test may incur significant cost, risk, and discomfort during follow-up sigmoidoscopy, barium enema, or colonoscopy.

(4) A false-positive test may lead to further unnecessary testing. Classifying a healthy patient as diseased based on a falsely positive diagnostic test can cause psychologic distress and may lead to risks from unnecessary therapy.

TABLE 1–1. CRITERIA FOR USE OF SCREENING PROCEDURES.

Characteristics of population
1. Sufficiently high prevalence of disease.
2. Likely to be compliant with subsequent tests and treatments.
Characteristics of disease
1. Significant morbidity and mortality.
2. Effective and acceptable treatment available.
3. Presymptomatic period detectable.
4. Improved outcome from early treatment.
Characteristics of test
1. Good sensitivity and specificity.
2. Low cost and risk.
3. Confirmatory test available and practical.

(5) A diagnostic or screening test may identify cases of disease that would not otherwise have been recognized and that would not have affected the patient. For example, early-stage, low-grade prostate cancer detected by PSA screening in an 84-year-old man with known severe congestive heart failure will probably not become symptomatic or require treatment during his lifetime.

(6) An individual test such as MRI of the head can cost more than $1400, and diagnostic tests as a whole account for approximately one-fifth of health care expenditures in the USA.

PERFORMANCE OF DIAGNOSTIC TESTS

Factors affecting both the patient and the specimen are important. The most crucial element in a properly conducted laboratory test is an appropriate specimen.

Patient Preparation

Preparation of the patient is important for certain tests—eg, a fasting state is needed for optimal glucose and triglyceride measurements; posture and sodium intake must be strictly controlled when measuring renin and aldosterone levels; and strenuous exercise should be avoided before taking samples for creatine kinase determinations, since vigorous muscle activity can lead to falsely abnormal results.

Specimen Collection

Careful attention must be paid to patient identification and specimen labeling. Knowing when the specimen was collected may be important. For instance, aminoglycoside levels cannot be interpreted appropriately without knowing whether the specimen was drawn just before ("trough" level) or after ("peak" level) drug administration. Drug levels cannot be interpreted if they are drawn during the drug's distribution phase (eg, digoxin levels drawn during the first 6 hours after an oral dose). Substances that have a circadian variation (eg, cortisol) can be interpreted only in the context of the time of day the sample was drawn.

During specimen collection, other principles should be remembered. Specimens should not be drawn above an intravenous line, as this may contaminate the sample with intravenous fluid. Excessive tourniquet time will lead to hemoconcentration and an increased concentration of protein-bound substances such as calcium. Lysis of cells during collection of a blood specimen will result in spuriously increased serum levels of substances concentrated in cells (eg, lactate dehydrogenase and potassium). Certain test specimens may require special handling or storage (eg, blood gas specimens). Delay in delivery of specimens to the laboratory can result in ongoing cellular metabolism and therefore spurious results for some studies (eg, low blood glucose).

TEST CHARACTERISTICS

Table 1–2 lists the general characteristics of useful diagnostic tests. Most of the principles detailed below can be applied not only to laboratory and radiologic tests but also to elements of the history and physical examination.

Accuracy

The accuracy of a laboratory test is its correspondence with the true value. An inaccurate test is one that differs from the true value even though the results may be reproducible (Figures 1–1A and 1–1B). In the clinical laboratory, accuracy of tests is maximized by calibrating laboratory equipment with reference material and by participation in external quality control programs.

Precision

Test precision is a measure of a test's reproducibility when repeated on the same sample. An imprecise test is one that yields widely varying results on repeated measurements (Figure 1–1B). The precision of diagnostic tests, which is monitored in clinical laboratories by using control material, must be good enough to distinguish clinically relevant changes in a patient's status from the analytic variability of the test. For instance, the manual white blood cell differential count is not precise

TABLE 1–2. PROPERTIES OF USEFUL DIAGNOSTIC TESTS.

1. Test methodology has been described in detail so that it can be accurately and reliably reproduced.
2. Test accuracy and precision have been determined.
3. The reference range has been established appropriately.
4. Sensitivity and specificity have been reliably established by comparison with a gold standard. The evaluation has used a range of patients, including those who have different but commonly confused disorders and those with a spectrum of mild and severe, treated and untreated disease. The patient selection process has been adequately described so that results will not be generalized inappropriately.
5. Independent contribution to overall performance of a test panel has been confirmed if a test is advocated as part of a panel of tests.

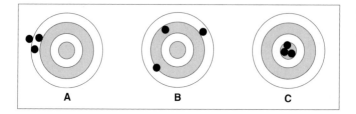

Figure 1–1. Relationship between accuracy and precision in diagnostic tests. The center of the target represents the true value of the substance being tested. Figure **(A)** represents a diagnostic test which is precise but inaccurate; on repeated measurement, the test yields very similar results, but all results are far from the true value. Figure **(B)** shows a test which is imprecise and inaccurate; repeated measurement yields widely different results, and the results are far from the true value. Figure **(C)** shows an ideal test, one that is both precise and accurate.

enough to detect important changes in the distribution of cell types, because it is calculated by subjective evaluation of a small sample (100 cells). Repeated measurements by different technicians on the same sample result in widely different results. Automated differential counts are more precise because they are obtained from machines that use objective physical characteristics to classify a much larger sample (10,000 cells).

Reference Range

Reference ranges are method- and laboratory-specific. In practice, they often represent test results found in 95% of a small population presumed to be healthy; by definition, then, 5% of healthy patients will have a positive (abnormal) test (Figure 1–2). As a result, slightly abnormal results should be interpreted critically—they may be either truly abnormal or falsely abnormal. The practitioner should be aware also that the more tests ordered, the greater the chance of obtaining a falsely abnormal result. For a healthy person subjected to 20 independent tests, there is a 64% chance that one test result will lie outside the reference range (Table 1–3). Conversely, values within the reference range may not rule out the actual presence of disease since the reference range does not establish the distribution of results in patients with disease.

It is important to consider also whether published reference ranges are appropriate for the patient being evaluated, since some ranges depend on age, sex, weight, diet, time of day, activity status, or posture. For instance, the reference ranges for hemoglobin concentration are age-

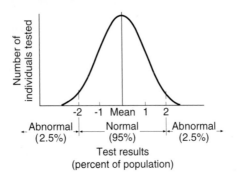

Figure 1–2. The reference range is usually defined as within 2 standard deviations of the mean test result (shown as –2 and 2) in a small population of healthy volunteers. Note that in this example, test results are normally distributed; however, many biologic substances will have distributions that are skewed.

and sex-dependent. Chapter 3 contains the reference ranges for commonly used chemistry and hematology tests. Test performance characteristics such as sensitivity and specificity are needed to interpret results and are discussed below.

Interfering Factors

The results of diagnostic tests can be altered by external factors, such as ingestion of drugs; and internal factors, such as abnormal physiologic states.

External interferences can affect test results in vivo or in vitro. In vivo, alcohol increases γ-glutamyl transpeptidase, and diuretics can affect

TABLE 1–3. RELATIONSHIP BETWEEN THE NUMBER OF TESTS AND THE PROBABILITY THAT A HEALTHY PERSON WILL HAVE ONE OR MORE ABNORMAL RESULTS.

Number of Tests	Probability That One or More Results Will Be Abnormal
1	5%
6	26%
12	46%
20	64%

sodium and potassium concentrations. Cigarette smoking can induce hepatic enzymes and thus reduce levels of substances such as theophylline that are metabolized by the liver. In vitro, cephalosporins may produce spurious serum creatinine levels due to interference with a common laboratory method.

Internal interferences result from abnormal physiologic states interfering with the test measurement. As an example, patients with gross lipemia may have spuriously low serum sodium levels if the test methodology used includes a step in which serum is diluted before sodium is measured. Because of the potential for test interference, clinicians should be wary of unexpected test results and should investigate reasons other than disease that may explain abnormal results, including laboratory error.

Sensitivity and Specificity

Clinicians should use measures of test performance such as sensitivity and specificity to judge the quality of a diagnostic test for a particular disease. Test **sensitivity** is the likelihood that a diseased patient has a positive test. If all patients with a given disease have a positive test (ie, no diseased patients have negative tests), the test sensitivity is 100%. A test with high sensitivity is useful to exclude a diagnosis because a highly sensitive test will render few results that are falsely negative. To exclude infection with the AIDS virus, for instance, a clinician might choose a highly sensitive test such as the HIV antibody test.

A test's **specificity** is the likelihood that a healthy patient has a negative test. If all patients who do not have a given disease have negative tests (ie, no healthy patients have positive tests), the test specificity is 100%. A test with high specificity is useful to confirm a diagnosis, because a highly specific test will have few results that are falsely positive. For instance, to make the diagnosis of gouty arthritis, a clinician might choose a highly specific test, such as the presence of negatively birefringent needle-shaped crystals within leukocytes on microscopic evaluation of joint fluid.

To determine test sensitivity and specificity for a particular disease, the test must be compared against a "gold standard," a procedure that defines the true disease state of the patient. For instance, the sensitivity and specificity of the ventilation/perfusion scan for pulmonary embolus are obtained by comparing the results of scans with the gold standard, pulmonary arteriography. Application of the gold standard examination to patients with positive scans establishes specificity. Failure to apply the gold standard examination following negative scans may result in an overestimation of sensitivity, since false negatives will not be identified. However, for many disease states (eg, pancreatitis), such a gold standard either does not exist or is very difficult or expensive to apply. Therefore, reliable estimates of test sensitivity and specificity are sometimes difficult to obtain.

Sensitivity and specificity can also be affected by the population from which these values are derived. For instance, many diagnostic tests are evaluated first using patients who have severe disease and control groups who are young and well. Compared with the general population, this study group will have more results that are truly positive (because patients have more advanced disease) and more results that are truly negative (because the control group is healthy). Thus, test sensitivity and specificity will be higher than would be expected in the general population, where more of a spectrum of health and disease are found. Clinicians should be aware of this **spectrum bias** when generalizing published test results to their own practice.

Test sensitivity and specificity depend on the threshold above which a test is interpreted to be abnormal (Figure 1–3). If the threshold is lowered, sensitivity is increased at the expense of lowered specificity, or vice versa.

Figure 1–4 shows how test sensitivity and specificity can be calculated using test results from patients previously classified by the gold standard as diseased or nondiseased.

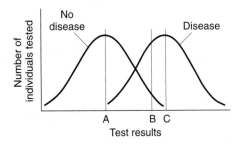

Figure 1–3. Hypothetical distribution of test results for healthy and diseased individuals. The position of the "cutoff point" between "normal" and "abnormal" (or "negative" and "positive") test results determines the test's sensitivity and specificity. If point "A" is the cutoff point, the test would have 100% sensitivity but low specificity. If point "C" is the cutoff point, the test would have 100% specificity but low sensitivity. For most tests, the cutoff point is determined by the reference range, ie, the range of test results that are within 2 standard deviations of the mean (point "B"). In some situations, the cutoff is altered to enhance either sensitivity or specificity.

Figure 1–4. Calculation of sensitivity, specificity, and probability of disease after a positive test (posttest probability). (TP, true positive; FP, false positive; FN, false negative; TN, true negative.)

The performance of two different tests can be compared by plotting the sensitivity and (1 minus the specificity) of each test at various reference range cutoff values. The resulting **receiver operator characteristic (ROC) curve** will often show which test is better; a clearly superior test will have an ROC curve that always lies above and to the left of the inferior test curve, and, in general, the better test will have a larger area under the ROC curve. For instance, Figure 1–5 shows the ROC curves for prostate-specific antigen (PSA) and prostatic acid phosphatase (PAP) in the diagnosis of prostate cancer. PSA is a superior test because it has higher sensitivity and specificity for all cutoff values.

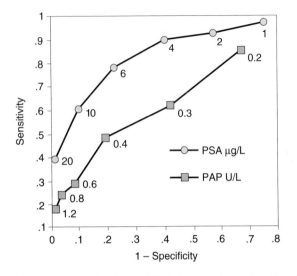

Figure 1–5. Receiver operator characteristic (ROC) curves for prostate-specific antigen (PSA) and prostatic acid phosphatase (PAP) in the diagnosis of prostate cancer. For all cutoff values, PSA has higher sensitivity and specificity; therefore, it is a better test based on these performance characteristics. *(Modified and reproduced, with permission, from Nicoll D et al: Routine acid phosphatase testing for screening and monitoring prostate cancer no longer justified. Clin Chem 1993;39:2540.)*

USE OF TESTS IN DIAGNOSIS AND MANAGEMENT

The value of a test in a particular clinical situation depends not only on the test's sensitivity and specificity but also on the probability that the patient has the disease before the test result is known **(pretest probability).** The results of a valuable test will substantially change the probability that the patient has the disease **(posttest probability).** Figure 1–4 shows how posttest probability can be calculated from the known sensitivity and specificity of the test and the estimated pretest probability of disease (or disease prevalence).

The pretest probability of disease has a profound effect on the posttest probability of disease. As demonstrated in Table 1–4, when a test with 90% sensitivity and specificity is used, the posttest probability can vary from 1% to 99% depending on the pretest probability of disease. Furthermore, as the pretest probability of disease decreases, it becomes less likely that someone with a positive test actually has the disease and more likely that the result represents a false positive.

TABLE 1–4. INFLUENCE OF PRETEST PROBABILITY ON THE POSTTEST PROBABILITY OF DISEASE WHEN A TEST WITH 90% SENSITIVITY AND 90% SPECIFICITY IS USED.

Pretest Probability	Posttest Probability
0.01	0.08
0.50	0.90
0.99	0.999

As an example, suppose the clinician wishes to calculate the posttest probability of prostate cancer using the PSA test and a cut-off value of 4 ng/mL. Using the data shown in Figure 1–5, sensitivity is 90% and specificity is 60%. The clinician estimates the pretest probability of disease given all the evidence and then calculates the posttest probability using the approach shown in Figure 1–5. The pretest probability that an otherwise healthy 50-year-old man has prostate cancer is equal to the prevalence of prostate cancer in that age group (probability = 10%) and the posttest probability is only 20%—ie, even though the test is positive, there is still an 80% chance that the patient does not have prostate cancer (Figure 1–6A). If the clinician finds a prostate nodule on rectal examination, the pretest probability of prostate cancer rises to 50% and the posttest probability using the same test is 69% (Figure 1–6B). Finally, if the clinician estimates the pretest probability to be 98% based on a prostate nodule, bone pain, and lytic lesions on spine x-rays, the posttest probability using PSA is 99% (Figure 1–6C). This example illustrates that pretest probability has a profound effect on posttest probability and that tests provide more information when the diagnosis is truly uncertain (pretest probability about 50%) than when the diagnosis is either unlikely or nearly certain.

ODDS-LIKELIHOOD RATIOS

An easier way to calculate the posttest probability of disease is to use the odds-likelihood approach. Sensitivity and specificity are combined into one entity called the likelihood ratio (LR).

$$LR = \frac{\text{Probability of result in diseased persons}}{\text{Probability of result in nondiseased persons}}$$

Every test has two likelihood ratios, one corresponding to a positive test (LR^+) and one corresponding to a negative test (LR^-):

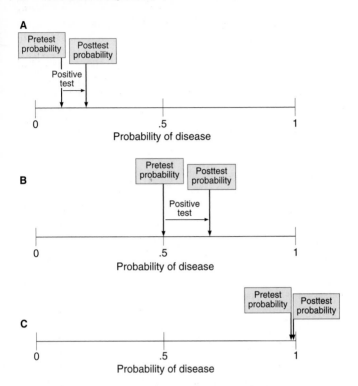

Figure 1–6. Effect of pretest probability and test sensitivity and specificity on the posttest probability of disease. (See text for explanation.)

$$LR^+ = \frac{\text{Probability that test is positive in diseased persons}}{\text{Probability that test is positive in nondiseased persons}}$$

$$= \frac{\text{Sensitivity}}{1 - \text{Specificity}}$$

$$LR^- = \frac{\text{Probability that test is negative in diseased persons}}{\text{Probability that test is negative in nondiseased persons}}$$

$$= \frac{1 - \text{Sensitivity}}{\text{Specificity}}$$

Lists of likelihood ratios can be found in some textbooks, journal articles, and computer programs (see Table 1–5 for sample values). Likelihood ratios can be used to make quick estimates of the usefulness of a contemplated diagnostic test in a particular situation. The simplest method for calculating posttest probability from pretest probability and likelihood ratios is to use a nomogram (Figure 1–7). The clinician places a straightedge through the points that represent the pretest probability and the likelihood ratio and then reads the posttest probability where the straightedge crosses the posttest probability line.

TABLE 1–5. LIKELIHOOD RATIOS (LR) FOR DIAGNOSTIC TESTS.

Test	Disease	LR+	LR−
Amylase (↑)	Pancreatitis	9.1	0.2
Anti-dsDNA (↑)	SLE	37	0.28
Antinuclear antibody	SLE	4.5	0.13
Carcinoembryonic antigen	Dukes A colon cancer	1.6	0.87
Creatine kinase MB	Myocardial infarction	32	0.05
Esophagogastroduodenoscopy (+)	Upper GI bleeding	18	0.11
ESR > 30 mm/h	Temporal arteritis	3.3	0.01
Exercise echocardiography (new wall motion abnormalities)	Coronary artery disease	6.2	0.23
Exercise ECG (ST depression > 1 mm)	Coronary artery disease	5.9	0.39
Ferritin	Iron deficiency anemia	85	0.15
Free T$_4$ (↑)	Hyperthyroidism	19	0.05
Free thyroxine index	Hyperthyroidism	6.8	0.06
Hepatitis A IgM antibody	Hepatitis A	99	0.01
Heterophil (+)	Infectious mononucleosis	97	0.03
Metanephrines (↑)	Pheochromocytoma	11	0.23
Pleural fluid protein > 3 g/dL	Exudative pleural effusion	10	0.12
Technetium Tc 99m pyrophosphate scan (highly focal uptake)	Myocardial infarction	> 360	0.64
Testosterone (↓)	Erectile dysfunction	32	0.03
TSH (↑)	Hypothyroidism	99	0.01
24-Hour urinary free cortisol (↑)	Hypercortisolism	10	0.07

Figure 1–7. Nomogram for determining posttest probability from pretest probability and likelihood ratios. To figure the posttest probability, place a straightedge between the pretest probability and the likelihood ratio for the particular test. The posttest probability will be where the straightedge crosses the posttest probability line. *(Adapted and reproduced, with permission, from Fagan TJ: Nomogram for Bayes's theorem. N Engl J Med 1975;293:257.)*

A more formal way of calculating posttest probabilities uses the likelihood ratio as follows:

$$\text{Pretest odds} \times \text{Likelihood ratio} = \text{Posttest odds}$$

To use this formulation, probabilities must be converted to odds, where the odds of having a disease are expressed as the chance of having the disease divided by the chance of not having the disease. For instance, a probability of 0.75 is the same as 3 : 1 odds (Figure 1–8).

To estimate the potential benefit of a diagnostic test, the clinician first estimates the pretest odds of disease given all available clinical information and then multiplies the pretest odds by the positive and negative likelihood ratios. The results are the **posttest odds,** or the odds that the patient has the disease if the test is positive or negative. To obtain the posttest probability, the odds are converted to a probability (Figure 1–8).

For example, if the clinician believes that the patient has a 60% chance of having a myocardial infarction (pretest odds of 3 : 2) and the creatine kinase MB test is positive ($LR^+ = 32$), then the posttest odds of having a myocardial infarction are

$$\text{Odds} = \frac{\text{Probability}}{1 - \text{Probability}}$$

Example: If probability = 0.75, then

$$\text{Odds} = \frac{0.75}{1 - 0.75} = \frac{0.75}{0.25} = \frac{3}{1} = 3:1$$

$$\text{Probability} = \frac{\text{Odds}}{\text{Odds} + 1}$$

Example: If odds = 3:1, then

$$\text{Probability} = \frac{3/1}{3/1 + 1} = \frac{3}{3 + 1} = 0.75$$

Figure 1–8. Formulas for converting between probability and odds.

$$\frac{3}{2} \times 32 = \frac{96}{2} \text{ or } 48:1 \text{ odds} \left(\frac{48/1}{48/1+1} = \frac{48}{48+1} = 96\% \text{ probability} \right)$$

If the CKMB test is negative ($LR^- = 0.05$), then the posttest odds of having a myocardial infarction are

$$\frac{3}{2} \times 0.05 = \frac{0.15}{2} \text{ odds} \left(\frac{0.15/2}{0.15/2+1} = \frac{0.15}{0.15+2} = 7\% \text{ probability} \right)$$

Sequential Testing

To this point, the impact of only one test on the probability of disease has been discussed, whereas during most diagnostic workups, clinicians obtain clinical information in a sequential fashion. To calculate the posttest odds after three tests, for example, the clinician might estimate the pretest odds and use the appropriate likelihood ratio for each test:

$$\text{Pretest odds} \times LR_1 \times LR_2 \times LR_3 = \text{Posttest odds}$$

When using this approach, however, the clinician should be aware of a major assumption: the chosen tests or findings must be **conditionally independent.** For instance, with liver cell damage, the aspartate aminotransferase (AST) and alanine aminotransferase (ALT) enzymes may be released by the same process and are thus not conditionally independent. If conditionally dependent tests are used in this sequential approach, an overestimation of posttest probability will result.

Threshold Approach to Decision Making

A key aspect of medical decision making is the selection of a treatment threshold, ie, the probability of disease at which treatment is indicated. Figure 1–9 shows a possible way of identifying a treatment threshold by considering the value (utility) of the four possible outcomes of the treat/don't treat decision.

A diagnostic test is useful only if it shifts the disease probability across the treatment threshold. For example, a clinician might decide to treat with antibiotics if the probability of streptococcal pharyngitis in a patient with a sore throat is greater than 25% (Figure 1–10A). If, after reviewing evidence from the history and physical examination, the clinician estimates the pretest probability of strep throat to be 15%, then a diagnostic test such as throat culture ($LR^+ = 7$) would be useful only if a positive test would shift the posttest probability above 25%. Use of the nomogram shown in Figure 1–7 indicates that the posttest

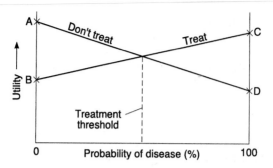

Figure 1–9. The "treat/don't treat" threshold. **(A)** Patient does not have disease and is not treated (highest utility). **(B)** Patient does not have disease and is treated (lower utility than A). **(C)** Patient has disease and is treated (lower utility than A). **(D)** Patient has disease and is not treated (lower utility than C).

probability would be 55% (Figure 1–10B); thus, ordering the test would be justified as it affects patient management. On the other hand, if the history and physical examination had suggested that the pretest probability of strep throat was 60%, the throat culture ($LR^- = 0.33$) would be indicated only if a negative test would lower the posttest probability below 25%. Using the same nomogram, the posttest probability after a negative test would be 33% (Figure 1–10C). Therefore, ordering the throat culture would not be justified.

This approach to decision making is now being applied in the clinical literature.

Decision Analysis

Up to this point, the discussion of diagnostic testing has focused on test characteristics and methods for using these characteristics to calculate the probability of disease in different clinical situations. Although useful, these methods are limited because they do not incorporate the many outcomes that may occur in clinical medicine or the values that patients and clinicians place on those outcomes. To incorporate outcomes and values with characteristics of tests, decision analysis can be used.

The basic idea of decision analysis is to model the options in a medical decision, assign probabilities to the alternative actions, assign values (utilities) to the various outcomes, and then calculate which decision gives the greatest value. To complete a decision analysis, the clinician would proceed as follows:

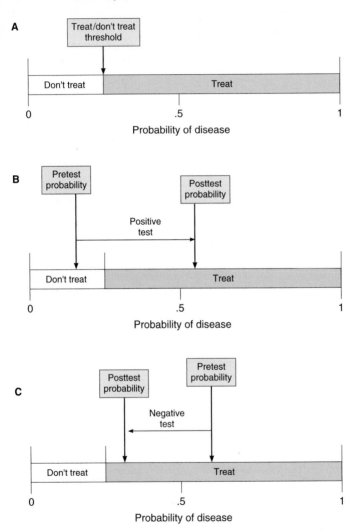

Figure 1–10. Threshold approach applied to test ordering. If the contemplated test will not change patient management, the test should not be ordered. (See text for explanation.)

(1) Draw a decision tree showing the elements of the medical decision.
(2) Assign probabilities to the various branches.
(3) Assign values (utilities) to the outcomes.
(4) Determine the expected utility (the product of probability and utility) of each branch.
(5) Select the decision with the highest expected utility.

Figure 1–11 shows a decision tree where the decision to be made is whether to treat without testing, perform a test and then treat based on the test result, or perform no tests and give no treatment. The clinician

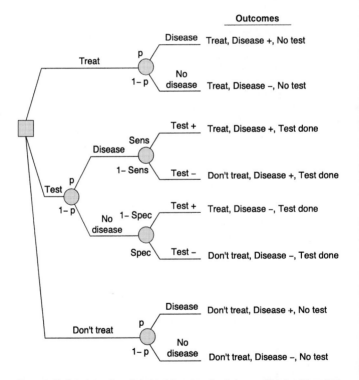

Figure 1–11. Generic tree for a clinical decision where the choices are (1) to treat the patient empirically, (2) to test and then treat if the test is positive, or (3) to withhold therapy. The square node is called a decision node, and the round nodes are called chance nodes. (p, pretest probability of disease; Sens, sensitivity; Spec, specificity.)

begins the analysis by building a decision tree showing the important elements of the decision. Once the tree is built, the clinician assigns probabilities to all the branches. In this case, all the branch probabilities can be calculated from (1) the probability of disease before the test (pretest probability), (2) the chance of a positive test if the disease is present (sensitivity), and (3) the chance of a negative test if the disease is absent (specificity). Next, the clinician assigns utility values to each of the outcomes.

After the expected utility is calculated, the clinician may identify which alternative has the highest value by this analysis.

Although time-consuming, decision analysis can help to structure complex clinical problems and to make difficult clinical decisions.

Evidence-Based Medicine

The focus over the past decade on evidence-based medicine stresses the examination of evidence from clinical research—rather than intuition and pathophysiologic reasoning—as a basis for clinical decision making. Evidence-based medicine relies on systematic reviews of the medical literature to inform clinical practice. Meta-analysis uses statistical techniques to combine evidence from different studies.

Clinical practice guidelines are systematically developed statements intended to assist practitioners and patients in making decisions about health care. Clinical algorithms and practice guidelines are now ubiquitous in medicine. Their utility and validity depend on the quality of the evidence that shaped the recommendations, on their being kept current, and on their acceptance and appropriate application by clinicians. While clinicians are concerned about the effect of guidelines on professional autonomy, many organizations are trying to use compliance with practice guidelines as a measure of quality of care.

Computer Access to Medical Information

The development of medical information science and computer technology now offer a vast amount of clinical information on CD-ROM or over the World Wide Web.

REFERENCES

Dekay ML, Asch DA: Is the defensive use of diagnostic tests good for patients, or bad? Med Decis Making 1998;18:19.

Detsky AS et al: Primer on medical decision analysis. (Five parts.) Med Decis Making 1997;17:123.

Jadad AR, Haynes RB: The Cochrane collaboration: Advances and challenges in improving evidence-based decision making. Med Decis Making 1998;18:2.

Maynard A: Evidence-based medicine: An incomplete method for informing treatment choices. Lancet 1997;349:126.

Panzer RJ, Black ER, Griner PF (editors): *Diagnostic Strategies for Common Medical Problems,* 2nd ed. American College of Physicians, 1999.

Sackett DL et al: *Clinical Epidemiology. A Basic Science for Clinical Medicine,* 2nd ed. Little, Brown, 1991.

Sox HC: The evaluation of diagnostic tests: Principles, problems, and new developments. Annu Rev Med 1996;47:463.

Tugwell P et al: Laboratory evaluation in the diagnosis of Lyme disease. Ann Intern Med 1997;127:1109. (Sensitivity, specificity, likelihood ratios, and pretest and posttest probabilities used to formulate guidelines for clinical diagnosis of Lyme disease.)

2

Laboratory Procedures in the Clinical Setting

Stephen J. McPhee, MD

This chapter presents information on how to perform common bedside laboratory procedures. Information on interpretation of results of body fluid analysis is included in some of the sections. Test results can be used for patient care only if the tests have been performed according to strict federal guidelines.

Contents *Page*

1. OBTAINING AND PROCESSING BODY FLUIDS

A. Safety Considerations

General Safety Considerations

Because all patient specimens are potentially infectious, the following precautions should be observed:

a. Universal body fluid and needle stick precautions must be observed at all times.

b. Disposable gloves and sometimes gown, mask, and goggles should be worn when collecting specimens.

c. Gloves should be changed and hands washed after contact with each patient. Dispose of gloves in an appropriate biohazard waste container.

d. Any spills should be cleaned up with 10% bleach solution.

Handling and Disposing of Needles and Gloves

a. Do not resheath needles.

b. Discard needles and gloves only into designated containers.

c. Do not remove a used needle from a syringe by hand. The needle may be removed using a specially designed waste collection system, or the entire assembly may (if disposable) be discarded as a unit into a designated container.

d. When obtaining blood cultures, it is hazardous and unnecessary to change needles.

e. Do not place phlebotomy or other equipment on the patient's bed.

B. Specimen Handling

Identification of Specimens

a. Identify the patient before obtaining the specimen. (If the patient is not known to you, ask for the name and check the wristband.)

b. Label each specimen container with the patient's name and identification number.

Specimen Tubes: Standard specimen tubes are now widely available and are easily identified by the color of the stopper (see also p 37):

a. Red-top tubes contain no anticoagulants or preservatives and are used for chemistry tests.

b. Marbled-top tubes contain material that allows ready separation of serum and clot by centrifugation.

c. Lavender-top tubes contain EDTA and are used for hematology tests (eg, blood or cell counts, differentials).

   d. Green-top tubes contain heparin and are used for tests that require plasma or anticoagulation.
   e. Blue-top tubes contain citrate and are used for coagulation tests.
   f. Gray-top tubes contain fluoride and are used for some chemistry tests (eg, glucose) if the specimen cannot be analyzed immediately.

Procedure

   a. When collecting multiple specimens, fill sterile tubes used for bacteriologic tests, then tubes without additives (ie, red-top tubes) before filling those with additives to avoid the potential for bacterial contamination, transfer of anticoagulants, etc. However, be certain to fill tubes containing anticoagulants before the blood specimen clots.
   b. The recommended order of filling tubes is (by type and color): (1) blood culture, (2) red top, (3) blue top, (4) green top, (5) lavender top.
   c. Fill each stoppered tube completely. Tilt each tube containing anticoagulant or preservative to mix thoroughly. Place any specimens on ice as required (eg, arterial blood). Deliver specimens to the laboratory promptly.
   d. For each of the major body fluids, Table 2–1 summarizes commonly requested tests and requirements for specimen handling and provides cross-references to tables and figures elsewhere in this book for help in interpretation of the results.

2. BASIC STAINING METHODS

A. Gram Stain

Preparation of Smear

   a. Obtain a fresh specimen of the material to be stained (eg, sputum) and smear a small amount on a glass slide. Thin smears give the best results (eg, press a sputum sample between two glass slides).
   b. Let the smear air-dry before heat-fixing, because heating a wet smear will usually distort cells and organisms.
   c. Heat-fix the smear by passing the clean side of the slide quickly through a Bunsen burner or other flame source (no more than three or four times). The slide should be warm, not hot.
   d. Let the slide cool before staining.

TABLE 2–1. BODY FLUID TESTS, HANDLING, AND INTERPRETATION.

Body Fluid	Commonly Requested Tests	Specimen Tube and Handling	Interpretation Guide
Arterial blood	pH, P_{O_2}, P_{CO_2}	Glass syringe. Evacuate air bubbles; remove needle; position rubber cap; place sample on ice; deliver immediately.	See acid-base nomogram p 337.
Ascitic fluid	Cell count, differential Protein, amylase Gram stain, culture Cytology (if neoplasm suspected)	Lavender top Red top Sterile Cytology	See ascitic fluid profiles, p 365.
Cerebrospinal fluid	Cell count, differential Gram stain, culture Protein, glucose VDRL or other studies (oligoclonal bands) Cytology (if neoplasm suspected)	Tube #1 Tube #2 Tube #3 Tube #4 Cytology	See cerebrospinal fluid profiles, p 369.
Pleural fluid	Cell count, differential Protein, glucose, amylase Gram stain, culture Cytology (if neoplasm suspected)	Lavender top Red top Sterile Cytology	See pleural fluid profiles, p 382.
Synovial fluid	Cell count, differential Protein, glucose Gram stain, culture Microscopic examination for crystals Cytology (if neoplasm [villonodular synovitis, metastatic disease] suspected)	Lavender top Red top Sterile Green top Cytology	See synovial fluid profiles, p 389, and Figure 2–6.
Urine	Urinalysis Dipstick Microscopic examination Gram stain, culture Cytology (if neoplasm suspected)	Clean tube Centrifuge tube Sterile Cytology	See Table 8–24, p 395. See Table 2–2, p 31. See Figure 2–3, p 34.

Staining Technique

    a. Put on gloves.

    b. Stain with crystal violet (10 seconds).

    c. Rinse with gently running water (5 seconds).

    d. Flood with Gram iodine solution (10–30 seconds).

    e. Rinse with gently running water (5 seconds).

　　f. Decolorize with acetone-alcohol solution until no more blue color leaches from the slide (5 seconds).
　　g. Rinse immediately with water (5 seconds).
　　h. Counterstain with safranin O (10 seconds).
　　i. Rinse with water (5 seconds).
　　j. Let the slide air-dry (or carefully blot with filter paper), then examine it under the microscope.

Microscopic Examination
　　a. Examine the smear first using the low-power lens for leukocytes and fungi. Screen for the number and color of polymorphonuclear cells (cell nuclei should be pink, not blue).
　　b. Examine using the high-power oil-immersion lens for microbial forms. Screen for intracellular organisms. Review the slide systematically for (1) fungi (mycelia, then yeast), (2) small gram-negative rods (bacteroides, haemophilus, etc) (3) gram-negative cocci (neisseria, etc), (4) gram-positive rods (listeria, etc), and (5) gram-positive cocci (streptococcus, staphylococcus, etc).
　　c. Label positive slides with the patient's name and identification number and save them for later review.
　　d. Figure 2–1 illustrates typical findings on a Gram-stained smear of sputum.

B. Wright Stain of Peripheral Blood Smear
Preparation of Smear
　　a. Obtain a fresh specimen of blood by pricking the patient's finger with a lancet. If alcohol is used to clean the fingertip, wipe it off first with a gauze pad.
　　b. Place a single drop of blood on a glass slide. Lay a second glass slide over the first one and rapidly pull it away lengthwise to leave a thin smear.
　　c. Let the smear air-dry. Do not heat-fix.

Staining Technique
　　a. Stain with fresh Wright stain (1 minute).
　　b. Gently add an equal amount of water and gently blow on the smear to mix the stain and water. Repeat by adding more water and blowing to mix. Look for formation of a shiny surface scum. Then allow the stain to set (3–4 minutes).
　　c. Rinse with gently running water (5 seconds).
　　d. Clean the back of the slide with an alcohol pad if necessary.

Microscopic Examination
　　a. Examine the smear first using the low-power lens to select a good area for study (red and white cells separated from one another).

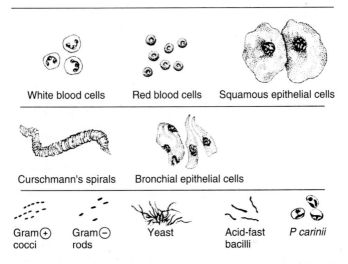

White blood cells   Red blood cells   Squamous epithelial cells

Curschmann's spirals   Bronchial epithelial cells

Gram⊕   Gram⊖   Yeast   Acid-fast   *P carinii*
cocci   rods   bacilli

Figure 2–1. Common findings on microscopic examination of the sputum. Most elements can be seen on Gram-stained smears except for acid-fast bacilli (auramine-rhodamine stain) and *Pneumocystis carinii* (Giemsa stain). *(Modified and reproduced, with permission from Krupp MA et al: Physician's Handbook, 21st ed. Originally published by Lange Medical Publications. Copyright © 1985 by The McGraw-Hill Companies, Inc.)*

    b. Then move to the high-power oil-immersion lens. Review the slide systematically for (1) platelet morphology, (2) white cells (differential types, morphology, toxic granulations and vacuoles, etc), and (3) red cells (size, shape, color, stippling, nucleation, etc).

    c. Label slides with the patient's name and identification number and save them for later review.

    d. See Figure 2–2 for examples of common peripheral blood smear abnormalities.

3. OTHER BEDSIDE LABORATORY PROCEDURES

A. Urinalysis

Collection and Preparation of Specimen

    a. Obtain a midstream urine specimen from the patient. The sample must be free of skin epithelium or bacteria, secretions, hair, lint, etc.

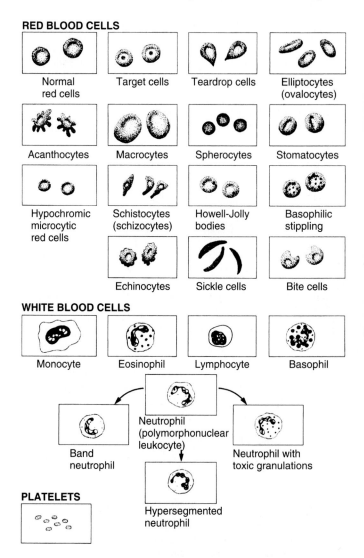

Figure 2–2. Common peripheral blood smear findings.

b. Examine the specimen while fresh (still warm). Otherwise, bacteria may proliferate, casts and crystals may dissolve, and particulate matter may settle out. (Occasionally, amorphous crystals precipitate out, obscuring formed elements. In cold urine, they are amorphous urate crystals; these may be dissolved by gently rewarming the urine. In alkaline urine, they are amorphous phosphate crystals; these may be dissolved by adding 1 mL of acetic acid.)

c. Place 10 mL in a tube and centrifuge at 2000–3000 rpm for 3–5 minutes.

d. Discard the supernatant. Resuspend the sediment in the few drops that remain by gently tilting the tube.

e. Place a drop on a glass slide, cover it with a coverslip, and examine under the microscope; no stain is needed. If bacterial infection is present, a single drop of methylene blue applied to the edge of the coverslip, or a Gram-stained smear of an air-dried, heat-fixed specimen, can assist in distinguishing gram-negative rods (eg, *E coli,* proteus, klebsiella) from gram-positive cocci (eg, enterococcus, *Staphylococcus saprophyticus*).

Procedural Technique

a. While the urine is being centrifuged, examine the remainder of the specimen by inspection and reagent strip ("dipstick") testing.

b. Inspect the specimen for color and clarity. Normally, urine is yellow or light orange. Dark orange urine is caused by ingestion of the urinary tract analgesic phenazopyridine (Pyridium, others); red urine, by hemoglobinuria, myoglobinuria, beets, senna, or rifampin therapy; green urine, by *Pseudomonas* infection or iodochlorhydroxyquin or amitriptyline therapy; brown urine, by bilirubinuria or fecal contamination; black urine, by intravascular hemolysis, alkaptonuria, melanoma, or methyldopa therapy; purplish urine, by porphyria; and milky white urine, by pus, chyluria, or amorphous crystals (urates or phosphates). Turbidity of urine is caused by pus, red blood cells, or crystals.

c. Reagent strips provide information about specific gravity, pH, protein, glucose, ketones, bilirubin, heme, nitrite, and esterase (Table 2–2). Dip a reagent strip in the urine and compare it with the chart on the bottle. Follow the timing instructions carefully. *Note:* Reagent strips cannot be relied on to detect some proteins (eg, globulins, light chains) or sugars (other than glucose).

d. Record the results.

TABLE 2–2. COMPONENTS OF THE URINE DIPSTICK.[1]

Test	Values	Lowest Detectable Range	Comments
Specific gravity	1.001–1.035	1.000–1.030	Highly buffered alkaline urine may yield low specific gravity readings. Moderate protein-uria (100–750 mg/dL) may yield high read-ings. Loss of concentrating or diluting capacity indicates renal dysfunction.
pH	5–9 units	5–8.5 units	Excessive urine on strip may cause protein reagent to run over onto pH area, yielding falsely low pH reading.
Protein	0	15–30 mg/dL albumin	False-positive readings can be caused by highly buffered alkaline urine. Reagent more sensitive to albumin than other proteins. A negative result does not rule out the presence of globulins, hemoglobin, Bence Jones proteins, or mucoprotein. 1+ = 30 mg/dL 3+ = 300 mg/dL 2+ = 100 mg/dL 4+ = ≥ 2000 mg/dL
Glucose	0	75–125 mg/dL	Test is specific for glucose. False-negative results occur with urinary ascorbic acid concentrations ≥ 50 mg/dL and with ketone body levels ≥ 50 mg/dL Test reagent reactivity also varies with specific gravity and temperature. Trace = 100 mg/dL 1 = 1000 mg/dL 1/4 = 250 mg/dL 2 = ≥ 2000 mg/dL 1/2 = 500 mg/dL
Ketone	0	5–10 mg/dL acetoacetate	Test does not react with acetone or b-hydroxy-butyric acid. (Trace) false-positive results may occur with highly pigmented urines or those containing levodopa metabolites or sulfhydryl-containing compounds (eg, mesna). Trace = 5 mg/dL Moderate = 40 mg/dL Small = 15 mg/dL Large = 80–160 mg/dL
Bilirubin	0	0.4–0.8 mg/dL	Indicates hepatitis (conjugated bilirubin). False-negative readings can be caused by ascorbic acid concentrations ≥ 25 mg/dL. False-positive readings can be caused by etodolac metabolites. Test is less sensitive than Ictotest Reagent tablets.

(*continued*)

TABLE 2–2 (CONT'D). COMPONENTS OF THE URINE DIPSTICK.[1]

Test	Values	Lowest Detectable Range	Comments
Blood	0[2]	0.015–0.062 mg/dL hemoglobin	Test equally sensitive to myoglobin and hemoglobin (including both intact erythrocytes and free hemoglobin). False-positive results can be caused by oxidizing contaminants (hypochlorite) and microbial peroxidase (urinary tract infection). Test sensitivity is reduced in urines with high specific gravity, captopril, or heavy proteinuria.
Nitrite	0	0.06–0.1 mg/dL nitrite ion	Test depends on the conversion of nitrate (derived from the diet) to nitrite by gramnegative bacteria in urine. Test specific for nitrite. False-negative readings can be caused by ascorbic acid. Test sensitivity is reduced in urines with high specific gravity.
Leukocytes (esterase)	0[3]	6–15 WBCs/hpf	Indicator of urinary tract infection. Test detects esterases contained in granulocytic leukocytes. Test sensitivity is reduced in urines with high specific gravity, elevated glucose concentrations ($\geq$ 4 g/dL), or presence of cephalexin, cephalothin, tetracycline, or high concentrations of oxalate.

[1] Package insert, revised 9/95. Bayer Diagnostics Reagent Strips for Urinalysis, Bayer Corporation.
[2] Except in menstruating females.
[3] Except in females with vaginitis.

Microscopic Examination

a. Examine the area under the coverslip under the low-power and high-dry lenses for cells, casts, crystals, and bacteria. (If a Gram stain is done, examine under the oil immersion lens.)

b. Cells may be red cells, white cells, squamous cells, transitional (bladder) epithelial cells, or atypical (tumor) cells. Red cells suggest upper or lower urinary tract infections (cystitis, prostatitis, pyelonephritis), glomerulonephritis, collagen vascular disease, trauma, renal calculi, tumors, drug reactions, and structural abnormalities (polycystic kidneys). White cells suggest inflammatory processes such as urinary tract infection (most common), collagen vascular disease, or interstitial nephritis. Red cell casts are considered pathognomonic of glomerulonephritis; white cell casts, of pyelonephritis; and fatty (lipid) casts, of nephrotic syndrome.

    c. The finding on a Gram-stained smear of unspun, clean, fresh urine of even one bacterium per field under the oil-immersion lens correlates fairly well with bacterial culture colony counts of greater than 100,000 organisms per μL.

    d. See Table 8–24, p 395, for a guide to interpretation of urinalysis; and Figure 2–3 for a guide to microscopic findings in urine.

B. Vaginal Fluid Wet Preparation
  Preparation of Smear and Staining Technique

    a. Place a small amount of vaginal discharge on a glass slide.

    b. Add 2 drops of sterile saline solution.

    c. Place a coverslip over the area to be examined.

  Microscopic Examination

    a. Examine under the microscope, using the high-dry lens and a low light source.

    b. Look for motile trichomonads (undulating protozoa propelled by four flagella). Look for clue cells (vaginal epithelial cells with large numbers of organisms attached to them, obscuring cell borders), pathognomonic of *Gardnerella vaginalis*-associated vaginosis.

    c. See Figure 2–4 for an example of a positive wet prep (trichomonads, clue cells) and Table 8–25, p 397 for the differential diagnosis of vaginal discharge.

C. Skin or Vaginal Fluid KOH Preparation
  Preparation of Smear and Staining Technique

    a. Obtain a skin specimen by using a No. 15 scalpel blade to scrape scales from the skin lesion onto a glass slide or to remove the top of a vesicle onto the slide. Or place a single drop of vaginal discharge on the slide.

    b. Place 1 or 2 drops of potassium hydroxide (10–20%) on top of the specimen on the slide. Lay a coverslip over the area to be examined.

    c. Heat the slide from beneath with a match or Bunsen burner flame until the slide contents begin to bubble.

    d. Clean carbon off the back side of the slide with an alcohol pad if necessary.

  Note: A fishy amine odor upon addition of KOH to a vaginal discharge is typical of bacterial vaginosis caused by *Gardnerella vaginalis.*

  Microscopic Examination

    a. Examine the smear under the high-dry lens for mycelial forms. Branched, septate hyphae are typical of dermatophytosis (eg, trichophyton, epidermophyton, microspo-

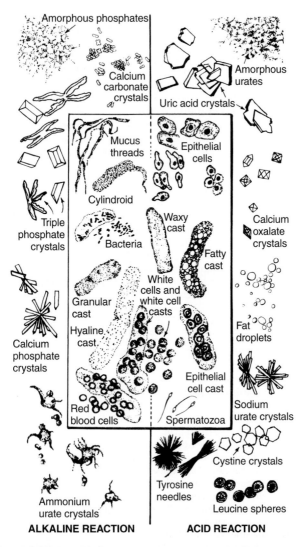

Figure 2–3. Microscopic findings on examination of the urine. *(Modified and reproduced, with permission from Krupp MA et al: Physician's Handbook, 21st ed. Originally published by Lange Medical Publications. Copyright © 1985 by The McGraw-Hill Companies, Inc.)*

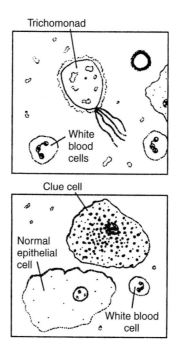

Figure 2–4. Wet preparation showing trichomonads, white blood cells, and "clue" cells.

rum species); branched, septate pseudohyphae with or without budding yeast forms are seen with candidiasis (candida species); and short, curved hyphae plus clumps of spores ("spaghetti and meatballs") are seen with tinea versicolor *(Malassezia furfur)*.
   b. See Figure 2–5 for an example of a positive KOH prep.

D. Synovial Fluid Examination for Crystals
Preparation of Smear
   a. No stain is necessary.
   b. Place a small amount of synovial fluid on a glass slide.
   c. Place a coverslip over the area to be examined.
Microscopic Examination
   a. Examine under a polarized light microscope with a red compensator, using the high-dry lens and a moderately bright light source.

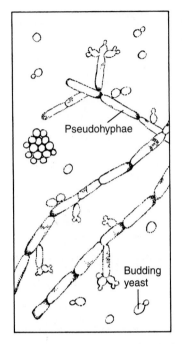

Figure 2–5. KOH preparation showing mycelial forms (pseudohyphae) and budding yeast typical of *Candida albicans.*

      b. Look for needle-shaped, negatively birefringent urate crystals (crystals parallel to the axis of the compensator appear yellow) in gout or rhomboidal, positively birefringent calcium pyrophosphate crystals (crystals parallel to the axis of the compensator appear blue) in pseudogout.

      c. See Figure 2–6 for examples of positive synovial fluid examinations for these two types of crystals.

E. Pulse Oximetry
Indications

To measure oxygen saturation in a noninvasive and often continuous fashion.

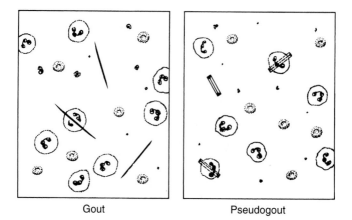

Gout   Pseudogout

Figure 2–6. Examination of synovial fluid for crystals, using a compensated, polarized microscope. In gout, crystals are needle-shaped, negatively birefringent, and composed of monosodium urate. In pseudogout, crystals are rhomboidal, positively birefringent, and composed of calcium pyrophosphate dihydrate. In both diseases, crystals can be found freefloating or within polymorphonuclear cells.

Contraindications

a. Hypotension, hypothermia, low perfusion states, severe or rapid desaturation, and severe anemia (hemoglobin < 5 g/dL) cause inaccurate readings.

b. Hyperbilirubinemia, methemoglobinemia, fetal hemoglobinemia, and carboxyhemoglobinemia can falsely elevate oxygen saturation measurements.

c. Excessive ambient light, simultaneous use of a blood pressure cuff, the presence of intravascular dyes (eg, methylene blue), and electrical interference (eg, MRI scanners, electrosurgery) can also cause erroneous readings.

Approach to the Patient

The patient should be positioned close to the pulse oximeter and should hold the probe site still. The sampling area should have good circulation and be free of skin irritation.

Procedural Technique

a. Plug the pulse oximeter into a grounded AC power outlet or make sure that sufficient battery power is available. Turn the oximeter on and wait until self-calibration is complete.

   b. Select the probe to be used and connect it to the pulse oximeter. The probe consists of a light source (a red light-emitting device [LED] in most cases) and a photodetector. Probes are available for the ear, finger, and, in neonates, the foot, ankle, palm, calf, and forearm.
   c. Attach the probe to the patient after cleansing the surrounding skin with an alcohol swab. Some probes come with double-sided adhesive disks that improve probe signal.
   d. Watch the waveform and pulse indicators to assess the quality of the signal. Readjust if a poor signal is present.
   e. Set alarm warnings on the device.
   f. Check the probe site at least every 4 hours. Care should be taken not to apply tension to the probe cables.

Possible Complications
   Allergic reaction to adhesives.

Comments
   Because of the curvilinear nature of the oxygen-hemoglobin dissociation curve, oxygen saturation (SaO_2) is not directly proportionate to oxygen partial pressure (PaO_2). Therefore, a relatively small change in oxygen saturation (eg, from 94% to 83%) can represent a large change in PaO_2 (eg, from 80 mm Hg to 50 mm Hg). In addition, the dissociation curve varies markedly from patient to patient and with pH, temperature, and altitude. To ensure accurate assessment of oxygenation, one should correlate pulse oximetry with arterial blood gas analysis.

REFERENCES
Gram Stain
Fournier AM: The Gram stain. Ann Intern Med 1998;128:776.
Hirschmann JV: The sputum Gram stain. J Gen Intern Med 1991;6:261.
Popescu A, Doyle RJ: The Gram stain after more than a century. Biotech Histochem 1996;71:145.
Reed WW et al: Sputum gram's stain in community-acquired pneumococcal pneumonia. A meta-analysis. West J Med 1996;165:197.

Urinalysis
Jou WW, Powers RD: Utility of dipstick urinalysis as a guide to management of adults with suspected infection or hematuria. South Med J 1998;91:266.
Lorincz AE et al: Urinalysis: current status and prospects for the future. Ann Clin Lab Sci 1999;29:169.

Misdraji J, Nguyen PL: Urinalysis. When—and when not—to order. Postgrad Med 1996;100:173.

Semeniuk H et al: Evaluation of the leukocyte esterase and nitrite urine dipstick screening tests for detection of bacteriuria in women with suspected uncomplicated urinary tract infections. J Clin Microbiol 1999;37:3051.

Vaginal Wet Prep

Ferris DG et al: Office laboratory diagnosis of vaginitis. Clinician-performed tests compared with a rapid nucleic acid hybridization test. J Fam Pract 1995;41:575.

Thihnkhamrop J: Vaginal fluid pH as a screening test for vaginitis. Int J Gynaecol Obstet 1999;66:143.

Wiesenfeld HC et al: The infrequent use of office-based diagnostic tests for vaginitis. Am J Obstet Gynecol 1999;181:39.

Synovial Fluid Examination

Schumacher HR: Crystal-induced arthritis: an overview. Am J Med 1996;100:46S.

Pulse Oximetry

Franklin ML: Transcutaneous measurement of partial pressure of oxygen and carbon dioxide. Respir Care Clin North Am 1995;1:11.

Grap MJ: Pulse oximetry. Crit Care Nurs 1998;18:94.

Jensen LA, Onyskiw JE, Prasad NG: Meta-analysis of arterial oxygen saturation monitoring by pulse oximetry in adults. Heart Lung 1998;27:387.

Ortiz FO et al: Accuracy of pulse oximetry in sickle cell disease. Am J Respir Crit Care Med 1999;159:447.

Sinex JE: Pulse oximetry: principles and limitations. Am J Emerg Med 1999;17:59.

Smatlak P et al: Clinical evaluation of noninvasive monitoring of oxygen saturation in critically ill patients. Am J Crit Care 1998;7:370.

3

Common Laboratory Tests: Selection and Interpretation

Diana Nicoll, MD, PhD, MPA, Stephen J. McPhee, MD,
and Michael Pignone, MD, MPH

HOW TO USE THIS SECTION

This section contains information about commonly used laboratory tests. It includes most of the blood, urine, and cerebrospinal fluid tests found in this book, with the exception of drug levels. Entries are in outline format and are arranged alphabetically.

Test/Reference Range/Collection

This first outline listing begins with the common test name, the specimen analyzed, and any test name abbreviation (in parentheses).

Below this in the first outline listing is the reference range for each test. The first entry is in conventional units, and the second entry (in [brackets]) is in SI units (Système International d'Unités). Any panic values for a particular test are placed here after the word "Panic." The reference ranges provided are from several large medical centers; consult your own clinical laboratory for those used in your institution.

This outline listing also shows which tube to use for collecting blood and other body fluids, how much the test costs (in relative symbolism; see below), and how to collect the specimen. Listed below are the common collection tubes and their contents:

Tube Top Color	Tube Contents	Typically Used In
Lavender	EDTA	Complete blood count
Marbled	Serum separator	Serum chemistry tests
Red	None	Blood banking (serum)
Blue	Citrate	Coagulation studies
Green	Heparin	Plasma studies
Yellow	Acid citrate	HLA typing
Navy	Trace metal free	Trace metals (eg, lead)
Gray	Inhibitor of glycolysis (sodium fluoride)	Lactic acid

The scale used for the cost of each test is:

Approximate Cost	Symbol Used in Tables
$1–20	$
$21–50	$$
$51–100	$$$
> $100	$$$$

Physiologic Basis

This outline listing contains physiologic information about the substance being tested. Information on classification and biologic importance, as well as interactions with other biologic substances and processes, is included.

Interpretation

This outline lists clinical conditions that affect the substance being tested. Generally, conditions with higher prevalence will be listed first. When the sensitivity of the test for a particular disease is known, that information will follow the disease name in parentheses, eg, "rheumatoid arthritis (83%)." Some of the common drugs that can affect the test substance in vivo will also be included in this outline listing.

Comments

This outline listing sets forth general information pertinent to the use and interpretation of the test and important in vitro interferences with the test procedure. Appropriate general references are also listed.

Test Name

The test name is placed as a header to the rest of the outline list to allow for quick referencing.

Test/Range/Collection	Physiologic Basis	Interpretation	Comments
ABO Grouping			
ABO grouping, serum and red cells (ABO) Red $ Properly identified and labeled blood specimens are critical.	The four blood groups A, B, O, and AB are determined by the presence of antigens A and B or their absence (O) on a patient's red blood cells. Antibodies are present in serum for which red cells lack antigen.	In the US white population, 45% are type O, 40% A, 11% B, 4% AB. In the African-American population, 49% are type O, 27% A, 20% B, 4% AB. In the US Asian population, 40% are type O, 28% A, 27% B, 5% AB. In the Native American population, 79% are type O, 16% A, 4% B, <1% AB.	For both blood donors and recipients, routine ABO grouping includes both red cell and serum testing, as checks on each other. Tube testing is as follows: patient's red cells are tested with anti-A and anti-B for the presence or absence of agglutination (forward or cell grouping), and patient's serum is tested against known A and B cells (reverse or serum grouping). *Technical Manual of the American Association of Blood Banks*, 11th ed. American Association of Blood Banks, 1993.
Acetaminophen			
Acetaminophen, serum (Tylenol; others) 10–20 mg/L [66–132 µmol/L] *Panic:* >50 mg/L Marbled $$ For suspected overdose, draw two samples at least 4 hours apart, at least 4 hours after ingestion. Note time of ingestion, if known. Order test stat.	In overdose, liver and renal toxicity are produced by the hydroxylated metabolite if it is not conjugated with glutathione in the liver.	**Increased in:** Acetaminophen overdose. Interpretation of serum acetaminophen level depends on time since ingestion. Levels drawn <4 hours after ingestion cannot be interpreted since the drug is still in the absorption and distribution phase. Use nomogram (Figure 8–1, p 336) to evaluate possible toxicity. Levels >150 mg/dL at 4 hours or >50 mg/dL at 12 hours after ingestion suggest toxicity. Nomogram inaccurate for chronic ingestions.	Do not delay acetylcysteine (Mucomyst) treatment (140 mg/kg orally) if stat levels are unavailable. Lancet 1971;1:519. Pediatrics 1975;55:871. Lancet 1976;2:109.

	Acetoacetate		Acetylcholine receptor antibody
Acetoacetate, serum or urine 0 mg/dL [μmol/L] Marbled or urine container $ Urine sample should be fresh.	Acetoacetate, acetone, and β-hydroxy-butyrate contribute to ketoacidosis when oxidative hepatic metabolism of fatty acids is impaired. Proportions in serum vary but are generally 20% acetoacetate, 78% β-hydroxybutyrate, and 2% acetone.	**Present in:** Diabetic ketoacidosis, alcoholic ketoacidosis, prolonged fasting, severe carbohydrate restriction with normal fat intake.	Nitroprusside test is semiquantitative; it detects acetoacetate and is sensitive down to 5–10 mg/dL. Trace = 5 mg/dL, small = 15 mg/dL, moderate = 40 mg/dL, large = 80 mg/dL [1 mg/dL = 100 μmol/L]. β-Hydroxybutyrate is not a ketone and is not detected by the nitroprusside test. Acetone is also not reliably detected by this method. Failure of test to detect β-hydroxy-butyrate in ketoacidosis may produce a seemingly paradoxical increase in ketones with clinical improvement as nondetectable β-hydroxybutyrate is replaced by detectable acetoacetate. Br Med J 1972;2:565.
Acetylcholine receptor antibody, serum Negative Marbled $$	Acetylcholine receptor antibodies are involved in the pathogenesis of myasthenia gravis. Sensitive radio-assay or ELISA is available based on inhibition of binding of ^{125}I alpha-bungarotoxin to the acetylcholine receptor.	**Positive in:** Myasthenia gravis. Sensitivity = 73%. Single fiber EMG may have best sensitivity.	Titer has been found to correlate with clinical severity. J Neurol Neurosurg Psychiatry 1993;56:496. Clin Chem 1993;39:2053. Muscle Nerve 1992;15:720.

Test/Range/Collection	Physiologic Basis	Interpretation	Comments
Adrenocorticotropic hormone, plasma (ACTH) 20–100 pg/mL [4–22 pmol/L] Heparinized plastic container $$$$ Send promptly to laboratory on ice. ACTH is unstable in plasma, is inactivated at room temperature, and adheres strongly to glass. Avoid all contact with glass.	Pituitary ACTH (release stimulated by hypothalamic corticotropin-releasing factor) stimulates cortisol release from the adrenal gland. There is feedback regulation of the system by cortisol. ACTH is secreted episodically and shows circadian variation, with highest levels at 6:00–8:00 AM; lowest levels at 9:00–10:00 PM.	**Increased in:** Pituitary (40–200 pg/mL) and ectopic (200–71,000 pg/mL) Cushing's syndrome, primary adrenal insufficiency (>250 pg/mL), adrenogenital syndrome with impaired cortisol production. **Decreased in:** Adrenal Cushing's syndrome (<20 pg/mL), pituitary ACTH (secondary adrenal) insufficiency (<50 pg/mL).	ACTH levels (RIA) can only be interpreted when measured with cortisol after standardized stimulation or suppression tests (see Adrenocortical insufficiency algorithm, p 338, and Cushing's syndrome algorithm, p 340). Postgrad Med 1998:104:61.
Alanine aminotransferase, serum (ALT, SGPT, GPT) 0–35 U/L [0–0.58 μkat/L] (laboratory-specific) Marbled $	Intracellular enzyme involved in amino acid metabolism. Present in large concentrations in liver, kidney; in smaller amounts, in skeletal muscle and heart. Released with tissue damage, particularly liver injury.	**Increased in:** Acute viral hepatitis (ALT > AST), biliary tract obstruction (cholangitis, choledocholithiasis), alcoholic hepatitis and cirrhosis (AST > ALT), liver abscess, metastatic or primary liver cancer; right heart failure, ischemia or hypoxia, injury to liver ("shock liver"), extensive trauma. Drugs that cause cholestasis or hepatotoxicity. **Decreased in:** Pyridoxine (vitamin B_6) deficiency.	ALT is the preferred enzyme for evaluation of liver injury. Screening ALT in low-risk populations has a low (12%) positive predictive value. Compr Ther 1994;20:50. Hosp Pract (Off Ed) Nov 1994;29:32. Dig Dis Sci 1993;38:2145.

(Column headers at top of table:) **Adrenocorticotropic hormone** | **Alanine aminotransferase**

Albumin		
Albumin, serum 3.4–4.7 g/dL [34–47 g/L] Marbled $	Major component of plasma proteins; influenced by nutritional state, hepatic function, renal function, and various diseases. Major binding protein. While there are more than 50 different genetic variants (alloalbumins), only occasionally does a mutation cause abnormal binding (eg, in familial dysalbuminemic hyperthyroxinemia).	**Increased in:** Dehydration, shock, hemoconcentration. **Decreased in:** Decreased hepatic synthesis (chronic liver disease, malnutrition, malabsorption, malignancy, congenital analbuminemia [rare]). Increased losses (nephrotic syndrome, burns, trauma, hemorrhage with fluid replacement, fistulas, enteropathy, acute or chronic glomerulonephritis). Hemodilution (pregnancy, CHF). Drugs: estrogens.	Serum albumin gives an indication of severity in chronic liver disease. Useful in nutritional assessment if there is no impairment in production or increased loss of albumin and is an independent risk factor for all-cause mortality in the elderly (age >70). There is a 10% reduction in serum albumin level in late pregnancy (related to hemodilution). J Med Genet 1994;31:355. Proc Natl Acad Sci U S A 1994;91:6476. JAMA 1994;272:1036. JAGS 1993;41:545.

	Aldosterone, plasma		
Test/Range/Collection	**Physiologic Basis**	**Interpretation**	**Comments**
Aldosterone, plasma *Salt-loaded* (120 meq Na+/d): Supine: 3–10 Upright: 5–30 ng/dL *Salt-depleted* (10 meq Na+/d): Supine: 12–36 Upright: 17–137 ng/dL [1 ng/dL = 27.7 pmol/L] Lavender or green $$$$ Early AM fasting specimen. Separate immediately and freeze.	Aldosterone is the major mineralocorticoid hormone and is a major regulator of extracellular volume and serum potassium concentration. For evaluation of hyperaldosteronism (associated with hypertension and hypokalemia), patients should be salt-loaded and recumbent when specimen is drawn. For evaluation of hypoaldosteronism (associated with hyperkalemia), patients should be salt-depleted and upright when specimen is drawn.	**Increased in:** Primary hyperaldosteronism (72%). **Decreased in:** Primary or secondary hypoaldosteronism.	Testing for hyperaldosteronism and hypoaldosteronism must be done using specific protocols, and results must be interpreted based on reference values from the laboratory performing the test. 24-hour urinary excretion of aldosterone is the most sensitive test for hyperaldosteronism. (See Aldosterone, urine, below.) The significance of an elevated plasma aldosterone level is difficult to interpret without simultaneous determination of plasma renin activity (PRA). In primary aldosteronism, plasma aldosterone is usually elevated while PRA is low; in secondary hyperaldosteronism, both plasma aldosterone and PRA are usually elevated. Am J Med 1983;74:641. Med Clin North Am 1988;72:1117. Mayo Clin Proc 1990;65:96.

	Aldosterone, urine	
Aldosterone, urine* *Salt-loaded* (120 meq Na+/d for 3–4 days): 1.5–12.5 µg/24 h *Salt-depleted* (20 meq Na+/d for 3–4 days): 18–85 µg/24 h [1 µg/24 h = 2.77 nmol/d] Bottle containing boric acid $$$$	Secretion of aldosterone is controlled by the renin-angiotensin system. Renin (synthesized and stored in juxtaglomerular cells of kidney) is released in response to both decreased perfusion pressure at the juxtaglomerular apparatus and negative sodium balance. Renin then hydrolyses angiotensinogen to angiotensin I, which is converted to angiotensin II, which then stimulates the adrenal gland to produce aldosterone.	**Increased in:** Primary and secondary hyperaldosteronism, some patients with essential hypertension. **Decreased in:** Primary hypoaldosteronism (eg, 18-hydroxylase deficiency), secondary hypoaldosteronism (hyporeninemic hypoaldosteronism).	Urinary aldosterone is the most sensitive test for primary hyperaldosteronism. Levels >14 µg/24 h after 3 days of salt-loading have a 96% sensitivity and 93% specificity for primary hyperaldosteronism. Only 7% of patients with essential hypertension have urinary aldosterone levels >14 µg/24 h after salt-loading. Neither serum potassium nor plasma renin activity (PRA) is a satisfactory screening test for hyperaldosteronism. Hypokalemia is present in only 73% of patients with hyperaldosteronism on a normal sodium diet, and in 86% after salt loading. Suppressed PRA has only a 64% sensitivity and 83% specificity for hyperaldosteronism. Am J Med 1983;74:641. Med Clin North Am 1988;72:1117. Mayo Clin Proc 1990;65:96. Endocrinol Metab Clin North Am 1994;23:271.

* To evaluate hyperaldosteronism, patient is salt-loaded and recumbent. Obtain 24-hour urine for aldosterone (and sodium to check that sodium excretion is >250 meq/day). To evaluate hypoaldosteronism, patient is salt-depleted and upright; check patient for hypotension before 24-hour urine collected.

Test/Range/Collection	Physiologic Basis	Interpretation	Comments
Alkaline phosphatase, serum 41–133 IU/L [0.7–2.2 µkat/L] (method- and age-dependent) Marbled $	Alkaline phosphatases are found in liver, bone, intestine, and placenta.	**Increased in:** Obstructive hepatobiliary disease, bone disease (physiologic bone growth, Paget's disease, osteomalacia, osteogenic sarcoma, bone metastases), hyperparathyroidism, rickets, benign familial hyperphosphatasemia, pregnancy (third trimester), GI disease (perforated ulcer or bowel infarct), hepatotoxic drugs. **Decreased in:** Hypophosphatasia.	Alkaline phosphatase performs well in measuring the extent of bone metastases in prostate cancer. Normal in osteoporosis. Alkaline phosphatase isoenzyme separation by electrophoresis or differential heat inactivation is unreliable. Use γ-glutamyl transpeptidase (GGT), which increases in hepatobiliary disease but not in bone disease, to infer origin of increased alkaline phosphatase (ie, liver or bone). Endocrinol Metab Clin North Am 1990;19:1. Int J Urol 1997;4:572.
Amebic serology, serum <1:64 titer Marbled $$	Test for presence of *Entamoeba histolytica* by detection of antibodies which develop 2–4 weeks after infection. Tissue invasion by the organism may be necessary for antibody production.	**Increased in:** Current or past infection with *E histolytica*. Amebic abscess (91%), amebic dysentery (84%), asymptomatic cyst carriers (9%), patients with other diseases and healthy people (2%).	In some endemic areas, as many as 44% of those tested have positive serologies. Preciptin or indirect hemagglutination (IHA) and recombinant antigen-based ELISA tests are available. N Engl J Med 1978;298:262. Ann Trop Parasitol 1993;87:31.

Ammonia			
Ammonia, plasma (NH₃) 18–60 μg/dL [11–35 μmol/L] Green $$ Separate plasma from cells immediately. Avoid hemolysis. Analyze immediately. Place on ice.	Ammonia is liberated by bacteria in the large intestine or by protein metabolism and is rapidly converted to urea in liver. In liver disease or portal-systemic shunting, the blood ammonia concentration increases. In acute liver failure, elevation of blood ammonia may cause brain edema; in chronic liver failure, it may be responsible for hepatic encephalopathy.	**Increased in:** Liver failure, hepatic encephalopathy (especially if protein consumption is high or if there is GI bleeding), fulminant hepatic failure, Reye's syndrome, portacaval shunting, cirrhosis, urea cycle metabolic defects, urea-splitting urinary tract infection with urinary diversion, and organic acidemias. Drugs: diuretics, acetazolamide, asparaginase, fluorouracil (5-FU) (transient), others. Spuriously increased by any ammonia-containing detergent on laboratory glassware. **Decreased in:** Decreased production by gut bacteria (kanamycin, neomycin). Decreased gut absorption (lactulose).	Correlates poorly with degree of hepatic encephalopathy. Test not useful in adults with known liver disease. Test is not as useful as CSF glutamine (see p 97). Klin Wochenschr 1990;68:175. Baillieres Clin Gastroenterol 1992;6:609. Proc Soc Exp Biol Med 1994;206:329.

	Amylase	Angiotensin-converting enzyme
Comments	Macroamylasemia is indicated by high serum but low urine amylase. Serum lipase is an alternative test for acute pancreatitis. Amylase isoenzymes are not of practical use because of technical problems. Gastroenterol Clin North Am 1990;19:793. J Gastroenterol 1994;29:189. Gastroenterologist 1994;2:119. Pancreas 1998;16:45.	Test is not useful as a screening test for sarcoidosis (low sensitivity). Specificity is compromised by positive tests in diseases more common than sarcoidosis. Some advocate measurement of ACE to follow disease activity in sarcoidosis. J Clin Pathol 1983;36:938.
Interpretation	**Increased in:** Acute pancreatitis (70–95%), pancreatic pseudocyst, pancreatic duct obstruction (cholecystitis, choledocholithiasis, pancreatic carcinoma, stone, stricture, duct sphincter spasm), bowel obstruction and infarction, mumps, parotitis, diabetic ketoacidosis, penetrating peptic ulcer, peritonitis, ruptured ectopic pregnancy, macroamylasemia. Drugs: azathioprine, hydrochlorothiazide. **Decreased in:** Pancreatic insufficiency, cystic fibrosis. Usually normal or low in chronic pancreatitis.	**Increased in:** Sarcoidosis (sensitivity = 63%, specificity = 93%, LRT = 9.0) (when upper limit of normal is 50), hyperthyroidism, acute hepatitis, primary biliary cirrhosis, diabetes mellitus, multiple myeloma, osteoarthritis, amyloidosis, Gaucher's disease, pneumoconiosis, histoplasmosis, miliary tuberculosis. Drugs: dexamethasone. **Decreased in:** Renal disease, obstructive pulmonary disease, hypothyroidism.
Physiologic Basis	Amylase hydrolyzes complex carbohydrates. Serum amylase is derived primarily from pancreas and salivary glands and is increased with inflammation or obstruction of these glands. Other tissues have some amylase activity, including ovaries, small and large intestine, and skeletal muscle.	ACE is a dipeptidyl carboxypeptidase that converts angiotensin I to the vasopressor, angiotensin II. ACE is normally present in the kidneys and other peripheral tissues. In granulomatous disease, ACE levels increase, derived from epithelioid cells within granulomas.
Test/Range/Collection	**Amylase,** serum 20–110 U/L [0.33–1.83 μkat/L] (laboratory-specific) Marbled $	**Angiotensin-converting enzyme,** serum (ACE) 12–35 U/L [<590 nkat/L] (method-dependent) Marbled $$

Antibody screen, serum Red $ Properly identified and labeled blood specimens are critical.	Detects antibodies to non-ABO red blood cell antigens in recipient's serum, using reagent red cells selected to possess antigens against which common antibodies can be produced. Further identification of the specificity of any antibody detected (using panels of red cells of known antigenicity) makes it possible to test donor blood for the absence of the corresponding antigen.	**Positive in:** Presence of alloantibody, autoantibody.	In practice, a type and screen (ABO and Rh grouping and antibody screen) is adequate workup for patients undergoing operative procedures unlikely to require transfusion. A negative antibody screen implies that a recipient can receive type-specific (ABO-Rh identical) blood with minimal risk. *Technical Manual of the American Association of Blood Banks*, 11th ed. American Association of Blood Banks, 1993.
Antidiuretic hormone, plasma (ADH) If serum osmolality >290 mosm/kg H_2O: 2–12 pg/mL If serum osmolality <290 mosm/kg H_2O: <2 pg/mL Lavender $$$$ Draw in two chilled tubes and deliver to lab on ice. Specimen for serum osmolality must be drawn at same time.	Antidiuretic hormone (vasopressin) is a hormone secreted from the posterior pituitary that acts on the distal nephron to conserve water and regulate the tonicity of body fluids. Water deprivation provides both an osmotic and a volume stimulus for ADH release by increasing plasma osmolality and decreasing plasma volume. Water administration lowers plasma osmolality and expands blood volume, inhibiting the release of ADH by the osmoreceptor and the atrial volume receptor mechanisms.	**Increased in:** Nephrogenic diabetes insipidus, syndrome of inappropriate antidiuretic hormone (SIADH). Drugs: nicotine, morphine, chlorpropamide, clofibrate, cyclophosphamide. **Normal relative to plasma osmolality in:** Primary polydipsia. **Decreased in:** Central (neurogenic) diabetes insipidus. Drugs: ethanol, phenytoin.	Test very rarely indicated. Measurement of serum and urine osmolality usually suffices. Test not indicated in diagnosis of SIADH. Patients with SIADH show decreased plasma sodium and decreased plasma osmolality, usually with high urine osmolality relative to plasma. These findings in a normovolemic patient with normal thyroid and adrenal function are sufficient to make the diagnosis of SIADH without measuring ADH itself. Semin Nephrol 1994;14:368.

Test/Range/Collection	Physiologic Basis	Interpretation	Comments
Antiglobulin test, direct (Direct Coombs, DAT) Negative Lavender or red $ Blood anticoagulated with EDTA is used to prevent in vitro uptake of complement components. A red top tube may be used, if necessary.	Direct antiglobulin test demonstrates in vivo coating of washed red cells with globulins, in particular IgG and C3d. Washed red cells are tested directly with antihuman globulin reagent. DAT is positive (shows agglutination) immediately when IgG coats red cells. Complement or IgA coating may only be demonstrated after incubation at room temperature.	**Positive in:** Autoimmune hemolytic anemia, hemolytic disease of the newborn, alloimmune reactions to recently transfused cells, and drug-induced hemolysis. Drugs: cephalosporins, levodopa, methadone, methyldopa, penicillin, phenacetin, quinidine.	A positive DAT implies in vivo red cell coating by immunoglobulins or complement. Such red cell coating may or may not be associated with immune hemolytic anemia. Polyspecific and anti-IgG reagents detect approximately 500 molecules of IgG per red cell, but autoimmune hemolytic anemia has been reported with IgG coating below this level. 10% of hospital patients have a positive DAT without clinical manifestations of immune-mediated hemolysis. A false-positive DAT is often seen in patients with hypergammaglobulinemia, eg, in some HIV-positive patients. *Technical Manual of the American Association of Blood Banks,* 11th ed. American Association of Blood Banks, 1993.
Antiglobulin test, indirect (Indirect Coombs) Negative Red $	Demonstrates presence in patient's serum of unexpected antibody to ABO and Rh-compatible red blood cells. First, the patient's serum is incubated in vitro with reagent red cells and washed to remove unbound globulins. Then antihuman globulin (AHG, Coombs) reagent is added. Agglutination of red cells indicates that serum contains antibodies to antigens present on the reagent red cells.	**Positive in:** Presence of alloantibody or autoantibody. Drugs: methyldopa.	The technique is used in antibody detection and identification and in the major cross-match prior to transfusion (see Type and Cross-Match, p 175). *Technical Manual of the American Association of Blood Banks,* 11th ed. American Association of Blood Banks, 1993.

	α_1-Antiprotease	Antistreptolysin O titer
α_1-Antiprotease (α_1-antitrypsin), serum 110–270 mg/dL [1.1–2.7 g/L] Marbled $$	α_1-Antiprotease is an α_1 globulin glycoprotein serine protease inhibitor (Pi) whose deficiency leads to excessive protease activity and panacinar emphysema in adults or liver disease in children (seen as ZZ and SZ phenotypes). Cirrhosis of the liver and liver cancer in adults are also associated with the Pi Z phenotype.	**Increased in:** Inflammation, infection, rheumatic disease, malignancy, and pregnancy because it is an acute phase reactant. **Decreased in:** Congenital α_1-antiprotease deficiency, nephrotic syndrome.	Smoking is a much more common cause of chronic obstructive pulmonary disease in adults than is α_1-antiprotease deficiency. N Engl J Med 1978;299:1045. N Engl J Med 1978;299:1099. Curr Opin Pulm Med 1996;2:155.
Antistreptolysin O titer, serum (ASO) Children <5 years: <85; 5–19 years: <170 Adults: <85 Todd units (laboratory-specific) Marbled $$	Detects the presence of antibody to the antigen streptolysin O produced by group A streptococci. Streptococcal antibodies appear about 2 weeks after infection. Titer rises to a peak at 4–6 weeks and may remain elevated for 6 months to 1 year. Test is based on the neutralization of the hemolytic activity of streptolysin O by antistreptolysin O antibodies in serum.	**Increased in:** Recent infection with group A beta-hemolytic streptococci: scarlet fever, erysipelas, streptococcal pharyngitis/tonsillitis (40–50%), rheumatic fever (80–85%), poststreptococcal glomerulonephritis. Some collagen-vascular diseases. Certain serum lipoproteins, bacterial growth products, or oxidized streptolysin O may result in inhibition of hemolysis and thus cause false-positive results.	Standardization of (Todd) units may vary significantly from laboratory to laboratory. ASO titers are not useful in management of acute streptococcal pharyngitis. In patients with rheumatic fever, test may be a more reliable indicator of recent streptococcal infection than throat culture. An increasing titer is more suggestive of acute streptococcal infection than a single elevated level. Even with severe infection, ASO titers will rise in only 70–80% of patients. N Engl J Med 1970;282:23,78. J Clin Epidemiol 1993;46:1181.

Test/Range/Collection	Physiologic Basis	Interpretation	Comments
		Antithrombin III	**Aspartate aminotransferase**
Antithrombin III (AT III), plasma 84–123% (qualitative) 22–39 mg/dL (quantitative) Blue $$ Transport to lab on ice. Plasma must be separated and frozen in a polypropylene tube within 2 hours.	Antithrombin III is a serine protease inhibitor that protects against thrombus formation by inhibiting thrombin and factors IXa, Xa, XIa, XIIa, plasmin, and kallikrein. It accounts for 70–90% of the anticoagulant activity of human plasma. Its activity is enhanced 100-fold by heparin. There are two types of assay: functional (qualitative) and immunologic (quantitative). Since the immunologic assay cannot rule out functional AT III deficiency, a functional assay should be ordered first. Functional assays test AT III activity in inhibiting thrombin or factor Xa. Given an abnormal functional assay, the quantitative immunologic test indicates whether there is decreased synthesis of AT III or intact synthesis of a dysfunctional protein.	**Increased by:** Oral anticoagulants. **Decreased in:** Congenital and acquired AT III deficiency (renal disease, chronic liver disease), oral contraceptive use, chronic disseminated intravascular coagulation, acute venous thrombosis (consumption), and heparin therapy.	Congenital and acquired AT III deficiency results in a hypercoagulable state, venous thromboembolism, and heparin resistance. Congenital AT III deficiency is present in 1:2000–1:5000 people and is autosomal codominant. Heterozygotes have AT III levels 20–60% of normal. Semin Thromb Hemost 1982;8:276. Thromb Haemost 1993;69:231.
Aspartate aminotransferase, serum (AST, SGOT, GOT) 0–35 IU/L [0–0.58 μkat/L] (laboratory-specific) Marbled $	Intracellular enzyme involved in amino acid metabolism. Present in large concentrations in liver, skeletal muscle, brain, red cells, and heart. Released into the bloodstream when tissue is damaged, especially in liver injury.	**Increased in:** Acute viral hepatitis (ALT > AST), biliary tract obstruction (cholangitis, choledocholithiasis), alcoholic hepatitis and cirrhosis (AST > ALT), liver abscess, metastatic or primary liver cancer; right heart failure, ischemia or hypoxia, injury to liver ("shock liver"), extensive trauma. Drugs that cause cholestasis or hepatotoxicity. **Decreased in:** Pyridoxine (vitamin B_6) deficiency.	Test is not indicated for diagnosis of myocardial infarction. AST/ALT ratio > 1 suggests cirrhosis in patients with hepatitis C. Compr Ther 1994;20:50. Hosp Pract (Off Ed) Nov 1994;29:32. Am J Gastroenterol 1998;93:44.

	B cell immunoglobulin heavy chain gene rearrangement	*bcr/abl* translocation
B cell immunoglobulin heavy chain gene rearrangement Whole blood, bone marrow, or frozen tissue Lavender $$$$	In general, the percentage of B lymphocytes with identical immunoglobulin heavy chain gene rearrangements is very low; in malignancies, however, the clonal expansion of one population leads to a large number of cells with identical B cell immunoglobulin heavy chain gene rearrangements. Southern blot is used to identify a monoclonal population.	**Positive in:** B cell neoplasms such as lymphoma.	Samples with > 10% of cells showing a given B cell rearrangement are considered positive. However, a large monoclonal population is consistent with—but not diagnostic of—malignancy. Arch Path Lab Med 1988;112:117.
bcr/abl translocation Blood Lavender $$$$	Approximately 95% of chronic myelogenous leukemia (CML) is associated with the "Philadelphia chromosome," a translocation that moves the *c-abl* proto-oncogene from chromosome 9 to the breakpoint cluster (*bcr*) region of chromosome 22. Southern blot is used to identify the translocation.	**Positive in:** Chronic myelogenous leukemia (sensitivity 95%) and acute lymphocytic leukemia (sensitivity 10–15%).	This assay will detect the 9;22 translocation if it has taken place in >10% of the cells. CML patients with bone marrow transplants can be monitored for recurrence of disease with this test. N Engl J Med 1988;319:990.

		Bilirubin	
Test/Range/Collection	Physiologic Basis	Interpretation	Comments
Bilirubin, serum 0.1–1.2 mg/dL [2–21 µmol/L] Direct (conjugated to glucuronide) bilirubin: 0.1–0.4 mg/dL [<7 µmol/L]; Indirect (unconjugated) bilirubin: 0.2–0.7 mg/dL [<12 µmol/L] Marbled $$	Bilirubin, a product of hemoglobin metabolism, is conjugated in the liver to mono- and diglucuronides and excreted in bile. Some conjugated bilirubin is bound to serum albumin, so-called D (delta) bilirubin. Elevated serum bilirubin occurs in liver disease, biliary obstruction, or hemolysis.	**Increased in:** Acute or chronic hepatitis, cirrhosis, biliary tract obstruction, toxic hepatitis, neonatal jaundice, congenital liver enzyme abnormalities (Dubin-Johnson, Rotor's, Gilbert's, Crigler-Najjar syndromes), fasting, hemolytic disorders. Hepatotoxic drugs.	Assay of total bilirubin includes conjugated (direct) and unconjugated (indirect) bilirubin plus delta bilirubin (conjugated bilirubin bound to albumin). It is usually clinically unnecessary to fractionate total bilirubin. The fractionation is unreliable by the diazo reaction and may underestimate unconjugated bilirubin. Only conjugated bilirubin appears in the urine, and it is indicative of liver disease; hemolysis is associated with increased unconjugated bilirubin. Persistence of delta bilirubin in serum in resolving liver disease means that total bilirubin does not effectively indicate the time course of resolution. Pediatrics 1992;89:80. Br J Hosp Med 1994;51:181. Pediatr Rev 1994;15:233.

Bleeding time		
Bleeding time 2–10 minutes $$ Test done by laboratory personnel. Simplate (presterilized device with spring-loaded blade) is used to make single cut 1 mm deep and 6 mm long on dorsal aspect of forearm after inflation of sphygmomanometer to 40 mm Hg. Filter paper is used to absorb blood from wound margins every 30 seconds, and time to cessation of bleeding is noted.	This is a test of platelet function, not a test of coagulation factors.	**Increased in:** Platelet disorders, thrombocytopenia, Bernard-Soulier syndrome, thrombasthenia. Also elevated in some forms of von Willebrand's disease, which is a disorder of factor VIII coagulant activity and not primarily a platelet disorder. Drugs: aspirin and other preparations containing aspirin.	Test is useful as a screening test (with aspirin challenge) for diagnosis of von Willebrand's disease and platelet disorders. Test adds no clinically useful information to the prediction of clinically significant bleeding beyond that obtained from the history, physical examination, and other laboratory tests—platelet count, blood urea nitrogen (BUN), prothrombin time (PT), and partial thromboplastin time (PTT). In patients with no history of bleeding and no intake of nonsteroidal anti-inflammatory drugs, an increased bleeding time does not correlate with actual surgical bleeding. Semin Thromb Hemost 1990;16:1. Blood 1994;84:3363. Med Clin North Am 1994;78:577.

Test/Range/Collection	Physiologic Basis	Interpretation	Comments
			Blood urea nitrogen
Blood urea nitrogen, serum (BUN) 8–20 mg/dL [2.9–7.1 mmol/L] Marbled $	Urea, an end product of protein metabolism, is excreted by the kidney. BUN is directly related to protein intake and nitrogen metabolism and inversely related to the rate of excretion of urea. Urea concentration in glomerular filtrate is the same as in plasma, but its tubular reabsorption is inversely related to the rate of urine formation. Thus, the BUN is a less useful measure of glomerular filtration rate than the serum creatinine (Cr).	**Increased in:** Renal failure (acute or chronic), urinary tract obstruction, dehydration, shock, burns, CHF, GI bleeding. Nephrotoxic drugs (eg, gentamicin). **Decreased in:** Hepatic failure, nephrotic syndrome, cachexia (low-protein and high-carbohydrate diets).	Urease assay method commonly used. BUN/Cr ratio (normally 12:1–20:1) is decreased in acute tubular necrosis, advanced liver disease, low protein intake, and following hemodialysis. BUN/Cr ratio is increased in dehydration, GI bleeding, and increased catabolism. Nursing 1994;24:88. Ann Emerg Med 1992;21:713.
			Brucella **antibody**
Brucella antibody, serum <1:80 titer Marbled $	Patients with acute brucellosis generally develop an agglutinating antibody titer of ≥ 1:160 within 3 weeks. The titer may rise during the acute infection, with relapses, brucellergin skin testing, or use of certain vaccines (see Interpretation). The agglutinin titer usually declines after 3 months or after successful therapy. Low titers may persist for years.	**Increased in:** *Brucella* infection (except *B canis*) (97% within 3 weeks of illness); recent brucellergin skin test; infections with *Francisella tularensis*, *Yersinia enterocolitica*, salmonella. Rocky mountain spotted fever; vaccinations for cholera and tularemia. **Normal in:** *B canis* infection.	This test will detect antibodies against all of the *Brucella* species except *B canis*. A fourfold or greater rise in titer in separate specimens drawn 1–4 weeks apart is indicative of recent exposure. Final diagnosis depends on isolation of organism by culture. J Clin Microbiol 1980;11:691. J Infect Dis 1989;159:219. Rev Infect Dis 1991;13:359.
			C-reactive protein
C-reactive protein, serum 0–2 mg/dL Marbled $	Marker of inflammation.	**Increased in:** Inflammatory states.	Elevated C-reactive protein level appears to be an independent risk factor for coronary heart disease events. Ann Intern Med 1999;130:933.

C1 esterase inhibitor		
C1 esterase inhibitor (C1 INH), serum Method-dependent Marbled $$	C1 esterase inhibitor (C1 INH) is an alpha-globulin, which controls the first stage of the classic complement pathway and inhibits thrombin, plasmin, and kallikrein. Deficiency results in spontaneous activation of C1, leading to consumption of C2 and C4. The functional assay involves the measurement of C1 INH as it inhibits the hydrolysis of a substrate ester by C1 esterase. Immunoassay of C1 INH is also available.	**Decreased in:** Hereditary angioedema (HAE) (85%) (15% of patients with HAE will have normal levels by immunoassay, but the protein is nonfunctional and levels determined by the functional assay will be low).	C1 esterase inhibitor deficiency is an uncommon cause of angioedema. There are two subtypes of hereditary angioedema. In one, the protein is absent; in the other, it is nonfunctional. Acquired angioedema has been attributed to massive consumption of C1 INH (presumably by tumor or lymphoma-related immune complexes) or to anti-C1 INH auto-antibody. When clinical suspicion exists, a serum C4 level screens for HAE. Low levels of C4 are present in all cases during an attack. C1 esterase inhibitor levels are not indicated unless either the C4 level is low or there is a very high clinical suspicion of HAE in a patient with normal C4 during an asymptomatic phase between attacks. In acquired C1 INH deficiency, the C1 level is also significantly decreased (often 10% of normal), whereas in HAE the C1 level is normal or only slightly decreased. Am J Med 1990;88:656. Ann Allergy 1991;67(2 Part 1):107. Med Clin North Am 1992;76:805. South Med J 1992;85:1084.

Test/Range/Collection	Physiologic Basis	Interpretation	Comments
C-peptide, serum 0.8–4.0 ng/mL [µg/L] Marbled $$$ Fasting sample preferred.	C-peptide is an inactive by-product of the cleavage of proinsulin to active insulin. Its presence indicates endogenous release of insulin. C-peptide is largely excreted by the kidney.	**Increased in:** Renal failure, ingestion of oral hypoglycemic drugs, insulinomas, B cell transplants. **Decreased in:** Factitious hypoglycemia due to insulin administration, pancreatectomy, type I diabetes mellitus (decreased or undetectable).	Test is most useful to detect factitious insulin injection (increased insulin, decreased C-peptide) or to detect endogenous insulin production in diabetic patients receiving insulin (C-peptide present). A molar ratio of insulin to C-peptide in peripheral venous blood >1.0 in a hypoglycemic patient is consistent with surreptitious or inadvertent insulin administration but not insulinoma. Arch Intern Med 1977;137:625. Am J Med 1989;86:335. Arch Intern Med 1993;153:650.
Calcitonin, plasma Male: <90 pg/mL [ng/L] Female: <70 pg/mL [ng/L] Green $$$ Fasting sample required. Place on ice.	Calcitonin is a 32-amino-acid polypeptide hormone secreted by the parafollicular C cells of the thyroid. It decreases osteoclastic bone resorption and lowers serum calcium levels.	**Increased in:** Medullary thyroid carcinoma (>500 pg/mL on two occasions), Zollinger-Ellison syndrome, pernicious anemia, pregnancy (at term), newborns, carcinoma (breast, lung, pancreas), chronic renal failure.	Test is useful to diagnose and monitor medullary thyroid carcinoma, although stimulation tests may be necessary (eg, pentagastrin test). Genetic testing is now available for the diagnosis of multiple endocrine neoplasia type II. (MEN II is the most common familial form of medullary thyroid carcinoma.) Mayo Clin Proc 1975;50:53. Ann Intern Med 1995;122:118.

Calcium, serum		
Calcium, serum (Ca²⁺) 8.5–10.5 mg/dL [2.1–2.6 mmol/L] **Panic:** <6.5 or >13.5 mg/dL Marbled $ Prolonged venous stasis during collection causes false increase in serum calcium.	Serum calcium is the sum of ionized calcium plus complexed calcium and calcium bound to proteins (mostly albumin). Level of ionized calcium is regulated by parathyroid hormone and vitamin D.	**Increased in:** Hyperparathyroidism, malignancies secreting parathyroid hormone–related protein (PTHrP) (especially squamous cell carcinoma of lung and renal cell carcinoma), vitamin D excess, milk-alkali syndrome, multiple myeloma, Paget's disease of bone with immobilization, sarcoidosis, other granulomatous disorders, familial hypocalciuria, vitamin A intoxication, thyrotoxicosis, Addison's disease. Drugs: antacids (some), calcium salts, chronic diuretic use (eg, thiazides), lithium, others. **Decreased in:** Hypoparathyroidism, vitamin D deficiency, renal insufficiency, pseudohypoparathyroidism, magnesium deficiency, hyperphosphatemia, massive transfusion, hypoalbuminemia.	Need to know serum albumin to interpret calcium level. For every decrease in albumin by 1 mg/dL, calcium should be corrected upward by 0.8 mg/dL. In 10% of patients with malignancies, hypercalcemia is attributable to coexistent hyperparathyroidism, suggesting that serum PTH levels should be measured at initial presentation of all hypercalcemic patients (see pp 134 and 354). Ann Intern Med 1990;112:499. Nursing 1993;23:69. Clin Endocrinol 1994;41:407.

	Calcium, ionized		
Test/Range/Collection	**Physiologic Basis**	**Interpretation**	**Comments**
Calcium, ionized, serum 4.4–5.4 mg/dL (at pH 7.4) [1.1–1.3 mmol/L] Whole blood specimen must be collected anaerobically and anticoagulated with standardized amounts of heparin. Tourniquet application must be brief. Specimen should be analyzed promptly. Marbled $$	Calcium circulates in three forms: as free Ca^{2+} (47%), protein-bound to albumin and globulins (43%), and as calcium-ligand complexes (10%) (with citrate, bicarbonate, lactate, phosphate, and sulfate). Protein binding is highly pH-dependent, and acidosis results in an increased free calcium fraction. Ionized Ca^{2+} is the form that is physiologically active. Ionized calcium is a more accurate reflection of physiologic status than total calcium in patients with altered serum proteins (renal failure, nephrotic syndrome, multiple myeloma, etc), altered concentrations of calcium-binding ligands, and acid-base disturbances. Measurement of ionized calcium is by ion-selective electrodes.	**Increased in:** ↓ blood pH. **Decreased in:** ↑ blood pH, citrate, heparin, EDTA.	Ionized calcium measurements are not needed except in special circumstances, eg, massive blood transfusion, liver transplantation, neonatal hypocalcemia, and cardiac surgery. Validity of test depends on sample integrity. Ann Clin Lab Sci 1991;21:297.

Calcium, urine

| **Calcium**, urine (U_{Ca}) | Ordinarily there is moderate urinary calcium excretion, the amount depending on dietary calcium, parathyroid hormone (PTH) level, and protein intake. Renal calculi occur much more often in hyperparathyroidism than in other hypercalcemic states. | **Increased in:** Hyperparathyroidism, osteolytic bone metastases, myeloma, osteoporosis, vitamin D intoxication, distal RTA, idiopathic hypercalciuria, thyrotoxicosis, Paget's disease, Fanconi's syndrome, hepatolenticular degeneration, schistosomiasis, sarcoidosis, malignancy (breast, bladder), osteitis deformans, immobilization. Drugs: acetazolamide, calcium salts, cholestyramine, corticosteroids, dihydrotachysterol, initial diuretic use (eg, furosemide), others. **Decreased in:** Hypoparathyroidism, pseudohypoparathyroidism, rickets, osteomalacia, nephrotic syndrome, acute glomerulonephritis, osteoblastic bone metastases, hypothyroidism, celiac disease, steatorrhea, hypocalciuric hypercalcemia, other causes of hypocalcemia. Drugs: aspirin, bicarbonate, chronic diuretic use (eg, thiazides, chlorthalidone), estrogens, indomethacin, lithium, neomycin, oral contraceptives. | Approximately one-third of patients with hyperparathyroidism have normal urine calcium excretion. The extent of calcium excretion can be expressed as a urine calcium (U_{Ca})/ urine creatinine (U_{Cr}) ratio. Normally, $$\frac{U_{Ca}\,(mg/dL)}{U_{Cr}\,(mg/dL)} < 0.14$$ and $$\frac{U_{Ca}\,(mmol/L)}{U_{Cr}\,(mmol/L)} < 0.40$$ Hypercalciuria is defined as a ratio >0.20 or >0.57, respectively. Test is useful in the evaluation of renal stones but is not usually needed for the diagnosis of hyperparathyroidism, which can be made using serum calcium (see above) and PTH measurements (see pp 134 and 354). It may be useful in hypercalcemic patients to rule out familial hypocalciuric hypercalcemia. In the diagnosis of hypercalciuria, U_{Ca}/U_{Cr} ratios in random single-voided urine specimens correlate well with 24-hour calcium excretions. *Arch Intern Med* 1991;151:1587. *Miner Electrolyte Metab* 1993;19:385. |
| 100–300 mg/24 h [2.5–7.5 mmol/24 h or 2.3–3.3 mmol/12 h] Urine bottle containing hydrochloric acid $$$ Collect 24-hour urine or 12-hour overnight urine. | | | |

Test/Range/Collection	Physiologic Basis	Interpretation	Comments
		Carbon dioxide	**Carboxyhemoglobin**
Carbon dioxide (CO_2), total, serum (bicarbonate) 22–28 meq/L [mmol/L] **Panic:** <15 or >40 meq/L [mmo/L] Marbled $ Do not leave exposed to air since this will cause falsely low CO_2 levels.	Bicarbonate-carbonic acid buffer is one of the most important buffer systems in maintaining normal body fluid pH. Total CO_2 is measured as the sum of bicarbonate concentration plus carbonic acid concentration plus dissolved CO_2. Since bicarbonate makes up 90–95% of the total CO_2 content, total CO_2 is a useful surrogate for bicarbonate concentration.	**Increased in:** Primary metabolic alkalosis, compensated respiratory acidosis, volume contraction, mineralocorticoid excess, congenital chloridorrhea. Drugs: diuretics (eg, thiazide, furosemide). **Decreased in:** Metabolic acidosis, compensated respiratory alkalosis. Fanconi's syndrome, volume overload. Drugs: acetazolamide, outdated tetracycline.	Total CO_2 determination is indicated for all seriously ill patients on admission. If arterial blood gas studies are done, total CO_2 test is redundant. Simultaneous measurement of pH and PCO_2 is required to fully characterize a patient's acid-base status.
Carboxyhemoglobin, whole blood (HbCO) < 9% [< 0.09] Lavender $$ Do not remove stopper.	Carbon monoxide (CO) combines irreversibly with hemoglobin at the sites that normally bind oxygen. This produces a decrease in oxygen saturation and a shift in the oxyhemoglobin dissociation curve, resulting in decreased release of oxygen to the tissues.	**Increased in:** Carbon monoxide poisoning. Exposure to automobile exhaust or smoke from fires. Cigarette smokers can have up to 9% carboxyhemoglobin, nonsmokers have <2%.	Test (if available within minutes, together with O_2 saturation by oximeter) is useful in evaluation of CO poisoning. PO_2 is usually normal in CO poisoning. Test measures carboxyhemoglobin spectrophotometrically. N Engl J Med 1989;321:1474.

Carcinoembryonic antigen		
Carcinoembryonic antigen, serum (CEA) 0–2.5 ng/mL [μg/L] Marbled $$	CEA is an oncofetal antigen, a glyco-protein associated with certain malignancies, particularly epithelial tumors.	**Increased in:** Colon cancer (72%), lung cancer (76%), pancreatic cancer (91%), stomach cancer (61%), cigarette smok-ers, benign liver disease (acute 50% and chronic 90%), benign GI disease (peptic ulcer, pancreatitis, colitis). Ele-vations >20 ng/mL are generally asso-ciated with malignancy. For breast cancer recurrence (using 5 ng/mL cut-off), sensitivity = 44.4% and specificity = 95.5%.	**Screening:** Test is not sensitive or spe-cific enough to be useful in cancer screening. **Monitoring after surgery:** Test is used to follow progression of colon cancer after surgery (elevated CEA levels suggest recurrence 3–6 months before other clinical indicators), although such monitoring has not yet been shown to improve survival rates. If monitoring is done, the same assay method must be used consistently in order to eliminate any method-dependent variability. JAMA 1983;270:943. Ann Intern Med 1991;115:623. Br Cancer Treat 1995;37:209.

	CD4/CD8 ratio		
Test/Range/Collection	Physiologic Basis	Interpretation	Comments
CD4/CD8 ratio, whole blood Ratio: 0.8–2.9 CD4: 359–1725 cells/μL (29–61%) CD8: 177–1106 cells/μL (18–42%) Lavender $$$ If an absolute CD4 count is required, also request a CBC and differential.	Lymphocyte identification depends on specific cell surface antigens (clusters of differentiation, CD), which can be detected with monoclonal antibodies using flow cytometry. CD4 cells are predominantly helper-inducer cells of the immunologic system. They react with peptide class II major histocompatibility complex antigens and augment B cell responses and T cell lymphokine secretion. CD4 cells are the major target of HIV-1. CD8 cells can be divided into suppressor cells, which decrease B cell responses, and cytotoxic T cells.	**Increased in:** Rheumatoid arthritis, type I diabetes mellitus, SLE without renal disease, primary biliary cirrhosis, atopic dermatitis, Sézary syndrome, psoriasis, chronic autoimmune hepatitis. **Decreased in:** AIDS/HIV infection, SLE with renal disease, acute CMV infection, burns, graft-versus-host disease, sunburn, myelodysplasia syndromes, acute lymphocytic leukemia in remission, recovery from bone marrow transplantation, herpes infection, infectious mononucleosis, measles, ataxia-telangiectasia, vigorous exercise.	Progressive decline in the number and function of CD4 lymphocytes seems to be the most characteristic immunologic defect in AIDS. Absolute CD4 measurement is particularly useful (more useful than the CD4/CD8 ratio) in determining eligibility for therapy (usually when CD4 < 500 cells/μL) and in monitoring the progress of the disease. Most AIDS-defining infections occur when the CD4 count drops below 200 cells/μL. Absolute CD4 count depends, analytically, on the reliability of the white blood cell differential count, as well as on the percentage of CD4 cells identified using the appropriate monoclonal antibody. Hematol Oncol Clin North Am 1991;5:215. Arch Intern Med 1994;154:1561.

	Centromere antibody		Ceruloplasmin, serum
Centromere antibody, serum (ACA) Negative Marbled $$	Anticentromere antibodies are antibodies to nuclear proteins of the kinetochore plate.	**Positive in:** CREST (70–90%), scleroderma (10–15%), Raynaud's disease (10–30%).	In patients with connective tissue disease, the predictive value of a positive test is >95% for scleroderma or related disease (CREST, Raynaud's disease). Diagnosis of CREST is made clinically (calcinosis, Raynaud's disease, esophageal dysmotility, sclerodactyly, and telangiectasia). In the absence of clinical findings, the test has low predictive value. (See also Autoantibodies table, p 367.) Rheum Dis Clin North Am 1992;18:483. Ann Rheum Dis 1993;52:586. Clin Rheumatol 1994;13:427. Ann Rheum Dis 1995;54:148.
Ceruloplasmin, serum 20–35 mg/dL [200–350 mg/L] Marbled $$	Ceruloplasmin, a 120,000–160,000 MW α_2-glycoprotein synthesized by the liver, is the main (95%) copper-carrying protein in human serum.	**Increased in:** Acute and chronic inflammation, pregnancy. Drugs: oral contraceptives, phenytoin. **Decreased in:** Wilson's disease (hepatolenticular degeneration) (95%), CNS disease other than Wilson's (15%), liver disease other than Wilson's (23%), malabsorption, malnutrition, primary biliary cirrhosis, nephrotic syndrome, severe copper deficiency, Menkes' disease (X-linked inherited copper deficiency).	Slitlamp examination for Kayser-Fleischer rings and serum ceruloplasmin level recommended for diagnosis of Wilson's disease. Serum copper level is very rarely indicated. Screening all patients with liver disease is ineffective. 5% of patients with Wilson's disease have low-normal levels of ceruloplasmin. Q J Med 1987;65:959. J Hepatol 1997;27:358.

	Chloride

Test/Range/Collection	Physiologic Basis	Interpretation	Comments
Chloride, serum (Cl⁻) 98–107 meq/L [mmol/L] Marbled $	Chloride, the principal inorganic anion of extracellular fluid, is important in maintaining normal acid-base balance and normal osmolality. If chloride is lost (as HCl or NH₄Cl), alkalosis ensues; if chloride is ingested or retained, acidosis ensues.	**Increased in:** Renal failure, nephrotic syndrome, renal tubular acidosis, dehydration, overtreatment with saline, hyperparathyroidism, diabetes insipidus, metabolic acidosis from diarrhea (loss of HCO₃), respiratory alkalosis, hyperadrenocorticism. Drugs: acetazolamide (hyperchloremic acidosis), androgens, hydrochlorothiazide, salicylates (intoxication). **Decreased in:** Vomiting, diarrhea, gastrointestinal suction, renal failure combined with salt deprivation, overtreatment with diuretics, chronic respiratory acidosis, diabetic ketoacidosis, excessive sweating, SIADH, salt-losing nephropathy, acute intermittent porphyria, water intoxication, expansion of extracellular fluid volume, adrenal insufficiency, hyperaldosteronism, metabolic alkalosis. Drugs: chronic laxative or bicarbonate ingestion, corticosteroids, diuretics.	Test is helpful in assessing normal and increased anion gap metabolic acidosis and in distinguishing hypercalcemia due to primary hyperparathyroidism (high serum chloride) from that due to malignancy (normal serum chloride). Exp Clin Endocrinol 1991;98:179. Crit Care Med 1992;20:227.

Cholesterol			
Cholesterol, serum Desirable <200 Borderline 200–239 High risk >240 mg/dL [Desirable <5.2 Borderline 5.2–6.1 High risk >6.2 mmol/L] Marbled $ Fasting preferred for LDL cholesterol. HDL and total cholesterol can be measured nonfasting.	Cholesterol level is determined by lipid metabolism, which is in turn influenced by heredity, diet, and liver, kidney, thyroid, and other endocrine organ functions. Total cholesterol (TC) = low density lipoprotein (LDL) cholesterol + high density lipoprotein (HDL) cholesterol + (triglycerides [TG] / 5) (valid only if TG < 400). Since LDL cholesterol is the clinically important entity, it is calculated as $$LDL = TC - HDL - \frac{TG}{5}$$ This calculation is valid only if specimen is obtained fasting (in order to obtain relevant triglyceride level).	**Increased in:** Primary disorders: polygenic hypercholesterolemia, familial hypercholesterolemia (deficiency of LDL receptors), familial combined hyperlipidemia, familial dysbetalipoproteinemia. Secondary disorders: hypothyroidism, uncontrolled diabetes mellitus, nephrotic syndrome, biliary obstruction, anorexia nervosa, hepatoma, Cushing's syndrome, acute intermittent porphyria. Drugs: corticosteroids. **Decreased in:** Severe liver disease (acute hepatitis, cirrhosis, malignancy), hyperthyroidism, severe acute or chronic illness, malnutrition, malabsorption (eg, HIV), extensive burns, familial (Gaucher's disease, Tangier disease), abetalipoproteinemia, intestinal lymphangiectasia.	It is important to treat the cause of secondary hypercholesterolemia (eg, hypothyroidism). Need to check total cholesterol and HDL cholesterol because cardiovascular risk may be increased with relatively modest total cholesterol elevation if HDL cholesterol is low. National Cholesterol Education Program Expert Panel has published clinical recommendations for cholesterol management (see JAMA 1993 reference). Arch Intern Med 1988;148:36. JAMA 1993;260:3015. Med Clin North Am 1994;78:117. Circulation 1995;91:908. JAMA 1998;279:1615.

	Chorionic gonadotropin, β-subunit, quantitative	

Test/Range/Collection	Physiologic Basis	Interpretation	Comments
Chorionic gonadotropin, β-subunit, quantitative, serum (β-hCG) Males and nonpregnant females: undetectable or <2 mIU/mL [IU/L] Marbled $$	Human chorionic gonadotropin is a glycoprotein made up of two subunits (α and β). Human glycoproteins such as LH, FSH, and TSH share the α subunit of hCG, but the β subunit is specific for hCG. hCG is produced by trophoblastic tissue, and its detection in serum or urine is the basis for pregnancy testing. Serum hCG can be detected as early as 24 hours after implantation at a concentration of 5 mIU/mL. During normal pregnancy, serum levels double every 2–3 days and are 50–100 mIU/mL at the time of the first missed menstrual period. Peak levels are reached 60–80 days after the last menstrual period (LMP) (30,000–100,000 mIU/mL), and levels then decrease to a plateau of 5,000–10,000 mIU/mL at about 120 days after LMP and persist until delivery.	**Increased in:** Pregnancy (including ectopic pregnancy), hyperemesis gravidarum, trophoblastic tumors (hydatidiform mole, choriocarcinoma of uterus), some germ cell tumors (teratomas of ovary or testicle, seminoma), ectopic hCG production by other malignancies (stomach, pancreas, lung, colon, liver). Failure of elevated serum levels to decrease after surgical resection of trophoblastic tumor indicates metastatic tumor; levels rising from normal indicate tumor recurrence. **Decreasing over time:** Threatened abortion.	Routine pregnancy testing is done by *qualitative* serum or urine hCG test. Test will be positive (>50 mIU/mL) in most pregnant women at the time of or shortly after the first missed menstrual period. *Quantitative* hCG testing is indicated for (1) the evaluation of suspected ectopic pregnancy (where levels are lower than in normal pregnancy at the same gestational age) if the routine pregnancy test is negative; (2) the evaluation of threatened abortion. In both situations, hCG levels fail to demonstrate the normal early pregnancy increase. Test is also indicated for following the course of trophoblastic and germ cell tumors. Hum Reprod 1992;7:701. West J Med 1993;159:195. Urology 1994;44:392.

	Clostridium difficile enterotoxin		Clotting time, activated
***Clostridium difficile* enterotoxin**, stool Negative (≤1 : 10 titer) Urine or stool container $$$ Must be tested within 12 hours of collection as toxin (B) is labile.	*Clostridium difficile*, a motile, gram-positive rod, is the major recognized agent of antibiotic-associated diarrhea, which is toxigenic in origin (see Antibiotic-associated colitis, p 224). There are two toxins (A and B) produced by *C difficile*. Cell culture is used to detect the cytopathic effect of the toxins, whose identity is confirmed by neutralization with specific antitoxins. Toxin A (more weakly cytopathic in cell culture) is enterotoxic and produces enteric disease. Toxin B (more easily detected in standard cell culture assays) fails to produce intestinal disease.	**Positive in:** Antibiotic-associated diarrhea (15–25%), antibiotic-associated colitis (50–75%), and pseudomembranous colitis (90–100%). About 3% of healthy adults and 10–20% of hospitalized patients have *C difficile* in their colonic flora. There is also a high carrier rate of *C difficile* and its toxin in healthy neonates.	Definitive diagnosis of disease caused by *C difficile* toxin is by endoscopic detection of pseudomembranous colitis. Direct examination of stool for leukocytes, gram-positive rods, or blood is not helpful. Culture of *C difficile* is not routinely performed, as it would isolate numerous nontoxigenic *C difficile* strains. Rev Infect Dis 1990;12:S243. Eur J Clin Microbiol 1996;15:561.
Clotting time, activated, whole blood (ACT) 114–186 seconds Special black tube $$ Performed at patient bedside. Avoid traumatic venipuncture, which may cause contamination with tissue juices and decrease clotting time.	A bedside or operating room test that assesses heparinization by measuring time taken for whole blood to clot.	**Prolonged in:** Heparin therapy, severe deficiency of clotting factors (except factors VII and XIII), functional platelet disorders, afibrinogenemia, circulating anticoagulants. **Normal in:** Thrombocytopenia, factor VII deficiency, von Willebrand's disease.	Many consider this test unreliable. Reproducibility of prolonged ACTs is poor. Increasingly, the ACT has been used in the operating room, dialysis units, critical care centers and during interventional cardiology/radiology procedures to monitor anticoagulation and titrate heparin dosages. At centers without experience, should not be used to regulate therapeutic heparin dosage adjustments; use partial thromboplastin time (PTT) instead. Am J Crit Care 1993;2(1):81. Clin Cardiol 1994;17(7):357.

Test/Range/Collection	Physiologic Basis	Interpretation	Comments
Coccidioides antibodies			
Coccidioides antibodies, serum or CSF Negative Marbled $$	Screens for presence of antibodies to *Coccidioides immitis*. Some centers use the mycelial-phase antigen, coccidioidin, to detect antibody. IgM antibodies appear early in disease in 75% of patients, begin to decrease after week 3, and are rarely seen after 5 months. They may persist in disseminated cases, usually in the immunocompromised. IgG antibodies appear later in the course of the disease. Meningeal disease may have negative serum IgG and require CSF IgG antibody titers.	**Positive in:** Infection by coccidioides (90%). **Negative in:** Coccidioidin skin testing, many patients with chronic cavitary coccidioides; 5% of meningeal coccidioides is negative by CSF complement fixation (CF) test.	Diagnosis is based upon culture and serologic testing. Precipitin and CF tests detect 90% of primary symptomatic cases. Precipitin test is most effective in detecting early primary infection or an exacerbation of existing disease. Test is diagnostic but not prognostic. CF test becomes positive later than precipitin test, and titers can be used to assess severity of infection. Titers rise as the disease progresses and decline as the patient improves. Enzyme immunoassay now available; data suggest good performance. N Engl J Med 1995;332:1077. Am J Clin Pathol 1997;107:148.
Cold agglutinins			
Cold agglutinins, plasma < 1:20 titer Lavender or blue $$ Specimen should be kept at 37 °C.	Detects antibodies that agglutinate red blood cells in the cold (strongly at 4°C, weakly at 24°C, and weakly or not at all at 37°C). These antibodies are present in primary atypical pneumonias due to *Mycoplasma pneumoniae*, in certain autoimmune hemolytic anemias, and in normal persons (not clinically significant).	**Increased in:** Chronic cold agglutinin disease, lymphoproliferative disorders (eg, Waldenström's macroglobulinemia), autoimmune hemolytic anemia, collagen-vascular diseases, *M pneumoniae* pneumonia, infectious mononucleosis, mumps orchitis, cytomegalovirus, tropical diseases (eg, trypanosomiasis).	In *Mycoplasma* pneumonia, titers rise early, are maximal at 3–4 weeks after onset, and then disappear rapidly. These antibodies are usually IgM anti-I antibodies distinct from antibodies to *M pneumoniae*. A rise in cold agglutinin antibody titer is suggestive of recent mycoplasma infection but is found in other diseases. N Engl J Med 1977;297:583.

	Complement C3	Complement C4
Complement C3, serum 64–166 mg/dL [640–1660 mg/L] Marbled $$	The classic and alternative complement pathways converge at the C3 step in the complement cascade. Low levels indicate activation by one or both pathways. Most diseases with immune complexes will show decreased C3 levels. Test is usually performed as an immunoassay (by radial immunodiffusion or nephelometry).	**Increased in:** Many inflammatory conditions as an acute phase reactant, active phase of rheumatic diseases (eg, rheumatoid arthritis, SLE), acute viral hepatitis, myocardial infarction, cancer, diabetes mellitus, pregnancy, sarcoidosis, amyloidosis, thyroiditis. **Decreased by:** Decreased synthesis (protein malnutrition, congenital deficiency, severe liver disease), increased catabolism (immune complex disease, membranoproliferative glomerulonephritis [75%], SLE, Sjögren's syndrome, rheumatoid arthritis, disseminated intravascular coagulation, paroxysmal nocturnal hemoglobinuria, autoimmune hemolytic anemia, gram-negative bacteremia), increased loss (burns, gastroenteropathies).	Complement C3 levels may be useful in following the activity of immune complex diseases. The best test to detect inherited deficiencies is CH50. N Engl J Med 1987;316:1525.
Complement C4, serum 15–45 mg/dL [150–450 mg/L] Marbled $$	C4 is a component of the classic complement pathway. Depressed levels usually indicate classic pathway activation. Test is usually performed as an immunoassay and not a functional assay.	**Increased in:** Various malignancies (not clinically useful). **Decreased by:** Decreased synthesis (congenital deficiency), increased catabolism (SLE, rheumatoid arthritis, proliferative glomerulonephritis, hereditary angioedema, and increased loss (burns, protein-losing enteropathies).	Low C4 accompanies acute attacks of hereditary angioedema, and C4 is used as a first-line test for the disease. C1 esterase inhibitor levels are not indicated for the evaluation of hereditary angioedema unless C4 is low. Congenital C4 deficiency occurs with an SLE-like syndrome. N Engl J Med 1987;316:1525. Am J Med 1990;88:656.

Test/Range/Collection	Physiologic Basis	Interpretation	Comments
Complement CH50, plasma or serum (CH50) 22–40 U/mL (laboratory-specific) Marbled $$$	The quantitative assay of hemolytic complement activity depends on the ability of the classic complement pathway to induce hemolysis of red cells sensitized with optimal amounts of anti-red cell antibodies. For precise titrations of hemolytic complement, the dilution of serum that will lyse 50% of the indicator red cells is determined as the CH50. This arbitrary unit depends on the conditions of the assay and is therefore laboratory-specific.	**Decreased with:** >50–80% deficiency of classic pathway complement components (congenital or acquired deficiencies). **Normal in:** Deficiencies of the alternative pathway complement components.	This is a functional assay of biologic activity. Sensitivity to decreased levels of complement components depends on exactly how the test is performed. It is used to detect congenital and acquired severe deficiency disorders of the classic complement pathway. N Engl J Med 1987;316:1525.
Cortisol, plasma or serum 8:00 AM: 5–20 μg/dL [140–550 nmol/L] Marbled, lavender, or green $$	Release of corticotropin-releasing factor (CRF) from the hypothalamus stimulates release of ACTH from the pituitary, which in turn stimulates release of cortisol from the adrenal. Cortisol provides negative feedback to this system. Test measures both free cortisol and cortisol bound to cortisol-binding globulin (CBG). Morning levels are higher than evening levels.	**Increased in:** Cushing's syndrome, acute illness, surgery, trauma, septic shock, depression, anxiety, alcoholism, starvation, chronic renal failure, increased CBG (congenital, pregnancy, estrogen therapy). **Decreased in:** Addison's disease; decreased CBG (congenital, liver disease, nephrotic syndrome).	Cortisol levels are useful only in the context of standardized suppression or stimulation tests. (See Cosyntropin stimulation test, p 77, and Dexamethasone suppression tests, p 83). Circadian fluctuations in cortisol levels limit usefulness of single measurements. Analysis of diurnal variation of cortisol is not useful diagnostically. Crit Care Clin 1991;7:23. Endocrinol Metab Clin North Am 1994;23:511.

	Cortisol (urinary free)	Cosyntropin stimulation test
Cortisol (urinary free), urine 10–110 μg/24 h [30–300 nmol/d] Urine bottle containing boric acid. $$$ Collect 24-hour urine.	Urinary free cortisol measurement is useful in the initial evaluation of suspected Cushing's syndrome (see Cushing's syndrome algorithm, p 340).	**Increased in:** Cushing's syndrome, acute illness, stress. **Not Increased in:** Obesity.	This test replaces both the assessment of 17-hydroxycorticosteroids and the 17-ketogenic steroids in the initial diagnosis of Cushing's syndrome. Not useful for the diagnosis of adrenal insufficiency. A shorter (12-hour) overnight collection and measurement of the ratio of urine free cortisol to urine creatinine appears to perform nearly as well as a 24-hour collection for urine free cortisol. Ann Intern Med 1992;116:211. Clin Endocrinol 1998;48:503.
Cosyntropin stimulation test, serum or plasma Marbled, green, or lavender $$$ First draw a cortisol level. Then administer cosyntropin (1 μg or 0.25 mg IV). Draw another cortisol level in 30 minutes.	Cosyntropin (synthetic ACTH preparation) stimulates the adrenal to release cortisol. A normal response is a doubling of basal levels or an increment of 7 μg/dL (200 nmol/L) to a level above 18 μg/dL (>504 nmol/L). A poor cortisol response to cosyntropin indicates adrenal insufficiency (see Adrenocortical insufficiency algorithm, Fig. 8-3, p 338).	**Decreased in:** Adrenal insufficiency, pituitary insufficiency, AIDS.	Test does not distinguish primary from secondary (pituitary) adrenal insufficiency, since in secondary adrenal insufficiency the atrophic adrenal may be unresponsive to cosyntropin. Test may not reliably detect pituitary insufficiency. Metyrapone test (p 127) may be useful to assess the pituitary-adrenal axis. Crit Care Clin 1991;7:23. Resp Med 1991;85:511. J Clin Endocrinol Metab 1998;83:2726.

	Creatine kinase		
Test/Range/Collection	**Physiologic Basis**	**Interpretation**	**Comments**
Creatine kinase, serum (CK) 32–267 IU/L [0.53–4.45 μkat/L] (method-dependent) Marbled $	Creatine kinase splits creatine phosphate in the presence of ADP to yield creatine and ATP. Skeletal muscle, myocardium, and brain are rich in the enzyme. CK is released by tissue damage.	**Increased in:** Myocardial infarction, myocarditis, muscle trauma, rhabdomyolysis, muscular dystrophy, polymyositis, severe muscular exertion, malignant hyperthermia, hypothyroidism, cerebral infarction, surgery, Reye's syndrome, tetanus, generalized convulsions, alcoholism, IM injections, DC countershock. Drugs: clofibrate, HMG-Co A reductase inhibitors.	CK is as sensitive a test as aldolase for muscle damage, so aldolase is not needed. During a myocardial infarction (MI), serum CK level rises rapidly (within 3–5 hours); elevation persists for 2–3 days post-myocardial infarction. Total CK is not specific enough for use in diagnosis of MI, but a normal total CK has a high negative predictive value. A more specific test is needed for diagnosis of MI (eg, CK-MB or cardiac troponin I. Cardiac troponin I and CK-MB or CK-MB mass concentration are better markers for myocardial infarction. Br Heart J 1994;72:112.

Creatine kinase MB		
Creatine kinase MB, serum (CKMB) enzyme activity <16 IU/L [<0.27 μkat/L] or <4% of total CK or <7 μg/L mass units (laboratory-specific) Marbled $$	CK consists of 3 isoenzymes, made up of 2 subunits, M and B. The fraction with the greatest electrophoretic mobility is CK1 (BB); CK2 (MB) is intermediate and CK3 (MM) moves slowest towards the anode. Skeletal muscle is characterized by isoenzyme MM and brain by isoenzyme BB. Myocardium has approximately 40% MB isoenzyme. Assay techniques include isoenzyme separation by electrophoresis (isoenzyme activity units) or immunoassay using antibody specific for MB fraction (mass units).	**Increased in:** Myocardial infarction, cardiac trauma, certain muscular dystrophies, and polymyositis. Slight persistent elevation reported in a few patients on hemodialysis.	CKMB is a relatively specific test for MI. It appears in serum approximately 4 hours after infarction, peaks at 12–24 hours, and declines over 48–72 hours. CKMB mass concentration is a more sensitive marker of MI than CKMB isoenzymes or total CK within 4–12 hours after infarction. Cardiac troponin I levels are useful in the late (after 48 hours) diagnosis of MI since, unlike CKMB, levels remain elevated for 5–7 days. Within 48 hours, sensitivity and specificity of troponin I are similar to CKMB. Specificity of troponin I is higher than CKMB in patients with skeletal muscle injury or renal failure, or postoperatively. Cardiac troponin I is therefore the preferred test. Estimation of CKMM and CKBB is not clinically useful. Use total CK. Br Heart J 1994;72:112. Clin Chem 1994;40(7 Pt1):1291. N Engl J Med 1994;330:670. N Engl J Med 1994;331:561.

Test/Range/Collection	Physiologic Basis	Interpretation	Comments
			Creatinine
Creatinine, serum (Cr) 0.6–1.2 mg/dL [50–100 μmol/L] Marbled $	Endogenous creatinine is excreted by filtration through the glomerulus and by tubular secretion. Creatinine clearance is an acceptable clinical measure of glomerular filtration rate (GFR), though it sometimes overestimates GFR (eg, in cirrhosis). For each 50% reduction in GFR, serum creatinine approximately doubles.	**Increased in:** Acute or chronic renal failure, urinary tract obstruction, nephrotoxic drugs, hypothyroidism. **Decreased in:** Reduced muscle mass.	In alkaline picrate method, substances other than Cr (eg, acetoacetate, acetone, β-hydroxybutyrate, α-ketoglutarate, pyruvate, glucose) may give falsely high results. Therefore, patients with diabetic ketoacidosis may have spuriously elevated Cr. Cephalosporins may spuriously increase or decrease Cr measurement. Increased bilirubin may spuriously decrease Cr. Clin Chem 1990;36:1951. Ann Pharmacother 1993;27:622.

Creatinine clearance		
Creatinine clearance, (Cl_{Cr}) Adults: 90–130 mL/min/1.73 m² BSA $$ Collect carefully timed 24-hour urine and simultaneous serum/plasma creatinine sample. Record patient's weight and height.	Widely used test of glomerular filtration rate (GFR). Theoretically reliable, but often compromised by incomplete urine collection. Creatinine clearance is calculated from measurement of urine creatinine (U_{Cr} [mg/dL]), plasma/serum creatinine (P_{Cr} [mg/dL]), and urine flow rate (V [mL/min]) according to the formula: $$Cl_{Cr}(mL/min) = \frac{U_{Cr} \times V}{P_{Cr}}$$ where $$V(mL/min) = \frac{24\text{-hour urine volume(mL)}}{1440}$$ Creatinine clearance is often "corrected" for body surface area (BSA [m²]) according to the formula: $$\frac{Cl_{Cr}}{(corrected)} = \frac{Cl_{Cr}}{(uncorrected)} \times \frac{1.73}{BSA}$$	**Increased in:** High cardiac output, exercise, acromegaly, diabetes mellitus (early stage), infections, hypothyroidism. **Decreased in:** Acute or chronic renal failure, decreased renal blood flow (shock, hemorrhage, dehydration, CHF). Drugs: nephrotoxic drugs.	Serum Cr may, in practice, be a more reliable indicator of renal function than 24-hour Cl_{Cr} unless urine collection is carefully monitored. An 8-hour collection provides results similar to those obtained by a 24-hour collection. Cl_{Cr} will overestimate GFR to the extent that Cr is secreted by the renal tubules (eg, in cirrhosis). Cl_{Cr} can be estimated from the serum creatinine using the following formula: $$Cl_{Cr}\text{(mL/min)} = \frac{(140 - Age) \times Wt(kg)}{72 \times P_{Cr}}$$ Crit Care Med 1993;21:1487. Pharmacotherapy 1993;13:135. Arch Intern Med 1994;154:201.

Test/Range/Collection	Physiologic Basis	Interpretation	Comments
	Cryoglobulins		
Cryoglobulins, serum <0.12 mg/mL Marbled $ Must be immediately transported to lab at 37°C	Cryoglobulins are immunoglobulins (IgG, IgM, IgA, or light chains) which precipitate on exposure to the cold. Type I cryoglobulins (25%) are monoclonal proteins, most commonly IgM, occasionally IgG, and rarely IgA or Bence Jones protein, seen in multiple myeloma and Waldenström's macroglobulinemia. Type II (25%) are mixed cryoglobulins with a monoclonal component (usually IgM but occasionally IgG or IgA) that complexes with autologous normal IgG in the cryoprecipitate. Type III (50%) are mixed polyclonal cryoglobulins (IgM and IgG).	**Increased in:** Immunoproliferative disorders (multiple myeloma, Waldenström's macroglobulinemia, chronic lymphocytic leukemia, lymphoma), collagenvascular disease (SLE, polyarteritis nodosa, rheumatoid arthritis), hemolytic anemia, essential mixed cryoglobulinemia, hepatitis B and C infection.	All types of cryoglobulins may cause cold-induced symptoms, including Raynaud's phenomenon, vascular purpura, and urticaria. Patients with type II and III cryoglobulinemia often have immune complex disease, with vascular purpura, arthritis, and nephritis. Typing of cryoglobulins by electrophoresis is not necessary for diagnosis or clinical management. About 50% of essential mixed cryoglobulinemia patients have evidence of hepatitis C infection. Am J Med 1980;68:757. JAMA 1982;248:2670. Am J Med 1994;96:124.
	Cryptococcal antigen		
Cryptococcal antigen, serum or CSF Negative Marbled (serum) or glass or plastic tube (CSF) $$	The capsular polysaccharide of *Cryptococcus neoformans* potentiates opportunistic infections by the yeast. The cryptococcal antigen test used is often a latex agglutination test.	**Increased in:** Cryptococcal infection.	False-positive and false-negative results have been reported. False-positives due to rheumatoid factor can be reduced by pretreatment of serum using pronase before testing. Sensitivity and specificity of serum cryptococcal antigen titer for cryptococcal meningitis are 91% and 83%, respectively. Ninety-six percent of cryptococcal infections occur in AIDS patients. Infect Immun 1994;62:1507. J Clin Microbiol 1994;32:2158. J Med Assoc Thai 1999;82:65.

	Cytomegalovirus antibody	Dexamethasone suppression test (low-dose)
Cytomegalovirus antibody, serum (CMV) Negative Marbled $$$	Detects the presence of antibody to CMV, either IgG or IgM. CMV infection is usually acquired during childhood or early adulthood. By age 20–40 years, 40–90% of the population has CMV antibodies.	**Increased in:** Previous or active CMV infection. False-positive CMV IgM tests occur when rheumatoid factor or infectious mononucleosis is present.	Serial specimens exhibiting a greater than fourfold titer rise suggest a recent infection. Active CMV infection must be documented by viral isolation. Useful for screening of potential organ donors and recipients. Detection of CMV IgM antibody in the serum of a newborn usually indicates congenital infection. Detection of CMV IgG antibody is not diagnostic, since maternal CMV IgG antibody passed via the placenta can persist in newborn's serum for 6 months. Rev Infect Dis 1988;10:S468.
Dexamethasone suppression test (single low-dose, overnight), serum 8:00 AM serum cortisol level: <5 μg/dL [<140 nmol/L] $$ Give 1 mg dexamethasone at 11:00 PM. At 8:00 AM, draw serum cortisol level.	In normal patients, dexamethasone suppresses the 8:00 AM serum cortisol level to below 5 μg/dL. Patients with Cushing's syndrome have 8:00 AM levels >10 μg/dL (>276 nmol/L).	**Positive in:** Cushing's syndrome (98% sensitivity, 98% specificity in lean outpatients), obese patients (13%), hospitalized or chronically ill patients (23%).	Good screening test for Cushing's syndrome. If this test is abnormal, use high-dose test (see below) to determine etiology. (See also Cushing's syndrome algorithm, p 340.) Patients taking phenytoin may fail to suppress because of enhanced dexamethasone metabolism. Depressed patients may also fail to suppress morning cortisol level. Ann Clin Biochem 1997; 34(Part 3):222.

Test/Range/Collection	Physiologic Basis	Interpretation	Comments
Dexamethasone suppression test (high-dose, overnight), serum 8:00 AM serum cortisol level: <5 µg/dL [<140 nmol/L] $$ Give 8 mg dexamethasone dose at 11:00 PM. At 8:00 AM, draw cortisol level.	Suppression of plasma cortisol levels to < 50% of baseline with dexamethasone indicates Cushing's disease (pituitary-dependent ACTH hypersecretion) and differentiates this from adrenal and ectopic Cushing's syndrome (see Cushing's syndrome algorithm, p 340).	**Positive in:** Cushing's disease (88–92% sensitivity; specificity 57–100%).	Test indicated only after a positive low-dose dexamethasone suppression test. Sensitivity and specificity depend on sampling time and diagnostic criteria. The ovine corticotropin-releasing hormone (CRH) stimulation test and bilateral sampling of the inferior petrosal sinuses combined with CRH administration are being evaluated for the definitive diagnosis of Cushing's disease. Measurement of urinary 17-hydroxy-corticosteroids has been replaced in this test by measurement of serum cortisol. Ann Intern Med 1986;104:180. Ann Intern Med 1990;112:434. J Clin Endocrinol Metab 1994;78:418. N Engl J Med 1994;331:629. Medicine 1995;74:74. Ann Intern Med 1994;121:318.
Double-stranded-DNA antibody (ds-DNA Ab), serum <1:10 titer Marbled $$	IgG or IgM antibodies directed against host double-stranded DNA.	**Increased in:** Systemic lupus erythematosus (60–70% sensitivity, 95% specificity) based on >1:10 titer. **Not increased in:** Drug-induced lupus.	High titers are seen only in SLE. Titers of ds-DNA antibody correlate well with disease activity and with occurrence of glomerulonephritis. (See also Autoantibodies table, p 367.) West J Med 1987;147:210. Clin Immunol Immunopathol 1988;47:121.

Test/Specimen	Physiologic Basis	Interpretation	Comments
Epstein-Barr virus antibodies, serum (EBV Ab) Negative Marbled $$	Antiviral capsid antibodies (anti-VCA) (IgM) often reach their peak at clinical presentation and last up to 3 months; anti-VCA IgG antibodies last for life. Early antigen antibodies (anti-EA) are next to develop, are most often positive at 1 month after presentation, typically last for 2–3 months, and may last up to 6 months in low titers. Anti-EA may also be found in some patients with Hodgkin's disease, chronic lymphocytic leukemia, and some other malignancies. Anti-EB nuclear antigen (anti-EBNA) antibody begins to appear in a minority of patients in the third or fourth week but is uniformly present by 6 months.	**Increased in:** EB virus infection, infectious mononucleosis. Antibodies to the diffuse (D) form of antigen (detected in the cytoplasm and nucleus of infected cells) are greatly elevated in nasopharyngeal carcinoma. Antibodies to the restricted (R) form of antigen (detected only in the cytoplasm of infected cells) are greatly elevated in Burkitt's lymphoma.	Most useful in diagnosing infectious mononucleosis in patients who have the clinical and hematologic criteria for the disease but who fail to develop the heterophile agglutinins (10%) (see Heterophile agglutination, p 107). EBV antibodies cannot be used to diagnose "chronic" mononucleosis. Chronic fatigue syndrome is not caused by EBV. The best indicator of primary infection is a positive anti-VCA IgM (check for false-positives caused by rheumatoid factor). Rose NR et al (editors): *Manual of Clinical Laboratory Immunology,* 4th ed. American Society for Microbiology, 1992. J Clin Microbiol 1996;34:3240.
Erythrocyte count, whole blood (RBC count) $4.2–5.6 \times 10^6/\mu L$ [$\times 10^{12}/L$] Lavender $	Erythrocytes are counted by automated instruments using electrical impedance or light scattering.	**Increased in:** Secondary polycythemia (hemoconcentration), polycythemia vera. Spurious increase with increased white blood cells. **Decreased in:** Anemia. Spurious decrease with autoagglutination.	Lab Med 1983;14:509.

Test/Range/Collection	Physiologic Basis	Interpretation	Comments
Erythrocyte sedimentation rate, whole blood (ESR) Male: <10 Female: <15 mm/h (laboratory-specific) Lavender $ Test must be run within 2 hours after sample collection.	In plasma, erythrocytes (red blood cells [RBCs]) usually settle slowly. However, if they aggregate for any reason (usually because of plasma proteins called acute phase reactants, eg, fibrinogen) they settle rapidly. Sedimentation of RBCs occurs because their density is greater than plasma. ESR measures the distance in mm that erythrocytes fall during 1 hour.	**Increased in:** Infections (osteomyelitis, pelvic inflammatory disease [75%]), inflammatory disease (temporal arteritis, polymyalgia rheumatica, rheumatic fever), malignant neoplasms, paraproteinemias, anemia, pregnancy, chronic renal failure, GI disease (ulcerative colitis, regional ileitis). For endocarditis, sensitivity = 93%. **Decreased in:** Polycythemia, sickle cell anemia, spherocytosis, anisocytosis, hypofibrinogenemia, hypogammaglobulinemia, congestive heart failure, microcytosis. Drugs: high-dose corticosteroids.	There is a good correlation between ESR and C-reactive protein, but ESR is less expensive. Test is useful and indicated only for diagnosis and monitoring of temporal arteritis and polymyalgia rheumatica. The test is not sensitive or specific for other conditions. ESR is higher in women, blacks, and older persons. Low value is of no diagnostic significance. Am J Med 1985;78:1001. Ann Intern Med 1986;104:515.
Erythropoietin, serum (EPO) 5–20 mIU/mL [4–26 IU/L] Marbled $$$	Erythropoietin is a glycoprotein hormone produced in the kidney that induces red blood cell production by stimulating proliferation, differentiation, and maturation of erythroid precursors. Hypoxia is the usual stimulus for production of EPO. In conditions of bone marrow hyporesponsiveness, EPO levels are elevated. In chronic renal failure, EPO production is decreased.	**Increased in:** Anemias associated with bone marrow hyporesponsiveness (aplastic anemia, iron deficiency anemia), secondary polycythemia (high-altitude hypoxia, COPD, pulmonary fibrosis), erythropoietin-producing tumors (cerebellar hemangioblastomas, pheochromocytomas, renal tumors), pregnancy, polycystic kidney disease. **Decreased in:** Anemia of chronic disease, renal failure, inflammatory states, primary polycythemia (polycythemia vera) (39%).	Test is not very useful in differentiating polycythemia vera from secondary polycythemia. Since virtually all patients with severe anemia due to chronic renal failure respond to EPO therapy, pretherapy EPO levels are not indicated. Patient receiving EPO as chronic therapy should have iron deficiency screening routinely. Curr Opin Nephrol Hypertens 1994;3:620. Haematologica 1997;82:406.

	Ethanol	Factor V (Leiden) mutation
Ethanol, serum (EtOH) 0 mg/dL [mmol/L] Marbled $$ Do not use alcohol swab. Do not remove stopper.	Measures serum level of ethyl alcohol (ethanol).	Present in: Ethanol ingestion.	Whole blood alcohol concentrations are about 15% lower than serum concentrations. Each 0.1 mg/dL of ethanol contributes about 22 mosm/kg to serum osmolality. Legal intoxication in many states is defined as >80 mg/dL (>17 mmol/L). N Engl J Med 1976;294:757.
Factor V (Leiden) mutation Blood Lavender or blue $$$$	The Leiden mutation is a single nucleotide base substitution leading to an amino acid substitution (glutamine replaces arginine) at one of the sites where coagulation factor V is cleaved by activated protein C. The mutation causes factor V to be partially resistant to protein C, which is involved in inhibiting coagulation. Factor V mutations may be present in up to half of the cases of unexplained venous thrombosis and are seen in 95% of patients with activated protein C resistance.	Positive in: Hypercoagulability secondary to factor V mutation (specificity approaches 100%).	The presence of mutation is only a risk factor for thrombosis, not an absolute marker for disease. Homozygotes have a 50- to 100-fold increase in risk of thrombosis (relative to the general population) and heterozygotes have a 7-fold increase in risk. The current PCR and reverse dot blot assay only detects the Leiden mutation of factor V; other mutations may yet be discovered. N Engl J Med 1995;332:912. Nature 1994;369:64. Ann Intern Med 1999;130:643.

Test/Range/Collection	Physiologic Basis	Interpretation	Comments
Factor VIII assay, plasma 40–150% of normal, (varies with age) Blue $$$ Deliver immediately to laboratory on ice. Stable for 2 hours.	Measures activity of factor VIII (antihemophilic factor), a key factor of the intrinsic clotting cascade.	**Increased in:** Inflammatory states (acute phase reactant), last trimester of pregnancy, oral contraceptives. **Decreased in:** Hemophilia A, von Willebrand's disease, disseminated intravascular coagulation, acquired factor VIII antibodies.	Normal hemostasis requires at least 25% of factor VIII activity. Symptomatic hemophiliacs usually have levels ≤5%. Disease levels are defined as severe (<1%), moderate (1–5%), and mild (>5%). Factor VIII assays are used to guide replacement therapy in patients with hemophilia. Semin Hematol 1967;4:93.
Fecal fat, stool Random: <60 droplets of fat/high power field 72 hour: < 7 g/d $$$ Qualitative: random stool sample is adequate. Quantitative: dietary fat should be at least 50–150 g/d for 2 days before collection. Then all stools should be collected for 72 hours and refrigerated.	In healthy people, most dietary fat is completely absorbed in the small intestine. Normal small intestinal lining, bile acids, and pancreatic enzymes are required for normal fat absorption.	**Increased in:** Malabsorption from small bowel disease (regional enteritis, celiac disease, tropical sprue), pancreatic insufficiency, diarrhea with or without fat malabsorption.	A random, qualitative fecal fat (socalled Sudan stain) is only useful if positive. Furthermore, it does not correlate well with quantitative measurements. Sudan stain appears to detect triglycerides and lipolytic by-products, whereas 72-hour fecal fat measures fatty acids from a variety of sources, including phospholipids, cholesteryl esters, and triglycerides. The quantitative method can be used to measure the degree of fat malabsorption initially and then after a therapeutic intervention. A normal quantitative stool fat reliably rules out pancreatic insufficiency and most forms of generalized small intestine disease. Gastroenterol Clin North Am 1989; 18:467. Gastroenterology 1992;102:1936.

Fecal occult blood		
Fecal occult blood, stool Negative $ Patient should be on a special diet free of exogenous peroxidase activity (meat, fish, turnips, horseradish), GI irritants (aspirin, non-steroidal anti-inflammatory drugs), and iron. To avoid false-negatives, patients should avoid taking vitamin C. Patient collects two specimens from three consecutive bowel movements.	Measures blood in the stool using gum guaiac as an indicator reagent. In the Hemoccult test, gum guaiac is impregnated in a test paper that is smeared with stool using an applicator. Hydrogen peroxide is used as a developer solution. The resultant phenolic oxidation of guaiac in the presence of blood in the stool yields a blue color.	**Positive in:** Upper GI disease (peptic ulcer, gastritis, variceal bleeding, esophageal and gastric cancer), lower GI disease (diverticulosis, colonic polyps, colon carcinoma, inflammatory bowel disease, vascular ectasias, hemorrhoids).	Although fecal occult blood testing is an accepted screening test for colon carcinoma, the sensitivity and specificity of an individual test are low. The utility of fecal occult blood testing after digital rectal examination has not been well studied. Three randomized controlled trials have shown reductions in colon cancer mortality with yearly (33% reduction) or biennial (15–21% reduction) testing. About 1000 fifty-year-olds must be screened for 10 years to save one life. BMJ 1998;317:559. Ann Intern Med 1997;126:811.

	Ferritin

Test/Range/Collection	Interpretation	Physiologic Basis	Comments
Ferritin, serum Males 16–300 ng/mL [μg/L] Females 4–161 ng/mL [μg/L] Marbled $$	**Increased in:** Iron overload (hemochromatosis [sensitivity 85%, specificity 95%], hemosiderosis), acute or chronic liver disease, alcoholism, various malignancies (eg, leukemia, Hodgkin's disease), chronic inflammatory disorders (eg, rheumatoid arthritis, adult Still's disease), thalassemia minor, hyperthyroidism, HIV infection, non-insulin-dependent diabetes mellitus, and postpartum state. **Decreased in:** Iron deficiency (60–75%).	Ferritin is the body's major iron storage protein. The serum ferritin level correlates with total body iron stores. The test is used to detect iron deficiency, to monitor response to iron therapy, and, in iron overload states, to monitor iron removal therapy. It is also used to predict homozygosity for hemochromatosis in relatives of affected patients. In the absence of liver disease, it is a more sensitive test for iron deficiency than serum iron and iron-binding capacity (transferrin saturation).	Serum ferritin is clinically useful in distinguishing between iron deficiency anemia (serum ferritin levels diminished) and anemia of chronic disease or thalassemia (levels usually normal or elevated). Test of choice for diagnosis of iron deficiency anemia. Ferritin (ng/mL) LR for Iron Deficiency >100 0.08 45–100 0.54 35–45 1.83 25–35 2.54 15–25 8.83 ≤15 52.0 Liver disease will increase serum ferritin levels and mask the diagnosis of iron deficiency. Am J Hematol 1993;42:177. Br J Haematol 1993;85:787. J Intern Med 1994;236:315. J Gen Intern Med 1992;7:145

Test / Specimen	Physiologic Basis	Interpretation	Comments
α-Fetoprotein, serum (AFP) 0–15 ng/mL [µg/L] Marbled $$ Avoid hemolysis.	α-Fetoprotein is a glycoprotein produced both early in fetal life and by some tumors.	**Increased in:** Hepatocellular carcinoma (72%), massive hepatic necrosis (74%), viral hepatitis (34%), chronic active hepatitis (29%), cirrhosis (11%), regional enteritis (5%), benign gynecologic diseases (22%), testicular carcinoma (embryonal) (70%), teratocarcinoma (64%), teratoma (37%), ovarian carcinoma (57%), endometrial cancer (50%), cervical cancer (53%), pancreatic cancer (23%), gastric cancer (18%), colon cancer (5%). **Negative in:** Seminoma.	The test is not sensitive or specific enough to be used as a general screening test for hepatocellular carcinoma. However, screening may be justified in populations at very high risk for hepatocellular cancer. In hepatocellular cancer or germ cell tumors associated with elevated AFP, the test may be helpful in detecting recurrence after therapy. AFP is also used to screen pregnant women at 15–20 weeks gestation for possible fetal neural tube defects. AFP level in maternal serum or amniotic fluid is compared with levels expected at a given gestational age. N Engl J Med 1987;317:342. Clin Chem 1992;38(8B Part 2):1523. West J Med 1993;159:312.
Fibrin D-dimers, plasma Negative Blue $$	Plasmin acts on fibrin to form various fibrin degradation products. The D-dimer level can be used as a measure of activation of the fibrinolytic system.	**Increased in:** Disseminated intravascular coagulation (DIC), other thrombotic disorders, pulmonary embolism, venous or arterial thrombosis.	Fibrin D-dimer assay has replaced the Fibrin(ogen) Split Products test as a screen for DIC, because the D-dimer assay can distinguish fibrin degradation products (in DIC) from fibrinogen degradation products (in primary fibrinogenolysis). Since the presence of fibrin D-dimer is not specific for DIC, the definitive diagnosis of DIC must depend on other tests, including the platelet count and serum fibrinogen level. Ann Intern Med 1998;129:1006.

Test/Range/Collection	Physiologic Basis	Interpretation	Comments
Fibrinogen (functional), plasma 175–433 mg/dL [1.75–4.3 g/L] *Panic:* <75 mg/dL Blue $$	Fibrinogen is synthesized in the liver and has a half-life of about 4 days. Thrombin cleaves fibrinogen to form insoluble fibrin monomers, which polymerize to form a clot.	**Increased in:** Inflammatory states (acute phase reactant), use of oral contraceptives, pregnancy. **Decreased in:** Decreased hepatic synthesis, increased consumption (disseminated intravascular coagulation [DIC], thrombolysis). Hereditary: Afibrinogenemia (rare), hypofibrinogenemia, dysfibrinogenemia.	Hypofibrinogenemia is an important diagnostic laboratory feature of DIC. Diagnosis of dysfibrinogenemia depends upon the discrepancy between measurable antigenic and low functional (clottable) fibrinogen levels. Blood 1982;60:284. Ann Intern Med 1993;118:956.
Fluorescent treponemal antibody-absorbed (FTA-ABS), serum Nonreactive Marbled $$	Detects specific antibodies against *Treponema pallidum.* Patient's serum is first diluted with nonpathogenic treponemal antigens (to bind nonspecific antibodies). The absorbed serum is placed on a slide that contains fixed *T pallidum.* Fluorescein-labeled antihuman gamma globulin is then added to bind to and visualize (under a fluorescence microscope) the patient's antibody on treponemes.	**Reactive in:** Syphilis: primary (95%), secondary (100%), late (96%), late latent (100%); also rarely positive in collagen-vascular diseases in the presence of antinuclear antibody.	Used to confirm a reactive nontreponemal screening:serologic test for syphilis such as RPR or VDRL (see pp 150 and 179, respectively). Once positive, the FTA-ABS may remain positive for life. However, one study found that at 36 months after treatment, 24% of patients had nonreactive FTA-ABS tests. In a study of HIV-infected men with a prior history of syphilis, 38% of patients with AIDS or ARC had loss of reactivity to treponemal tests, compared with 7% of HIV-seropositive asymptomatic men and 0% of HIV-seronegative men. Ann Intern Med 1986;104:368. J Infect Dis 1990;162:862. Ann Intern Med 1991;114:1005.

Test / Specimen / Cost	Physiologic Basis	Interpretation	Comments / References
Folic acid (RBC), whole blood 165–760 ng/mL [370–1720 nmol/L] Lavender $$$	Folate is a vitamin necessary for methyl group transfer in thymidine formation, and hence DNA synthesis. Deficiency can result in megaloblastic anemia.	**Decreased in:** Tissue folate deficiency (from dietary folate deficiency), B_{12} deficiency (50–60%, since cellular uptake of folate depends on B_{12}).	Red cell folate level correlates better than serum folate level with tissue folate deficiency. A low red cell folate level may indicate either folate or B_{12} deficiency. A therapeutic trial of folate (and not red cell or serum folate testing) is indicated when the clinical and dietary history is strongly suggestive of folate deficiency and the peripheral smear shows hypersegmented polymorphonuclear leukocytes. However, the possibility of vitamin B_{12} deficiency must always be considered in the setting of megaloblastic anemia, since folate therapy will treat the hematologic, but not the neurologic, sequelae of vitamin B_{12} deficiency. Blood 1983;61:624.
Follicle-stimulating hormone, serum (FSH) Male: 1–10 mIU/mL Female: (mIU/mL) Follicular 4–13 Luteal 2–13 Midcycle 5–22 Postmenopausal 20–138 (laboratory-specific) Marbled $$	FSH is stimulated by the hypothalamic hormone GnRH and is then secreted from the anterior pituitary in a pulsatile fashion. Levels rise during the preovulatory phase of the menstrual cycle and then decline. Elevation of FSH is the most sensitive indicator of onset of menopause.	**Increased in:** Primary (ovarian) gonadal failure, ovarian or testicular agenesis, castration, postmenopause, Klinefelter's syndrome, drugs. **Decreased in:** Hypothalamic disorders, pituitary disorders, pregnancy, anorexia nervosa. Drugs: corticosteroids, oral contraceptives.	Test indicated in the workup of amenorrhea in women (see Amenorrhea algorithm, p 339), delayed puberty, impotence, and infertility in men. Impotence workup should begin with serum testosterone measurement. Basal FSH levels in premenopausal women depend on age, smoking history, and menstrual cycle length and regularity. Br Med J 1987;294:815. Endocrinol Metab Clin North Am 1992;21:921. JAMA 1993;270:83. J Clin Endocrinol Metab 1994;79:1105.

Test/Range/Collection	Physiologic Basis	Interpretation	Comments
Free erythrocyte protoporphyrin, whole blood (FEP) <35 μg/dL (method-dependent) Lavender $$$	Protoporphyrin is produced in the next to last step of heme synthesis. In the last step, iron is incorporated into protoporphyrin to produce heme. Enzyme deficiencies, lack of iron, or presence of interfering substances (lead) can disrupt this process and cause elevated FEP.	**Increased in:** Decreased iron incorporation into heme (iron deficiency, infection, and lead poisoning), erythropoietic protoporphyria.	FEP can be used to screen for lead poisoning in children provided that iron deficiency has been ruled out. Test does not discriminate between uroporphyrin, coproporphyrin, and protoporphyrin, but protoporphyrin is the predominant porphyrin measured. Clin Pediatr 1991;30:74. Am J Dis Child 1993;147:66.
Fructosamine, serum 1.6–2.6 mmol/L Marbled $	Glycation of albumin produces fructosamine, a less expensive marker of glycemic control than HbA$_{1c}$.	**Increased in:** diabetes mellitus.	Fructosamine correlates well with fasting plasma glucose (r = 0.74) but cannot be used to predict precisely the HbA$_{1c}$. Acta Diabetologica 1998;35:48.
Gamma-glutamyl transpeptidase, serum (GGT) 9–85 U/L [0.15–1.42 μkat/L] (laboratory-specific) Marbled $	GGT is an enzyme present in liver, kidney, and pancreas. It is induced by alcohol intake and is an extremely sensitive indicator of liver disease, particularly alcoholic liver disease.	**Increased in:** Liver disease: acute viral or toxic hepatitis, chronic or subacute hepatitis, alcoholic hepatitis, cirrhosis, biliary tract obstruction (intrahepatic or extrahepatic), primary or metastatic liver neoplasm, mononucleosis. Drugs (by enzyme induction): phenytoin, carbamazepine, barbiturates, alcohol.	GGT is useful in follow-up of alcoholics undergoing treatment since the test is sensitive to modest alcohol intake. GGT is elevated in 90% of patients with liver disease. GGT is used to confirm hepatic origin of elevated serum alkaline phosphatase. Alcohol Clin Exp Res 1990;14:250. Am J Gastroenterol 1992;87:991.

	Gastrin	Glucose
Test / Specimen	**Gastrin, serum** <300 pg/mL [ng/L] Marbled $$ Overnight fasting required.	**Glucose, serum** 60–110 mg/dL [3.3–6.1 mmol/L] **Panic:** <40 or >500 mg/dL Marbled $ Overnight fasting usually required.
Physiology	Gastrin is secreted from G cells in the stomach antrum and stimulates acid secretion from the gastric parietal cells. Values fluctuate throughout the day but are lowest in the early morning.	Normally, the glucose concentration in extracellular fluid is closely regulated so that a source of energy is readily available to tissues and so that no glucose is excreted in the urine.
Interpretation	**Increased in:** Gastrinoma (Zollinger-Ellison syndrome) (80–93% sensitivity), antral G cell hyperplasia, hypochlorhydria, achlorhydria, chronic atrophic gastritis, pernicious anemia. Drugs: antacids, cimetidine, and other H_2 blockers; omeprazole and other proton pump inhibitors. **Decreased in:** Antrectomy with vagotomy.	**Increased in:** Diabetes mellitus, Cushing's syndrome (10–15%), chronic pancreatitis (30%). Drugs: corticosteroids, phenytoin, estrogen, thiazides. **Decreased in:** Pancreatic islet cell disease with increased insulin, insulinoma, adrenocortical insufficiency, hypopituitarism, diffuse liver disease, malignancy (adrenocortical, stomach, fibrosarcoma), infant of a diabetic mother, enzyme deficiency diseases (eg, galactosemia). Drugs: insulin, ethanol, propranolol; sulfonylureas, tolbutamide, and other oral hypoglycemic agents.
Comments	Gastrin is the first-line test for determining whether a patient with active ulcer disease has a gastrinoma. Gastric analysis is not indicated. Before interpreting an elevated level, be sure that the patient is not taking antacids, H_2 blockers, or proton pump inhibitors. Both fasting and post-secretin infusion levels may be required for diagnosis. Endocrinol Metab Clin North Am 1993;22:823. Lancet 1996;347:270.	Diagnosis of diabetes mellitus requires a fasting plasma glucose of >126 mg/dL on more than one occasion. Hypoglycemia is defined as a glucose of <50 mg/dL in men and <40 mg/dL in women. While random serum glucose levels correlate with home glucose monitoring results (weekly mean capillary glucose values), there is wide fluctuation within individuals. Thus, glycosylated hemoglobin levels are favored to monitor glycemic control. JAMA 1999;281:1203.

Test/Range/Collection	Physiologic Basis	Interpretation	Comments
Glucose tolerance test			
Glucose tolerance test, serum Fasting: <110 1-hour: <200 2-hour: <140 mg/dL [Fasting: <6.4 1-hour: <11.0 2-hour: <7.7 mmol/L] Marbled $$ Subjects should receive a 150- to 200-g/d carbohydrate diet for at least 3 days prior to test. A 75-g glucose dose is dissolved in 300 mL of water for adults (1.75 g/kg for children) and given after an overnight fast. Serial determinations of plasma or serum venous blood glucoses are obtained at baseline, at 1 hour, and at 2 hours.	The test determines the ability of a patient to respond appropriately to a glucose load.	**Increased glucose rise (decreased glucose tolerance) in:** Diabetes mellitus, impaired glucose tolerance, gestational diabetes, severe liver disease, hyperthyroidism, stress (infection), increased absorption of glucose from GI tract (hyperthyroidism, gastrectomy, gastroenterostomy, vagotomy, excess glucose intake), Cushing's syndrome, pheochromocytoma. Drugs: diuretics, oral contraceptives, glucocorticoids, nicotinic acid, phenytoin. **Decreased glucose rise (flat glucose curve) in:** Intestinal disease (celiac sprue, Whipple's disease), adrenal insufficiency (Addison's disease), hypopituitarism, pancreatic islet cell tumors or hyperplasia.	Test is not generally required for diagnosis of diabetes mellitus. In screening for gestational diabetes, the glucose tolerance test is performed between 24 and 28 weeks of gestation. After a 50-g oral glucose load, a 2-hour postprandial blood glucose is measured as a screen. If the result is > 140 mg/dL, then the full test with 100-g glucose load is done using the following reference ranges: Fasting: <105 1-hour: <190 2-hour: <165 3-hour: <145 mg/dL Routine screening for gestational diabetes has not been found to be cost-effective, and is not recommended by the Canadian Task Force on the Periodic Health Examination. J Fam Pract 1993;37:27. Diabetes Care 1999;22(Suppl 1):55.

	G6PD screen		Glutamine
Glucose-6-phosphate dehydrogenase screen, whole blood (G6PD) 4–8 units/g Hb [0.07–0.14 µkat/L] Green or blue $$	G6PD is an enzyme in the hexose monophosphate shunt that is essential in generating reduced glutathione and NADPH, which protect hemoglobin from oxidative denaturation. Numerous G6PD isoenzymes have been identified. Most African-Americans have G6PD-A(+) isoenzyme. 10–15% have G6PD-A(−), which has only 15% of normal enzyme activity. It is transmitted in an X-linked recessive manner. Some Mediterranean people have the B− variant that has extremely low enzyme activity (1% of normal).	**Increased in:** Young erythrocytes (reticulocytosis). **Decreased in:** G6PD deficiency.	In deficient patients, hemolytic anemia can be triggered by oxidant agents: antimalarial drugs (eg, chloroquine), nalidixic acid, nitrofurantoin, dapsone, phenacetin, vitamin C, and some sulfonamides. Any African-American about to be given an oxidant drug should be screened for G6PD deficiency. (Also screen people from certain Mediterranean areas: Greece, Italy, etc.) Hemolytic episodes can also occur in deficient patients who eat fava beans, in patients with diabetic acidosis, and in infections. G6PD deficiency may be the cause of hemolytic disease of newborns in Asians and Mediterraneans. Ann Intern Med 1985;103:245.
Glutamine, CSF Glass or plastic tube 6–15 mg/dL ***Panic:*** >40 mg/dL $$$	Glutamine is synthesized in the brain from ammonia and glutamic acid. Elevated CSF glutamine is associated with hepatic encephalopathy.	**Increased in:** Hepatic encephalopathy.	Test is not indicated if albumin, alanine aminotransferase (ALT), bilirubin, and alkaline phosphatase are normal or if there is no clinical evidence of liver disease. Hepatic encephalopathy is essentially ruled out if the CSF glutamine is normal. Arch Intern Med 1971;127:1033. Science 1974;183:81.

	Glycohemoglobin		
Test/Range/Collection	**Physiologic Basis**	**Interpretation**	**Comments**
Glycohemoglobin; glycated (glycosylated) hemoglobin, serum (HbA$_{1c}$) 3.9–6.9% (method-dependent) Lavender $$	During the life span of each red blood cell, glucose combines with hemoglobin to produce a stable glycated hemoglobin. The level of glycated hemoglobin is related to the mean plasma glucose level during the prior 1–3 months. There are three glycated A hemoglobins, HbA$_{1a}$, HbA$_{1b}$, and HbA$_{1c}$. Some assays quantitate HbA$_{1c}$; some quantitate total HbA$_{1}$; and some quantitate all glycated hemoglobins, not just A.	**Increased in:** Diabetes mellitus, splenectomy. Falsely high results can occur depending on the method used and may be due to presence of hemoglobin F or uremia. **Decreased in:** Any condition that shortens red cell life span (hemolytic anemias, congenital spherocytosis, acute or chronic blood loss, sickle cell disease, hemoglobinopathies).	Test is not currently recommended for diagnosis of diabetes mellitus, though it performs well. It is used to monitor long-term control of blood glucose level. Reference ranges are method-specific. Development and progression of chronic complications of diabetes are related to the degree of altered glycemia. Measurement of HbA$_{1c}$ can improve metabolic control by leading to changes in diabetes treatment. Diabetes Care 1994;17:938. JAMA 1996;246:1246.

	Growth hormone	**Haptoglobin**
Growth hormone, serum (GH) 0–5 ng/mL [µg/L] Marbled $$$	Growth hormone is a single-chain polypeptide of 191 amino acids that induces the generation of somatomedins, which directly stimulate collagen and protein synthesis. GH levels are subject to wide fluctuations during the day.	**Increased in:** Acromegaly (90% have GH levels >10 ng/mL), Laron dwarfism (defective GH receptor), starvation. Drugs: dopamine, levodopa. **Decreased in:** Pituitary dwarfism, hypopituitarism.	Nonsuppressibility of GH levels to <2 ng/mL after 100 g oral glucose and elevation of IGF-1 levels are the two most sensitive tests for acromegaly. Random determinations of GH are rarely useful in the diagnosis of acromegaly. For the diagnosis of hypopituitarism or growth hormone deficiency in children, an insulin hypoglycemia test has been used. Failure to increase GH levels to > 5 ng/mL after insulin (0.1 unit/kg) is consistent with GH deficiency. Endocrinol Metab Clin North Am 1992;21:649. Clin Endocrinol 1997;46:531. Lancet 1998;352:1455.
Haptoglobin, serum 46–316 mg/dL [0.5–2.2 g/L] Marbled $$	Haptoglobin is a glycoprotein synthesized in the liver that binds free hemoglobin.	**Increased in:** Acute and chronic infection (acute phase reactant), malignancy, biliary obstruction, ulcerative colitis, myocardial infarction, and diabetes mellitus. **Decreased in:** Newborns and children, posttransfusion intravascular hemolysis, autoimmune hemolytic anemia, liver disease (10%). May be decreased following uneventful transfusion (10%) for unknown reasons.	Low haptoglobin is considered an indicator of hemolysis, but it is of uncertain clinical predictive value because of the greater prevalence of other conditions associated with low levels and because of occasional normal individuals who have very low levels. It thus has low specificity. High-normal levels probably rule out significant intravascular hemolysis. JAMA 1980;243:1909. Clin Chem 1987;33:1265.

Helicobacter pylori antibody

Test/Range/Collection	Physiologic Basis	Interpretation	Comments
Helicobacter pylori antibody, serum Negative Marbled $$	*Helicobacter pylori* is a gram-negative spiral bacterium that is found on gastric mucosa. It induces acute and chronic inflammation in the gastric mucosa and a positive serologic antibody response. Serologic testing for *H pylori* antibody (IgG) is by ELISA.	**Increased (positive) in:** Histologic (chronic or chronic active) gastritis due to *H pylori* infection (with or without peptic ulcer disease). Sensitivity 98%, specificity 48%. Asymptomatic adults: 15–50%.	95% of patients with duodenal ulcers and > 70% of patients with gastric ulcers have chronic infection with *H pylori* along with associated histologic gastritis. All patients with peptic ulcer disease and positive *H pylori* serology should be treated to eradicate *H pylori* infection. The prevalence of *H pylori*-positive serologic tests in asymptomatic adults is approximately 35% overall but is >50% in patients over age 60. Fewer than one in six adults with *H pylori* antibody develop peptic ulcer disease. Treatment of asymptomatic adults is not currently recommended. The role of *H pylori* in patients with chronic dyspepsia is controversial. There is currently no role for treatment of such patients except in clinical trials. After successful eradication, serologic titers fall over a 3- to 6-month period but remain positive in up to 50% of patients at 1 year. Gastroenterol Clin North Am 1993;22:105. Gut 1994;35:19. Ann Intern Med 1994;120:977. JAMA 1994;272:65. Can J Infect Dis 1998;9:277.

	Hematocrit		Hemoglobin A$_2$
Hematocrit, whole blood (Hct) Male: 39–49% Female: 35–45% (age-dependent) Lavender $	The hematocrit represents the percentage of whole blood volume composed of erythrocytes. Laboratory instruments calculate the Hct from the erythrocyte count (RBC) and the mean corpuscular volume (MCV) by the formula: $$Hct = RBC \times MCV$$	**Increased in:** Hemoconcentration (as in dehydration, burns, vomiting), polycythemia, extreme physical exercise. **Decreased in:** Macrocytic anemia (liver disease, hypothyroidism, vitamin B$_{12}$ deficiency, folate deficiency), normocytic anemia (early iron deficiency, anemia of chronic disease, hemolytic anemia, acute hemorrhage) and microcytic anemia (iron deficiency, thalassemia).	Conversion from hemoglobin (Hb) to hematocrit is roughly Hb $\times$ 3 = Hct. Hematocrit reported by clinical laboratories is not a spun hematocrit. The spun hematocrit may be spuriously high if the centrifuge is not calibrated, if the specimen is not spun to constant volume, or if there is "trapped plasma." In determining transfusion need, the clinical picture must be considered in addition to the hematocrit. Point-of-care instruments may not measure hematocrit accurately in all patients. JAMA 1988;259:2433. Arch Pathol Lab Med 1994;118:429. Clin Chem 1995;41:306.
Hemoglobin A$_2$, whole blood (HbA$_2$) 1.5–3.5% of total hemoglobin (Hb) Lavender $$	HbA$_2$ is a minor component of normal adult hemoglobin (< 3.5% of total Hb).	**Increased in:** β-Thalassemia major (HbA$_2$ levels 4–10% of total Hb), β-thalassemia minor (HbA$_2$ levels 4–8% of total Hb). **Decreased in:** Untreated iron deficiency, hemoglobin H disease.	Test is useful in the diagnosis of β-thalassemia minor (in absence of iron deficiency, which decreases HbA$_2$ and can mask the diagnosis). Quantitated by column chromatographic or automated HPLC techniques. Normal HbA$_2$ levels are seen in delta β-thalassemia or very mild β-thalassemias. Blood 1988;72:1107. J Clin Pathol 1993;46:852. Hematol Pathol 1994;8:25.

	Hemoglobin electrophoresis		
Test/Range/Collection	**Physiologic Basis**	**Interpretation**	**Comments**
Hemoglobin electrophoresis, whole blood HbA: > 95 HbA$_2$: 1.5–3.5% Lavender, blue, or green $$	Hemoglobin electrophoresis is used as a screening test. It is used to detect and differentiate hemoglobin variants. Separation of hemoglobins by electrophoresis is based on different rates of migration of charged hemoglobin molecules in an electric field.	↑HbS: HbA > HbS = Sickle cell trait (HbAS) or sickle α-thalassemia; HbS and F, no HbA = Sickle cell anemia (HbSS) or sickle β-thalassemia; HbS > HbA and F: Sickle β+-thalassemia. ↑HbC: HbA > HbC = HbC trait (HbAC); HbC and F, no HbA = HbC disease; HbC > HbA = HbC β+-thalassemia. ↑HbH: HbH disease. ↑HbA$_2$, F: See HbA$_2$, above, and HbF, below.	Evaluation of a suspected hemoglobinopathy should include electrophoresis of a hemolysate to detect an abnormal hemoglobin and quantitation of hemoglobins A$_2$ and F. Automated HPLC instruments are proving to be useful alternative methods for hemoglobinopathy screening. Molecular diagnosis aids in genetic counseling of patients with thalassemia and combined hemoglobinopathies. Semin Perinatol 1990;14:483. Clin Chem 1990;36:903.

	Physiologic Basis	Interpretation	Comments
Hemoglobin, fetal, whole blood (HbF) Adult: <2% (varies with age) Lavender, blue, or green $$	Fetal hemoglobin constitutes about 75% of total hemoglobin at birth and declines to 50% at 6 weeks, 5% at 6 months, and <1.5% by 1 year. During the first year, adult hemoglobin (HbA) becomes the predominant hemoglobin.	**Increased in:** Hereditary disorders: eg, β-thalassemia major (60–100% of total Hb is HbF), β-thalassemia minor (2–5% HbF), sickle cell anemia (1–3% HbF), hereditary persistence of fetal hemoglobin (10–40% HbF). Acquired disorders <10% HbF): aplastic anemia, megaloblastic anemia, leukemia. **Decreased in:** Hemolytic anemia of the newborn.	Semiquantitative acid elution test provides an estimate of fetal hemoglobin only and varies widely between laboratories. It is useful in distinguishing hereditary persistence of fetal hemoglobin (all RBCs show an increase in fetal hemoglobin) from β-thalassemia minor (only a portion of RBCs are affected). Enzyme-linked antiglobulin test is used to detect fetal red cells in the Rh(−) maternal circulation in suspected cases of Rh sensitization and to determine the amount of RhoGAM to administer (1 vial/15 mL fetal RBC). Prenatal diagnosis of hemoglobinopathies may be accomplished by quantitative hemoglobin levels by HPLC or molecular diagnostic techniques. J Clin Pathol 1972;25:738. Clin Chem 1992;38:1906.
Hemoglobin, total, whole blood (Hb) Male: 13.6–17.5 g/dL Female: 12.0–15.5 g/dL (age-dependent) [Male: 136–175 Female: 120–155 g/L] ***Panic:*** ≤7 g/dL Lavender $	Hemoglobin is the major protein of erythrocytes and transports oxygen from the lungs to peripheral tissues. It is measured by spectrophotometry on automated instruments after hemolysis of red cells and conversion of all hemoglobin to cyanmethemoglobin.	**Increased in:** Hemoconcentration (as in dehydration, burns, vomiting), polycythemia, extreme physical exercise. **Decreased in:** Macrocytic anemia (liver disease, hypothyroidism, vitamin B_{12} deficiency, folate deficiency), normocytic anemia (early iron deficiency, anemia of chronic disease, hemolytic anemia, acute hemorrhage, and microcytic anemia (iron deficiency, thalassemia).	Hypertriglyceridemia and very high white blood cell counts can cause false elevations of Hb. JAMA 1988;259:2433.

	Hemosiderin	Hepatitis A antibody
Test/Range/Collection	**Hemosiderin,** urine Negative Urine container $$ Fresh, random sample.	**Hepatitis A antibody,** serum (Anti-HAV) Negative Marbled $$
Physiologic Basis	Hemosiderin is a protein produced by the digestion of hemoglobin. Its presence in the urine indicates acute or chronic release of free hemoglobin into the circulation with accompanying depletion of the scavenging proteins, hemopexin and haptoglobin. Presence of hemosiderin usually indicates intravascular hemolysis or recent transfusion.	Hepatitis A is caused by a non-enveloped 27 nm RNA virus of the enterovirus-picornavirus group and is usually acquired by the fecal-oral route. IgM antibody is detectable within a week after symptoms develop and persists for 6 months. IgG appears 4 weeks later than IgM and persists for years (see Figure 8–7, p 343, for time course of serologic changes).
Interpretation	**Increased in:** Intravascular hemolysis: hemolytic transfusion reactions, paroxysmal nocturnal hemoglobinuria, microangiopathic hemolytic anemia, mechanical destruction of erythrocytes (heart valve hemolysis), sickle cell anemia, thalassemia major, oxidant drugs with G6PD deficiency (eg, dapsone). Hemochromatosis.	Positive in: Acute hepatitis A (IgM), convalescence from hepatitis A (IgG).
Comments	Hemosiderin can be qualitatively detected in urinary sediment using Prussian blue stain. Med Clin North Am 1992;76:649.	The most commonly used test for hepatitis A antibody is an immunoassay that detects total IgG and IgM antibodies. This test can be used to establish immune status. Specific IgM testing is necessary to diagnose acute hepatitis A. IgG antibody positivity is found in 40–50% of adults in USA and Europe (higher rates in developing nations). Testing for anti-HAV (IgG) may reduce cost of HAV vaccination programs. Arch Intern Med 1994;154:663.

		Hepatitis B surface antigen	Hepatitis B surface antibody	Hepatitis B core antibody
Hepatitis B surface antigen, serum (HBsAg) Negative Marbled $$	In hepatitis B virus infection, surface antigen is detectable 2–5 weeks before onset of symptoms, rises in titer, and peaks at about the time of onset of clinical illness. Generally it persists for 1–5 months, declining in titer and disappearing with resolution of clinical symptoms (see Figure 8–8, p 344, for time course of serologic changes).	**Increased in:** Acute hepatitis B, chronic hepatitis B (persistence of HBsAg for >6 months, positive HBcAb [total]), HBsAg-positive carriers. May be undetectable in acute hepatitis B infection. If clinical suspicion is high, HBcAb (IgM) test is then indicated.	First-line test for the diagnosis of acute or chronic hepatitis B. If positive, no other test is needed. HBeAg is a marker of extensive viral replication found only in HBsAg-positive sera. Persistently HBeAg-positive patients are more infectious than HBeAg-negative patients and more likely to develop chronic liver disease. Annu Rev Med 1981;32:1. Clin Microbiol Rev 1999;12:351.	
Hepatitis B surface antibody, serum (HBsAb, anti-HBs) Negative Marbled $$	Test detects antibodies to hepatitis B virus (HBV) which are thought to confer immunity to hepatitis B. Since several subtypes of hepatitis B exist, there is a possibility of subsequent infection with a second subtype.	**Increased in:** Hepatitis B immunity due to HBV infection or hepatitis B vaccination. **Absent in:** Hepatitis B carrier state, nonexposure.	Test indicates immune status. It is not useful for the evaluation of acute or chronic hepatitis. (See Figure 8–8, p 344, for time course of serologic changes.) Ann Intern Med 1985;103:201. Dig Dis Scie 1986;31:620 Clin Microbiol Rev 1999;12:351.	
Hepatitis B core antibody, total, serum (HBcAb, anti-HBc) Negative Marbled $$	HBcAB (IgG and IgM) will be positive (as IgM) about 2 months after exposure to hepatitis B. Its persistent positivity may reflect chronic hepatitis (IgM) or recovery (IgG). (See Figure 8–8, p 344, for time course of serologic changes.)	**Positive in:** Hepatitis B (acute and chronic), hepatitis B carriers (high levels), prior hepatitis B (immune) when IgG present in low titer with or without HBsAb. **Negative:** After hepatitis B vaccination.	HBcAb (total) is useful in evaluation of acute or chronic hepatitis only if HBsAg is negative. An HBcAb (IgM) test is then indicated only if the HBcAb (total) is positive. HBcAb (IgM) may be the only serologic indication of acute HBV infection. Dig Dis Sci 1985;30:1022. Mayo Clin Proc 1988;63:201. Clin Microbiol Rev 1999;12:351.	

Test/Range/Collection	Physiologic Basis	Interpretation	Comments
	Hepatitis Be antigen		
Hepatitis Be antigen/antibody (HBeAg/Ab), serum Negative Marbled $$	HBeAg is a soluble protein secreted by hepatitis B virus, related to HBcAg, indicating viral replication and infectivity. Two distinct serologic types of hepatitis B have been described, one with a positive HBeAg and the other with a negative HBeAg and a positive anti-HBe antibody.	**Increased (positive) in:** HBV (acute, chronic) hepatitis.	The assumption has been that loss of HBeAg and accumulation of HBeAb are associated with decreased infectivity. Testing has proved unreliable, and tests are not routinely needed as indicators of infectivity. All patients positive for HBsAg must be considered infectious. Anti-HBeAb is used to select patients for clinical trials of interferon therapy or liver transplantation. Proc Natl Acad Sci U S A 1991;88:4186. J Med Microbiol 1994;41:374.
	Hepatitis C antibody		
Hepatitis C antibody, serum (HCAb) Negative Marbled $$	Detects antibody to hepatitis C virus. Current screening test (ELISA) detects antibodies to proteins expressed by putative structural (HC31) and nonstructural (HC31, C100-3) regions of the HCV genome. The presence of these antibodies indicates that the patient has been infected with HCV, and may harbor infectious HCV, and may be capable of transmitting HCV. A recombinant immunoblot assay (RIBA) is available as a confirmatory test.	**Increased in:** Acute hepatitis C (only 20–50%; seroconversion may take 6 months or more), posttransfusion chronic non-A, non-B hepatitis (70–90%), sporadic chronic non-A, non-B hepatitis (30–80%), blood donors (0.5–1%), non-blood-donating general public (2–3%), hemophiliacs (75%), intravenous drug abusers (40–80%), hemodialysis patients (1–30%), male homosexuals (4%).	Sensitivity of current assays is 86%, specificity 99.5%. Seropositivity for hepatitis C documents previous exposure, not necessarily acute infection. Seronegativity in acute hepatitis does not exclude the diagnosis of hepatitis C, especially in immunosuppressed patients. Testing of donor blood for hepatitis C has significantly reduced the incidence of posttransfusion hepatitis. N Engl J Med 1989;321:1538. Hepatology 1993;18:497. Dis Mon 1994;40(3):117. Am Fam Physician 1999;59:79.

	Hepatitis D antibody	**Heterophile agglutination**
Hepatitis D antibody, serum (Anti-HDV) Negative Marbled $$	This antibody is a marker for acute or persisting infection with the delta agent, a defective RNA virus that can only infect HBsAg-positive patients. Hepatitis B virus (HBV) plus hepatitis D virus (HDV) infection may be more severe than HBV infection alone. Antibody to HDV ordinarily persists for about 6 months following acute infection. Further persistence indicates carrier status.	**Positive in:** Hepatitis D.	Test only indicated in HBsAg-positive patients. Chronic HDV hepatitis occurs in 80–90% of HBsAg carriers who are superinfected with delta, but in less than 5% of those who are co-infected with both viruses simultaneously. Hepatology 1985;5:188. Ann Intern Med 1989;110:779.
Heterophile aggluti-nation, serum (Monospot, Paul-Bunnell test) Negative Marbled $	Infectious mononucleosis is an acute saliva-transmitted infectious disease due to the Epstein-Barr virus (EBV). Heterophile (Paul-Bunnell) antibodies (IgM) appear in 60% of mononucle-osis patients within 1–2 weeks and in 80–90% within the first month. They are not specific for EBV but are found only rarely in other disorders. Titers are substantially diminished by 3 months after primary infection and are not detectable by 6 months.	**Positive in:** Infectious mononucleosis (90–95%). **Negative in:** Heterophile-negative mononucleosis: CMV, heterophile-negative EBV, toxoplasmosis, hepatitis viruses, HIV-1 seroconversion, listerio-sis, tularemia, brucellosis, cat scratch disease, Lyme disease, syphilis, rick-ettsial infections, medications (phenytoin, sulfasalazine, dapsone), collagen–vascular diseases (especially lupus), subacute infective endocarditis.	The three classic signs of infectious mononucleosis are lymphocytosis, a "significant number" (>10–20%) of atypical lymphocytes on Wright-stained peripheral blood smear, and positive heterophile test. If heterophile test is negative in the setting of hematologic and clinical evidence of illness, a repeat test in 1–2 weeks may be positive. EBV serology (anti-VCA and anti-EBNA) may also be indicated, especially in children and teenage patients who may have negative heterophile tests (see EBV antibodies, p 85). Hum Pathol 1974;5:551. Pediatrics 1985;75:1011. Clin Microbiol Rev 1988;1:300.

Histoplasma capsulatum antigen

Test/Range/Collection	Physiologic Basis	Interpretation	Comments
***Histoplasma capsulatum* antigen,** urine, serum, CSF (HPA) Negative Marbled (serum) $$ Deliver urine, CSF in a clean plastic or glass container tube.	Heat-stable *H capsulatum* polysaccharide is detected by radioimmunoassay or ELISA using alkaline phosphatase or horseradish peroxidase-conjugated antibodies.	**Increased in:** Disseminated histoplasmosis (90–97% in urine, 50–78% in blood, and approximately 42% in CSF), localized disease (16% in urine), blastomycosis (urine and serum), coccidioidomycosis (CSF).	RIA for *H capsulatum* var *capsulatum* polysaccharide antigen in urine is a useful test in diagnosis of disseminated histoplasmosis and in assessing efficacy of treatment or in detecting relapse, especially in AIDS patients and when serologic tests for antibodies may be negative. Because the test has low sensitivity in localized pulmonary disease, it is not useful for ruling out localized pulmonary histoplasmosis. HPA in bronchoalveolar lavage fluid has 70% sensitivity for the diagnosis of pulmonary histoplasmosis. N Engl J Med 1986;314:83. Am J Med 1989;87:396. Arch Intern Med 1989;149:302. Am Rev Respir Dis 1992;145:1421.

Histoplasma capsulatum precipitins	*Histoplasma capsulatum* CF antibody
Positive in: Previous, chronic, or acute histoplasma infection, recent histoplasmin skin testing. Cross-reactions at low levels in patients with blastomycosis and coccidioidomycosis.	**Increased in:** Previous, chronic, or acute histoplasma infection (75–80%), acute histoplasmin skin testing (20%), other fungal disease, leishmaniasis. Cross-reactions in patients with blastomycosis and coccidioidomycosis.
Histoplasmosis is usually seen in the Mississippi and Ohio River Valleys but may appear elsewhere. Test is useful as a screening test or as an adjunct to complement fixation test (see below) in diagnosis of systemic histoplasmosis. Rose NR et al (editors): *Manual of Clinical Laboratory Immunology,* 4th ed. American Society for Microbiology, 1992.	Elevated CF titers of >1:16 are suggestive of infection. Titers of >1:32 or rising titers are usually indicative of active infection. Histoplasmin skin test is not recommended for diagnosis since it interferes with subsequent serologic tests. About 3.5–12% of clinically normal persons have positive titers, usually less than 1:16. Hosp Pract (Off Ed) Feb 1991;26:41. Rose NR et al (editors): *Manual of Clinical Laboratory Immunology,* 4th ed. American Society for Microbiology, 1992.
***Histoplasma capsulatum* precipitins,** serum Negative Marbled $$	Histoplasmosis is the most common systemic fungal infection and typically starts as a pulmonary infection with influenza-like symptoms. This may heal, progress, or lie dormant with reinfection occurring at a later time. This test screens for presence of histoplasma antibody by detecting precipitin "H" and "M" bands. Positive H band indicates active infection, M band indicates acute or chronic infection or prior skin testing. Presence of both suggests active histoplasmosis.	Quantitates level of histoplasma antibody. Antibodies in primary pulmonary infections are generally found within 4 weeks after exposure and frequently are present at the time symptoms appear. Two types of CF test are available based on mycelial antigen and yeast phase antigen. The yeast phase test is considerably more sensitive. Latex agglutination (LA) and ELISA tests are also available but are less reliable.
***Histoplasma capsulatum* complement fixation (CF) antibody,** serum <1:4 titer Marbled $$ Submit paired sera, one specimen collected within 1 week after onset of illness and another 2 weeks later.		

Test/Range/Collection	Physiologic Basis	Interpretation	Comments
HIV antibody, serum Negative Marbled $$	This test detects antibody against the human immunodeficiency virus-1 (HIV-1), the etiologic agent of AIDS. HIV antibody test is considered positive only when a repeatedly reactive enzyme immunoassay (EIA) is confirmed by a Western blot analysis or immunofluorescent antibody test (IFA).	**Positive in:** HIV infection: EIA sensitivity >99% after first 2–4 months of infection, specificity 99%. When combined with confirmatory test, specificity is 99.995%.	A positive p24 antigen test in an HIV antibody-negative individual must be confirmed by a viral neutralization assay. While Western blot test is currently the most sensitive and specific assay for HIV serodiagnosis, it is highly dependent on the proficiency of the laboratory performing the test and on the standardization of the procedure. Ann Intern Med 1987;106:671. Arch Pathol Lab Med 1989;113:975. JAMA 1991;266:2861. Infect Dis Clin North Am 1993;7:203.
HLA typing, serum and blood (HLA) Marbled (2 mL) and Yellow (40 mL) $$$$ Specimens must be < 24 hours old. Refrigerate serum, but not blood in yellow tubes.	The human leukocyte antigen (HLA) system consists of four closely linked loci (HLA-A, -B, -C, and -DR) located on the short arm of chromosome 6. The most widely used technique for HLA typing is the microlymphocyte toxicity test. This is a complement-mediated serologic assay in which anti-HLA antibodies is added to peripheral blood lymphocytes. Cell death indicates that the lymphocytes carried the specific targeted antigen.	**Useful in:** Evaluation of transplant candidates and potential donors and for paternity and forensic testing.	While diseases associated with particular HLA antigens have been identified, HLA typing for the diagnosis of these diseases is not generally indicated. Cell 1984;36:1.

Test/Specimen	Physiologic Basis	Interpretation	Comments
HLA-B27 typing, whole blood Negative Yellow $$$ Specimens must be <24 hours old.	The HLA-B27 allele is found in approximately 8% of the US white population. It occurs less frequently in the African-American population.	There is an increased incidence of spondyloarthritis among patients who are HLA-B27-positive. HLA-B27 is present in 88% of patients with ankylosing spondylitis. It is also associated with the development of Reiter's syndrome (80%) following infection with *Shigella* or *Salmonella*.	The best diagnostic test for ankylosing spondylitis is a lumbar spine film and not HLA-B27 typing. HLA-B27 testing is not usually clinically indicated. Ann Intern Med 1980;92:208. Br J Rheumatol 1987;36:185.
5-Hydroxyindoleacetic acid, urine (5-HIAA) 2–8 mg/24 h [10–40 μmol/d] Urine bottle containing hydrochloric acid $$	Serotonin (5-hydroxytryptamine) is a neurotransmitter that is metabolized by monoamine oxidase (MAO) to 5-HIAA and then excreted into the urine. Serotonin is secreted by most carcinoid tumors, which arise from neuroendocrine cells in locations derived from the embryonic gut.	**Increased in:** Metastatic carcinoid tumor (foregut, midgut, and bronchial). Nontropical sprue (slight increase). Diet of bananas, walnuts, avocado, eggplant, pineapple, plums. Drugs: reserpine. **Negative in:** Rectal carcinoids (usually), renal insufficiency. Drugs: MAO inhibitors, phenothiazines. Test is often falsely positive because pretest probability is low. Using 5-HIAA/Cr ratio may improve performance.	Since most carcinoid tumors drain into the portal vein and serotonin is rapidly cleared by the liver, the carcinoid syndrome (flushing, bronchial constriction, diarrhea, hypotension, and cardiac valvular lesions) is a late manifestation of carcinoid tumors, appearing only after hepatic metastasis has occurred. N Engl J Med 1986;315:702. Clin Chem 1992;38:1730. Endocrinol Metab Clin North Am 1993;22:823. Clin Chem 1994;40:86. Ann Clin Lab Sci 1998;28:167.

Test/Range/Collection	Physiologic Basis	Interpretation	Comments
IgG index, serum and CSF 0.29–0.59 ratio Marbled (for serum) and glass/plastic tube (for CSF) $$$ Collect serum and CSF simultaneously.	This test compares CSF IgG and albumin levels to serum levels. An increased ratio allegedly reflects synthesis of IgG within the central nervous system.	**Increased in:** Multiple sclerosis (80–90%), neurosyphilis, subacute sclerosing panencephalitis, other inflammatory and infectious CNS diseases.	Test is reasonably sensitive but not specific for multiple sclerosis. (Compare with Oligoclonal bands, p 131.) Mayo Clin Proc 1989;64:577. J Clin Pathol 1996;49:24.
Immunoelectrophoresis, serum (IEP) Negative Marbled $$$	Immunoelectrophoresis is used to identify specific immunoglobulin (Ig) classes. Serum is separated electrophoretically and reacted with antisera of known specificity. Newer technique (immunofixation) is available and easier to interpret.	**Positive in:** Presence of identifiable monoclonal paraprotein: multiple myeloma, Waldenström's macroglobulinemia, Franklin's disease (heavy chain disease), lymphoma, leukemia, monoclonal gammopathy of undetermined significance. The most common form of myeloma is the IgG type.	Test is indicated to identify an Ig spike seen on serum protein electrophoresis, to differentiate a polyclonal from a monoclonal increase, and to identify the nature of a monoclonal increase. Test is not quantitative and is not sensitive enough to use for the evaluation of immunodeficiency. Order quantitative immunoglobulins for this purpose (see below). Hematol Oncol Clin North Am 1997;11:71. Arch Pathol Lab Med 1999;123:114. Arch Pathol Lab Med 1999;123:126.

The header row of the table:

| | IgG index | Immunoelectrophoresis |

Immunoglobulins		
Immunoglobulins, serum (Ig) IgA: 78–367 mg/dL IgG: 583–1761 mg/dL IgM: 52–335 mg/dL [IgA: 0.78–3.67 g/L] IgG: 5.83–17.6 g/L] IgM: 0.52–3.35 g/L] Marbled $$$	IgG makes up about 85% of total serum immunoglobulins and predominates late in immune responses. It is the only immunoglobulin to cross the placenta. IgM antibody predominates early in immune responses. Secretory IgA plays an important role in host defense mechanisms by blocking transport of microbes across mucosal surfaces.	↑ **IgG:** *Polyclonal:* Autoimmune diseases (eg, SLE, rheumatoid arthritis), sarcoidosis, chronic liver diseases, some parasitic diseases, chronic or recurrent infections. *Monoclonal:* Multiple myeloma (IgG type), lymphomas, or other malignancies. ↑ **IgM:** *Polyclonal:* Isolated infections such as viral hepatitis, infectious mononucleosis, early response to bacterial or parasitic infection. *Monoclonal:* Waldenström's macroglobulinemia, lymphoma. ↑ **IgA:** *Polyclonal:* Chronic liver disease, chronic infections (especially of the GI and respiratory tracts). *Monoclonal:* Multiple myeloma (IgA). ↓ **IgG:** Immunosuppressive therapy, genetic (SCID, Wiskott-Aldrich syndrome, common variable immunodeficiency). ↓ **IgM:** Immunosuppressive therapy. ↓↓ **IgA:** Inherited IgA deficiency (ataxia-telangiectasia, combined immuno-deficiency disorders).	Quantitative immunoglobulin levels are indicated in the evaluation of immunodeficiency or the quantitation of a paraprotein. IgG deficiency is associated with recurrent and occasionally severe pyogenic infections. The most common form of multiple myeloma is the IgG type. Science 1986;231:1241. Hematol Oncol Clin North Am 1997;11:71. Am Fam Physician 1999;5:1885.

Test/Range/Collection	Physiologic Basis	Interpretation	Comments
Inhibitor screen, plasma Negative Blue $$ Fill tube completely.	Test is useful for evaluating a prolonged partial thromboplastin time (PTT), prothrombin time (PT), or thrombin time. (Presence of heparin should first be excluded.) Patient's plasma is mixed with normal plasma and a PTT is performed. If the patient has a factor deficiency, the postmixing PTT will be normal. If an inhibitor is present, it will be prolonged.	**Positive in:** Presence of inhibitor: Antiphospholipid antibodies (lupus anticoagulant (LAC) or anticardiolipin antibodies), factor-specific antibodies. **Negative in:** Factor deficiencies.	LAC prolongs a PTT immediately and is the most common inhibitor. Poor sensitivity for lupus anticoagulant owing to relatively high phospholipid levels in this assay system. 1–4 hour incubation period may be needed to detect factor-specific antibodies with low in vitro affinities. About 15% of hemophilia A patients develop inhibitor against factor VIII. Semin Thromb Hemost 1994;20:79. Thromb Haemost 1996;16:146.
Insulin antibody, serum Negative Marbled $$$	Insulin antibodies develop in nearly all diabetics treated with insulin. Most antibodies are IgG and do not cause clinical problems. Occasionally, high-affinity antibodies can bind to exogenous insulin and cause insulin resistance.	**Increased in:** Insulin therapy, type I diabetics before treatment (secondary to autoimmune pancreatic B cell destruction).	Insulin antibodies interfere with most assays for insulin. Insulin antibody test is not sensitive or specific for the detection of surreptitious insulin use; use C-peptide level (see p 62.) Anti-insulin and islet cell antibodies are poor predictors of IDDM and only roughly correlate with insulin requirements in patients with diabetes. Diabetes 1996;45:1720. Diabetes Care 1996;19:146.

	Insulin, immunoreactive	Iron
Test / Specimen	**Insulin, immunoreactive, serum** 6–35 µU/mL [42–243 pmol/L] Marbled $$ Fasting sample required. Measure glucose concurrently.	**Iron, serum** (Fe^{2+}) 50–175 µg/dL [9–31 µmol/L] Marbled $ Avoid hemolysis.
Physiologic Basis	Measures levels of insulin, either endogenous or exogenous.	Plasma iron concentration is determined by absorption from the intestine; storage in the intestine, liver, spleen, bone marrow; rate of breakdown or loss of hemoglobin; and rate of synthesis of new hemoglobin.
Interpretation	**Increased in:** Insulin-resistant states (eg, obesity, type II diabetes mellitus, uremia, glucocorticoids, acromegaly), liver disease, surreptitious use of insulin or oral hypoglycemic agents, insulinoma (pancreatic islet cell tumor). **Decreased in:** Type I diabetes mellitus, hypopituitarism.	**Increased in:** Hemosiderosis (eg, multiple transfusions, excess iron administration), hemolytic anemia, pernicious anemia, aplastic or hypoplastic anemia, viral hepatitis, lead poisoning, thalassemia, hemochromatosis. Drugs: estrogens, ethanol, oral contraceptives. **Decreased in:** Iron deficiency, nephrotic syndrome, chronic renal failure, many infections, active hematopoiesis, remission of pernicious anemia, hypothyroidism, malignancy (carcinoma), postoperative state, kwashiorkor.
Comments	Measurement of serum insulin level has little clinical value except in the diagnosis of fasting hypoglycemia. An insulin-to-glucose ratio of >0.3 is presumptive evidence of insulinoma. C-peptide should be used as well as serum insulin to distinguish insulinoma from surreptitious insulin use, since C-peptide will be absent with exogenous insulin use (see C-peptide, p 62). Eur J Endocrinol 1998;138:86.	Absence of stainable iron on bone marrow aspirate differentiates iron deficiency from other causes of microcytic anemia (eg, thalassemia, sideroblastic anemia, some chronic disease anemias), but the procedure is invasive and expensive. Serum iron, iron-binding capacity, and transferrin saturation—or serum ferritin—may obviate the need for bone marrow examination. Serum iron, iron-binding capacity, and transferrin saturation are useful (see p 90) in screening family members for hereditary hemochromatosis. Recent transfusion will confound the test results. JAMA 1997;277:973. Ann Intern Med 1998;129:905. Ann Intern Med 1998;129:923.

	Iron-binding capacity		
Test/Range/Collection	Physiologic Basis	Interpretation	Comments
Iron-binding capacity, total, serum (TIBC) 250–460 µg/dL [45–82 µmol/L] Marbled $$	Iron is transported in plasma complexed to transferrin, which is synthesized in the liver. Total iron-binding capacity is calculated from transferrin levels measured immunologically. Each molecule of transferrin has two iron-binding sites, so its iron-binding capacity is 1.47 mg/g. Normally, transferrin carries an amount of iron representing about 16–60% of its capacity to bind iron (ie, % saturation of iron-binding capacity is 16–60%).	**Increased in:** Iron deficiency anemia, late pregnancy, infancy, hepatitis. Drugs: oral contraceptives. **Decreased in:** Hypoproteinemic states (eg, nephrotic syndrome, starvation, malnutrition, cancer), hyperthyroidism, chronic inflammatory disorders, chronic liver disease, other chronic disease.	Increased % transferrin saturation with iron is seen in iron overload (iron poisoning, hemolytic anemia, sideroblastic anemia, thalassemia, hemochromatosis, pyridoxine deficiency, aplastic anemia). Decreased % transferrin saturation with iron is seen in iron deficiency (usually saturation <16%). Transferrin levels can also be used to assess nutritional status. Recent transfusion will confound the test results. Clin Chem 1997;43:2408. Ann Intern Med 1998;129:925. Ann Intern Med 1998;129:962.

	Lactate dehydrogenase	Lactate dehydrogenase isoenzymes
Lactate dehydrogenase, serum (LDH) 88–230 U/L [1.46–3.82 µkat/L] (laboratory-specific) Marbled $ Hemolyzed specimens are unacceptable.	LDH is an enzyme that catalyzes the interconversion of lactate and pyruvate in the presence of NAD/NADH. It is widely distributed in body cells and fluids. Because LDH is highly concentrated in red blood cells (RBCs), spuriously elevated serum levels will occur if RBCs are hemolyzed during specimen collection.	**Increased in:** Tissue necrosis, especially in acute injury of cardiac muscle, RBCs, kidney, skeletal muscle, liver, lung, or skin. Commonly elevated in various carcinomas and in *Pneumocystis carinii* pneumonia (78–94%) and lymphoma in AIDS. Marked elevations occur in hemolytic anemias, vitamin B_{12} deficiency anemia, folate deficiency anemia, polycythemia vera, thrombotic thrombocytopenic purpura (TTP), hepatitis, cirrhosis, obstructive jaundice, renal disease, musculoskeletal disease, CHF. Drugs causing hepatotoxicity (eg, acetaminophen) or hemolysis. **Decreased in:** Drugs: clofibrate, fluoride (low dose).	LDH is elevated after myocardial infarction (for 2–7 days), in liver congestion (eg, in CHF), and in *P carinii* pneumonia. LDH is not a useful liver function test, and it is not specific enough for the diagnosis of hemolytic or megaloblastic anemias. Its main diagnostic use has been in myocardial infarction, when the creatine kinase-MB elevation has passed (see CK-MB, p 79, and Figure 8–17, p 353). LDH isoenzymes are preferred over total serum LDH in late diagnosis of MI, but both tests are now being replaced by cardiac troponin I levels. Arch Intern Med 1997;157:1441. Chest 1997;111:1187.
Lactate dehydrogenase isoenzymes, serum (LDH isoenzymes) LDH_1/LDH_2: < 0.85 Marbled $$ Hemolyzed specimens are unacceptable.	LDH consists of five isoenzymes separable by electrophoresis. The fraction with the greatest electrophoretic mobility is called LDH_1; the one with the least, LDH_5. LDH_1 is found in high concentrations in heart muscle, RBCs, and kidney cortex; LDH_5 in skeletal muscle and liver.	**Increased in:** LDH_1/LDH_2 >0.85 in myocardial infarction, hemolysis (hemolytic or megaloblastic anemia) or acute renal infarction. LDH_5 is increased in liver disease, congestive heart failure, skeletal muscle injury, and essential thrombocythemia.	The only clinical indication for LDH isoenzyme measurement has been to rule out myocardial infarction in patients presenting more than 24 hours after onset of symptoms (LDH_1/LDH_2 >0.85 is usually present within 12–48 hours). It may also be helpful if CK-MB results cannot be easily interpreted. The test is being replaced by measurement of cardiac troponin I (see CK-MB, p 79). Arch Intern Med 1997;157:1441.

Test/Range/Collection	Physiologic Basis	Interpretation	Comments
Lactate, venous blood 0.5–2.0 meq/L [mmol/L] Gray $$ Collect on ice in gray-top tube containing fluoride to inhibit in vitro glycolysis and lactic acid production.	Severe tissue anoxia leads to anaerobic glucose metabolism with production of lactic acid.	**Increased in:** Lactic acidosis, ethanol ingestion, sepsis, shock, liver disease, diabetic ketoacidosis, muscular exercise, hypoxia; regional hypoperfusion (bowel ischemia); prolonged use of a tourniquet (spurious elevation); type I glycogen storage disease, fructose 1,6-diphosphatase deficiency (rare), pyruvate dehydrogenase deficiency. Drugs: phenformin, metformin, isoniazid toxicity.	Lactic acidosis should be suspected when there is a markedly increased anion gap (>18 meq/L) in the absence of other causes (eg, renal failure, ketosis, ethanol, methanol, or salicylate). Lactic acidosis is characterized by lactate levels >5 mmol/L in association with metabolic acidosis. Tissue hypoperfusion is the most common cause. Blood lactate levels may indicate whether perfusion is being restored by therapy. Am J Med 1996;101:109. Ann Intern Med 1997;127:170. Medicine 1998;77:73. Semin Nephrol 1998;18:83.

	Lead	Lecithin/sphingomyelin ratio
	Subtle neurologic impairment may be detectable in children with lead levels of 15 µg/dL and in adults at 30 µg/dL; full-blown symptoms appear at >60 µg/dL. Most chronic lead poisoning leads to a moderate anemia with basophilic stippling of erythrocytes on peripheral blood smear. Acute poisoning is rare and associated with abdominal pain and constipation. Blood lead levels are useful in the diagnosis. Industrial workers' limit: <50 µg/dL. Pediatrics 1994;93:201. Pediatrics 1996;97:79. Ann Intern Med 1999;130:7.	Test identifies fetal lung maturity effectively only 60% of the time: ie, 40% of fetuses with an L/S ratio of <2.0 will not develop hyaline membrane disease. Precision of L/S ratio test is poor: results on a single sample may vary by ±25%. Test is not reliable to assess fetal lung maturity in offspring of diabetic mothers. Med Decis Making 1990;10:201. Clin Chem 1994;40:541. Am J Obstet Gynecol 1998;179;1640.
	Increased in: Lead poisoning, including abnormal ingestion (especially lead-containing paint, moonshine whiskey), occupational exposures (metal smelters, miners, welders, storage battery workers, auto manufacturers, ship builders, paint manufacturers, printing workers, pottery workers, gasoline refinery workers), retained bullets.	**Increased in:** Contamination of amniotic fluid by blood, meconium, or vaginal secretions that contain lecithin (false-positives). **Decreased in:** Fetal lung immaturity; 95% of normal fetuses.
	Lead salts are absorbed through ingestion, inhalation, or the skin. About 5–10% of ingested lead is found in blood and 95% of this is in erythrocytes. 80–90% is taken up by bone, where it is relatively inactive. Lead poisons enzymes by binding to protein disulfide groups, leading to cell death. Lead levels fluctuate. Several specimens may be needed to rule out lead poisoning.	This test is used to estimate lung maturity in fetuses at risk for hyaline membrane disease. As fetal pulmonary surfactant matures, there is a rapid rise in amniotic fluid lecithin content. To circumvent the dependency of lecithin concentrations on amniotic fluid volume and analytic recovery of lecithin, the assay examines the lecithin/sphingomyelin ratio.
Lead, whole blood (Pb) Child (<6 yrs): <10 mg/dL Child (>6 yrs): <25 mg/dL Adult: <40 µg/dL [Child (<6): <0.48 mmol/L Child (>6): <1.21 mol/L Adult: <1.93 µmol/L] Navy $$ Use trace metal-free navy blue top tube with heparin.		
Lecithin/sphingomyelin ratio, amniotic fluid (L/S ratio) >2.0 (method-dependent) $$$ Collect in a plastic tube.		

Test/Range/Collection	Physiologic Basis	Interpretation	Comments
		***Legionella* antibody**	**Leukocyte alkaline phosphatase**
***Legionella* antibody,** serum <1:32 titer Marbled $$$ Submit paired sera, one collected within 2 weeks of illness and another 2–3 weeks later.	*Legionella pneumophila* is a weakly staining gram-negative bacillus that causes Pontiac fever (acute influenza-like illness) and Legionnaire's disease (a pneumonia that may progress to a severe multi-system illness). It does not grow on routine bacteriologic culture media. Antibodies are detected by indirect immunofluorescent tests to serogroup 1 of *L pneumophila*. There are at least six serogroups of *L pneumophila* and at least 22 species of *Legionella*.	**Increased in:** Legionella infection (80% of patients with pneumonia have a fourfold rise in titer); cross-reactions with other infectious agents (*Yersinia pestis* [plague], *Francisella tularensis* [tularemia], *Bacteroides fragilis, Mycoplasma pneumoniae, Leptospira interrogans,* campylobacter serotypes).	A greater than fourfold rise in titer to >1:128 in specimens gathered more than 3 weeks apart indicates recent infection. A single titer of >1:256 is considered diagnostic. About 50–60% of cases of legionellosis may have a positive direct fluorescent antibody test. Culture can have a sensitivity of 50%. All three methods may increase sensitivity to 90%. This test is species-specific. Polyvalent antiserum is needed to test for all serogroups and species. Epidemiol Infect 1994;112:347. Clin Infect Dis 1996;23:656.
Leukocyte alkaline phosphatase, whole blood (LAP) 40–130 Based on 0–4+ rating of 100 PMNs Green $$ Blood smear from finger stick preferred. If collecting venous blood, make smear as soon as possible.	The test measures the amount of alkaline phosphatase in neutrophils in a semiquantitative fashion. Neutrophilic leukocytes on a peripheral blood smear are stained for alkaline phosphatase activity and then 100 are scored on a scale from 0 to 4+ on the basis of the intensity of the dye in their cytoplasm.	**Increased in:** Leukemoid reaction (eg, severe infections), polycythemia vera, myelofibrosis with myeloid metaplasia. **Decreased in:** Chronic myeloid leukemia, paroxysmal nocturnal hemoglobinuria.	Test may be helpful for distinguishing leukemoid reactions (high-normal or increased LAP) from chronic myeloid leukemia (decreased LAP), but it is poorly reproducible. Br J Haematol 1997;96:815.

Test	Description/Interpretation	Comments
Leukocyte (white blood cell) count, total (WBC count) 3.4–10 × 10³/µL [× 10⁶/L] *Panic:* <1.5 × 10³/µL Lavender $	Measure of the total number of leukocytes in whole blood. Counted on automated instruments using light scattering or electrical impedance after lysis of red blood cells. WBCs are distinguished from platelets by size.	**Increased in:** Infection, inflammation, hematologic malignancy, leukemia, lymphoma. Drugs: corticosteroids. **Decreased in:** Aplastic anemia (decreased production), B_{12} or folate deficiency (maturation defect), sepsis (decreased survival). Drugs: phenothiazines, chloramphenicol, aminopyrine.	A spurious increase may be seen when there are a large number of nucleated red cells. WBC count is a poor predictor of severity of disease in the diagnosis of appendicitis. Lab Med 1983;14:509. J Clin Pathol 1996;49:664. Am Surg 1998;64:983.
Lipase, serum 0–160 U/L [0–2.66 µkat/L] (laboratory-specific) Marbled $$	Lipases are responsible for hydrolysis of glycerol esters of long-chain fatty acids to produce fatty acids and glycerol. Lipases are produced in the liver, intestine, tongue, stomach, and many other cells. Assays are highly dependent on the substrate used.	**Increased in:** Acute, recurrent, or chronic pancreatitis, pancreatic pseudocyst, pancreatic malignancy, peritonitis, biliary disease, hepatic disease, diabetes mellitus (especially diabetic ketoacidosis), intestinal disease, gastric malignancy or perforation.	The sensitivity of lipase in acute pancreatitis is similar to that of amylase; lipase remains elevated longer than amylase. The specificity of lipase and amylase in acute pancreatitis is similar, though both are poor. Test sensitivity is not very good for chronic pancreatitis or pancreatic cancer. Lipase to amylase ratio is not useful in distinguishing alcoholic from non-alcoholic pancreatitis. Arch Pathol Lab Med 1991;115:325. Clin Chem 1991;37:447. Am J Gastroenterol 1995;90:67.

Test/Range/Collection	Physiologic Basis	Interpretation	Comments
Luteinizing hormone			**Luteinizing hormone**
Luteinizing hormone, serum (LH) Male: 1–10 mIU/mL Female: (mIU/mL) Follicular 1–18 Luteal 0.4–20 Midcycle peak 24–105 Postmenopausal 15–62 (laboratory-specific) Marbled $$	LH is stimulated by the hypothalamic hormone gonadotropin-releasing hormone (GnRH). It is secreted from the anterior pituitary and acts on the gonads. LH is the principal regulator of steroid biosynthesis in the ovary and testis.	**Increased in:** Primary hypogonadism, polycystic ovary syndrome, post-menopause. **Decreased in:** Pituitary or hypothalamic failure, anorexia nervosa, severe stress, malnutrition, Kallman's syndrome (gonadotropin deficiency associated with anosmia). Drugs: digoxin, oral contraceptives, phenothiazines.	Intact human chorionic gonadotropin (hCG) cross-reacts with LH in most immunoassays so that LH levels appear to be falsely elevated in pregnancy or in individuals with hCG-secreting tumors. Repeated measurement may be required to diagnose gonadotropin deficiencies. Measurement of total testosterone is the test of choice to diagnose polycystic ovary syndrome. Br J Obstet Gynaecol 1992;99:232. J Clin Endocrinol Metab 1994;78:1208. Obstet Gynecol 1994;84:613.
Lyme disease antibody			**Lyme disease antibody**
Lyme disease antibody, serum ELISA: negative Western blot: non-reactive Marbled $	Test detects the presence of antibody to *Borrelia burgdorferi,* the etiologic agent in Lyme disease, an inflammatory disorder transmitted by the ticks *Ixodes dammini, I pacificus,* and *I scapularis* in the northeastern and midwestern, western, and southeastern USA, respectively. Detects IgM antibody, which develops within 3–6 weeks after the onset of rash; or IgG, which develops within 6–8 weeks after the onset of disease. IgG antibody may persist for months.	**Positive in:** Lyme disease, asymptomatic individuals living in endemic areas, syphilis (*Treponema pallidum*), tick-borne relapsing fever (*Borrelia hermsii*). **Negative** during the first 5 weeks of infection or after antibiotic therapy.	Test is less sensitive in patients with only a rash. Since culture or direct visualization of the organism is difficult, serologic diagnosis (by ELISA) is indicated, though sensitivity and specificity and standardization of procedure between laboratories need improvement. Cross-reactions may occur with syphilis (should be excluded by RPR and treponemal antibody assays). N Engl J Med 1989;321:586. Ann Intern Med 1991;114:472. Ann Intern Med 1997;127:1106.

	Magnesium			Mean corpuscular hemoglobin		
Magnesium, serum (Mg^{2+}) 1.8–3.0 mg/dL [0.75–1.25 mmol/L] **Panic:** <0.5 or >4.5 mg/dL Marbled $	Magnesium is primarily an intracellular cation (second most abundant, 60% found in bone); it is a necessary cofactor in numerous enzyme systems, particularly ATPases. In extracellular fluid, it influences neuromuscular response and irritability. Magnesium concentration is determined by intestinal absorption, renal excretion, and exchange with bone and intracellular fluid.	**Increased in:** Dehydration, tissue trauma, renal failure, hypoadrenocorticism, hypothyroidism. Drugs: aspirin (prolonged use), lithium, magnesium salts, progesterone, triamterene. **Decreased in:** Chronic diarrhea, enteric fistula, starvation, chronic alcoholism, total parenteral nutrition with inadequate replacement, hypoparathyroidism (especially post parathyroid surgery), acute pancreatitis, chronic glomerulonephritis, hyperaldosteronism, diabetic ketoacidosis. Drugs: albuterol, amphotericin B, calcium salts, cisplatin, citrates (blood transfusion), cyclosporine, diuretics, ethacrynic acid.	Hypomagnesemia is associated with tetany, weakness, disorientation, and somnolence. A magnesium deficit may exist with little or no apparent change in serum level. There is a progressive reduction in serum magnesium level during normal pregnancy (related to hemodilution). Crit Care Med 1998;26:1949. Crit Care Med 1998;26:2048. Semin Nephrol 1998;18:58.		
Mean corpuscular hemoglobin, blood (MCH) 26–34 pg Lavender $	MCH indicates the amount of hemoglobin per red blood cell in absolute units. Low MCH can mean hypochromia or microcytosis or both. High MCH is evidence of macrocytosis.	**Increased in:** Macrocytosis. **Decreased in:** Microcytosis (iron deficiency, thalassemia). Hypochromia (lead poisoning, sideroblastic anemia, anemia of chronic disease).	MCH is calculated from measured values of hemoglobin (Hb) and red cell count (RBC) by the formula: $$MCH = \frac{Hb}{RBC}$$ Obstet Gynecol 1999;93:427.		

Test/Range/Collection	Physiologic Basis	Interpretation	Comments	Mean corpuscular hemoglobin concentration	Mean corpuscular volume
Mean corpuscular hemoglobin concentration, blood (MCHC) 31–36 g/dL [310–360 g/L] Lavender $	MCHC describes how fully the erythrocyte volume is filled with hemoglobin and is calculated from measurement of hemoglobin (Hb), mean corpuscular volume (MCV), and red cell count (RBC) by the formula: $$MCHC = \frac{Hb}{MCV \times RBC}$$	**Increased in:** Marked spherocytosis. Spuriously increased in autoagglutination, hemolysis (with spuriously high Hb or low MCV or RBC), lipemia. Cellular dehydration syndromes, xerocytosis. **Decreased in:** Hypochromic anemia (iron deficiency, thalassemia, lead poisoning), sideroblastic anemia, anemia of chronic disease. Spuriously decreased with high white blood cell count, low Hb, or high MCV or RBC.	Lab Med 1983;14:509.		
Mean corpuscular volume, blood (MCV) 80–100 fL Lavender $	Average volume of the red cell is measured by automated instrument, by electrical impedance, or by light scatter.	**Increased in:** Liver disease, megaloblastic anemia (folate, B$_{12}$ deficiencies), reticulocytosis, newborns. Spurious increase in autoagglutination, high white blood cell count. Drugs: methotrexate, phenytoin, zidovudine. **Decreased in:** Iron deficiency, thalassemia; decreased or normal in anemia of chronic disease.	MCV can be normal in combined iron and folate deficiency. In patients with two red cell populations (macrocytic and microcytic), MCV may be normal. MCV is an insensitive test in the evaluation of anemia. Patients with iron deficiency anemia or pernicious anemia commonly have a normal MCV. J Gen Intern Med 1990;5:187. Br J Haematol 1994;88:443. Am J Clin Pathol 1996;106:201.		

	Metanephrines	Methanol
Metanephrines, urine 0.3–0.9 mg/24 h [1.6–4.9 μmol/24 h] Urine bottle containing hydrochloric acid $$$ Collect 24-hour urine.	Catecholamines, secreted in excess by pheochromocytomas, are metabolized by the enzyme catechol-O-methyltransferase to metanephrines, and these are excreted in the urine.	**Increased in:** Pheochromocytoma (96% sensitivity, 98% specificity), neuroblastoma, ganglioneuroma. Drugs: monoamine oxidase inhibitors.	First-line test for diagnosis of pheochromocytoma (see Pheochromocytoma algorithm, p 355). Since <0.1% of hypertensives have a pheochromocytoma, routine screening of all hypertensives would yield a positive predictive value of <10%. Avoid overutilization of tests. Do not order urine vanillylmandelic acid, urine catecholamines, and plasma catecholamines at the same time. Plasma catecholamine levels are often spuriously increased when drawn in the hospital setting. Mayo Clin Proc 1990;65:88. Ann Intern Med 1995;123:101. Ann Intern Med 1996;125:331.
Methanol, whole blood Negative Green or lavender $$	Serum methanol levels >20 mg/dL are toxic and levels >40 mg/dL are life-threatening.	**Increased in:** Methanol intoxication.	Methanol intoxication is associated with metabolic acidosis and an osmolal gap. Methanol is commonly ingested in its pure form or in cleaning and copier solutions. Acute ingestion causes an optic neuritis that may result in blindness. Med Toxicol 1986;1:309. Ann Emerg Med 1995;26:202.

Test/Range/Collection	Physiologic Basis	Interpretation	Comments
Methemoglobin, whole blood (MetHb) <0.005 g/dL [<0.5 g/L] Lavender $$ Analyze promptly.	Methemoglobin has its heme iron in the oxidized ferric state and thus cannot combine with and transport oxygen. Methemoglobin can be assayed spectrophotometrically by measuring the decrease in absorbance at 630–635 nm due to the conversion of methemoglobin to cyanmethemoglobin with cyanide.	**Increased in:** Hemoglobin variants (HbM) (rare), methemoglobin reductase deficiency. Oxidant drugs such as sulfonamides (dapsone, sulfasalazine), nitrites and nitrates, aniline dyes, phenacetin, anesthetics such as benzocaine.	Levels of 1.5 g/dL (10% of total Hb) result in visible cyanosis. Patients with levels of about 35% have headache, weakness, and breathlessness. Levels in excess of 70% are usually fatal. Fetal methemoglobin is accurately measured using newer multiple-wavelength spectrophotometers. Am J Med Sci 1985;289:200. Am J Hematol 1993;42:7. Clin Chem 1998;44:1569.
Methylmalonic acid, serum 0–0.4 µmol/L Marbled $$	Elevation of serum methylmalonic acid in cobalamin deficiency results from impaired conversion of methylmalonyl-CoA to succinyl-CoA, a pathway involving methylmalonyl-CoA mutase as enzyme and adenosylcobalamin as coenzyme.	**Increased in:** Vitamin B_{12} (cobalamin) deficiency (95%), pernicious anemia, renal insufficiency, elderly (5–15%).	Explanation of high frequency (5–15%) of increased serum methylmalonic acid in the elderly with low or normal serum cobalamin is unclear. Only a small number have pernicious anemia confirmed. Normal levels can exclude vitamin B_{12} deficiency in the presence of low unexplained cobalamin levels found in lymphoid disorders. Test is usually normal in HIV patients who may have low vitamin B_{12} levels without cobalamin deficiency, because of low vitamin B_{12} binding protein. Semin Hematol 1999;36:29. Semin Hematol 1999;36:35. Am J Clin Nutr 1997;66:741.

Metyrapone test (overnight)		
Metyrapone test (overnight), plasma or serum 8 AM cortisol: <10 µg/dL [<280 nmol/L] 8 AM 11-deoxycortisol: >7 µg/dL [>202 nmol/L] Marbled, lavender, or green $$$ Give 2.0–2.5 g of metyrapone orally at 12:00 midnight. Draw serum cortisol and 11–deoxycortisol levels at 8:00 AM.	The metyrapone stimulation test assesses both pituitary and adrenal reserve and is mainly used to diagnose secondary adrenal insufficiency (see Adrenocortical Insufficiency algorithm, p 338). Metyrapone is a drug that inhibits adrenal 11 β-hydroxylase and blocks cortisol synthesis. The consequent fall in cortisol increases release of ACTH and hence production of steroids formed proximal to the block (eg, 11-deoxycortisol).	**Decreased in:** An 8 AM 11-deoxycortisol level ≤7 µg/dL indicates primary or secondary adrenal insufficiency.
		The metyrapone test can be useful in steroid-treated patients to assess the extent of suppression of the pituitary-adrenal axis. The use of an extended metyrapone test in the differential diagnosis of ACTH-dependent Cushing's syndrome (pituitary versus ectopic) has been questioned. Ann Intern Med 1994;121:318. Clin Endocrinol 1996;45:483. Clin Endocrinol 1997;47:145.

Test/Range/Collection	Physiologic Basis	Interpretation	Comments
β_2-Microglobulin		**β_2-Microglobulin**	
β_2-Microglobulin, serum (β_2-M) <0.2 mg/dL [<2.0 mg/L] Marbled $$$	β_2-Microglobulin is a portion of the HLA molecule on cell surfaces synthesized by all nucleated cell types and is present in all body fluids. It is increased in many conditions that are accompanied by high cell turnover.	**Increased in:** Any type of inflammation, autoimmune disorders, lymphoid malignancies, multiple myeloma, viral infections (HIV, CMV). Marked elevation in patients with amyloidosis and renal failure.	Of tests used to predict progression to AIDS in HIV-infected patients, CD4 cell number has the most predictive power, followed closely by β_2-microglobulin. Asymptomatic HIV patients with elevated β_2-microglobulin levels have a two- to threefold increased chance of disease progression. However, β_2-microglobulin does not provide information significantly more useful than the combination of serial CD4 count and serum IgA in predicting onset of AIDS. β_2-Microglobulin is of prognostic value in multiple myeloma: serum level increases with increasing tumor mass. AIDS 1994;8:911. Semin Hematol 1997;34(1 Suppl):29. J Am Soc Nephrol 1998;9:1723.

	Microhemagglutination-*Treponema pallidum*	Mitochondrial antibody
Micro-hemagglutination-*Treponema pallidum*, serum (MHA-TP) Nonreactive Marbled $$	The MHA-TP test measures specific antibody against *T pallidum* in a patient's serum by agglutination of *T pallidum* antigen-coated erythrocytes. Antibodies to nonpathogenic treponemes are first removed by binding to nonpathogenic treponemal antigens.	Test is used to confirm reactive serologic tests for syphilis (RPR or VDRL). Compared to FTA-ABS, MHA-TP is slightly less sensitive in all stages of syphilis and becomes reactive somewhat later in the disease. Because test usually remains positive for long periods of time regardless of therapy, it is not useful in assessing the effectiveness of therapy. In one study, 36 months after treatment of syphilis, 13% of patients had nonreactive MHA-TP tests. Ann Intern Med 1986;104:368. J Infect Dis 1990;162:862. Ann Intern Med 1991;114:1005. Clin Microbiol Rev 1995;8:1.
	Increased in: Syphilis: primary (64–87%), secondary (96–100%), late latent (96–100%), tertiary (94–100%); infectious mononucleosis, collagen-vascular diseases, hyperglobulinemia and dysglobulinemia.	
Mitochondrial anti-body, serum Negative Marbled $$	Qualitative measure of antibodies against hepatic mitochondria. Rabbit hepatocytes are incubated first with serum and then (after washing) with a fluorescein-tagged antibody to human immunoglobulin. Hepatocytes are then viewed for presence of cytoplasmic staining.	Primarily used to distinguish primary biliary cirrhosis (antibody present) from extrahepatic biliary obstruction (antibody absent). Hepatology 1986;6:381. Acta Med Scand 1986;220:241. Dig Dis 1992;10:85. Am J Gastroenterol 1999;94:47.
	Increased in: Primary biliary cirrhosis (87–98%), chronic active hepatitis (25–28%); lower titers in viral hepatitis, infectious mononucleosis, neoplasms, cryptogenic cirrhosis (25–30%).	

	Neutrophil cytoplasmic antibodies		
Test/Range/Collection	**Physiologic Basis**	**Interpretation**	**Comments**
Neutrophil cytoplasmic antibodies, serum (ANCA) Negative Marbled $$$	Measurement of autoantibodies in serum against cytoplasmic constituents of neutrophils. (See also Autoantibodies table, p 367.)	**Positive in:** Wegener's granulomatosis, systemic vasculitis, crescentic glomerulonephritis, paraneoplastic vasculitis, ulcerative colitis.	Test sensitivity for Wegener's granulomatosis ranges from 56% to 96%, depending on the population studied. Test specificity for Wegener's granulomatosis is claimed to be high (99%) when requiring diffuse cytoplasmic staining for a positive result, but interpretation is highly technique-dependent. In the patient with systemic vasculitis, elevated ANCA levels imply active disease and high likelihood of recurrence. However, ANCA levels can be persistently elevated and should be used in conjunction with other clinical indices in treatment decisions. N Engl J Med 1988;318:1651. Ann Intern Med 1989;111:28. Am J Kidney Dis 1995;25:380. Ann Intern Med 1995;123:925.

	Nuclear antibody		Oligoclonal bands
Nuclear antibody, serum (ANA) <1:20 Marbled $$	Heterogeneous antibodies to nuclear antigens (DNA and RNA, histone and nonhistone proteins). Nuclear antibody is measured in serum by layering the patient's serum over human epithelial cells and detecting the antibody with fluorescein-conjugated polyvalent antihuman immunoglobulin.	**Elevated in:** Patients over age 65 (35–75%, usually in low titers), systemic lupus erythematosus (98%), drug-induced lupus (100%), Sjögren's syndrome (80%), rheumatoid arthritis (30–50%), scleroderma (60%), mixed connective tissue disease (100%), Felty's syndrome, mononucleosis, hepatic or biliary cirrhosis, hepatitis, leukemia, myasthenia gravis, dermatomyositis, polymyositis, chronic renal failure.	A negative ANA test does not completely rule out SLE, but alternative diagnoses should be considered. Pattern of ANA staining may give some clues to diagnoses, but since the pattern also changes with serum dilution, it is not routinely reported. Only the rim (peripheral) pattern is highly specific (for SLE). Not useful as a screening test. Should be used only when there is clinical evidence of a connective tissue disease. West J Med 1987;147:210. Arch Intern Med 1996;156:1421. Clin Chem 1997;43:1981.
Oligoclonal bands, serum and CSF Negative Marbled and glass or plastic tube for CSF $$ Collect serum and CSF simultaneously.	Electrophoretic examination of IgG found in CSF may show oligoclonal bands not found in serum. This suggests local production in CSF of limited species of IgG.	**Positive in:** Multiple sclerosis (88%), CNS syphilis, subacute sclerosing panencephalitis, other CNS inflammatory diseases.	Test is indicated only when multiple sclerosis is suspected clinically. Test interpretation is very subjective. IgG index is a more reliable test analytically, but neither test is specific for multiple sclerosis. Neurology 1985;35:212. Mayo Clin Proc 1989;64:577. Am J Clin Pathol 1998;109:585.

Test/Range/Collection	Physiologic Basis	Interpretation	Comments
Osmolality, serum (Osm) 285–293 mosm/kg H_2O [mmol/kg H_2O] ***Panic:*** <240 or >320 mosm/kg H_2O Marbled $$	Test measures the osmotic pressure of serum by the freezing point depression method. Plasma and urine osmolality are more useful indicators of degree of hydration than BUN, hematocrit, or serum proteins. Serum osmolality can be estimated by the following formula: $$Osm = 2(Na^+) + \frac{BUN}{2.8} + \frac{Glucose}{18}$$ where Na^+ is in meq/L and BUN and glucose are in mg/dL.	**Increased in:** Diabetic ketoacidosis, nonketotic hyperosmolar hyperglycemic coma, hypernatremia secondary to dehydration (diarrhea, severe burns, vomiting, fever, hyperventilation, inadequate water intake, central or nephrogenic diabetes insipidus, or osmotic diuresis), hypernatremia with normal hydration (hypothalamic disorders, defective osmostat), hypernatremia with overhydration (iatrogenic or accidental excessive NaCl or $NaHCO_3$ intake), alcohol or other toxic ingestion (see Comments), hypercalcemia; tube feedings. Drugs: corticosteroids, mannitol, glycerin. **Decreased in:** Pregnancy (third trimester), hyponatremia with hypovolemia (adrenal insufficiency, renal losses, diarrhea, vomiting, severe burns, peritonitis, pancreatitis), hyponatremia with normovolemia, hyponatremia with hypervolemia (congestive heart failure, cirrhosis, nephrotic syndrome, SIADH, postoperative state). Drugs: chlorthalidone, cyclophosphamide, thiazides.	If the difference between calculated and measured serum osmolality is greater than 10 mosm/kg H_2O, suspect the presence of a low-molecular-weight toxin (alcohol, methanol, isoprophyl alcohol, ethylene glycol, acetone, ethyl ether, paraldehyde, or mannitol), ethanol being the most common. (See p 381 for further explanation.) Every 100 mg/dL of ethanol increases serum osmolality by 22 mosm/kg H_2O. While the osmolal gap may overestimate the blood alcohol level, a normal serum osmolality excludes ethanol intoxication. Clin Chem 1990;36:2004. J Emerg Med 1992;10:129. Pharmacotherapy 1993;13:60. Clin Chem 1998;44:1582.

Osmolality, serum

	Osmolality, urine	Oxygen, partial pressure
	Osmolality, urine (Urine Osm) Random: 100–900 mosm/kg H$_2$O [mmol/kg H$_2$O] Urine container $$	**Oxygen, partial pressure,** whole blood (Po$_2$) 83–108 mm Hg [11.04–14.36 kPa] Heparinized syringe $$$ Collect arterial blood in a heparinized syringe. Send to laboratory immediately on ice.
	Test measures renal tubular concentrating ability.	Test measures the partial pressure of oxygen (oxygen tension) in arterial blood. Partial pressure of oxygen is critical since it determines (along with hemoglobin and blood supply) tissue oxygen supply.
	Increased in: Hypovolemia. Drugs: anesthetic agents (during surgery), carbamazepine, chlorpropamide, cyclophosphamide, metolazone, vincristine. **Decreased in:** Diabetes insipidus, primary polydipsia, exercise, starvation. Drugs: acetohexamide, demeclocycline, glyburide, lithium, tolazamide.	**Increased in:** Oxygen therapy. **Decreased in:** Ventilation/perfusion mismatching (asthma, COPD, atelectasis, pulmonary embolism, pneumonia, interstitial lung disease, airway obstruction by foreign body, shock); alveolar hypoventilation (kyphoscoliosis, neuromuscular disease, head injury, stroke); right-to-left shunt (congenital heart disease). Drugs: barbiturates, opioids.
	With average fluid intake, normal random urine osmolality is 100–900 mosm/kg H$_2$O. After 12-hour fluid restriction, normal random urine osmolality is >850 mosm/kg H$_2$O. Am J Med 1982;72:308.	% saturation of hemoglobin (So$_2$) represents the oxygen content divided by the oxygen carrying capacity of hemoglobin. % saturation on blood gas reports is calculated not measured. It is calculated from Po$_2$ and pH using reference oxyhemoglobin dissociation curves for normal adult hemoglobin (lacking methemoglobin, carboxyhemoglobin, etc). At Po$_2$ <60 mm Hg, the oxygen saturation (and content) cannot be reliably estimated from the Po$_2$. Therefore, oximetry should be used to determine % saturation directly. JAMA 1990;264:244. Am J Clin Pathol 1995;(1 Suppl):579. Obstet Gynecol Surv 1998;53:645.

Test/Range/Collection	Physiologic Basis	Interpretation	Comments
Parathyroid hormone, serum (PTH) Intact PTH: 11–54 pg/mL [1.2–5.7 pmol/L] (laboratory-specific) Marbled $$$$ Fasting sample preferred; simultaneous measurement of serum calcium and phosphorus is also required.	PTH is secreted from the parathyroid glands. It mobilizes calcium from bone, increases distal renal tubular reabsorption of calcium, decreases proximal renal tubular reabsorption of phosphorus, and stimulates 1,25-hydroxy vitamin D synthesis from 25-hydroxy vitamin D by renal 1α-hydroxylase. The "intact" PTH molecule (84 amino acids) has a circulating half-life of about 5 minutes. Carboxyl terminal and mid-molecule fragments make up 90% of circulating PTH. They are biologically inactive, cleared by the kidney, and have half-lives of about 1–2 hours. The amino terminal fragment is biologically active and has a half-life of 1–2 minutes. Measurement of PTH by immunoassay depends on the specificity of the antibodies used.	**Increased in:** Primary hyperparathyroidism, secondary hyperparathyroidism due to renal disease, vitamin D deficiency. Drugs: lithium, furosemide, phosphates. **Decreased in:** Hypoparathyroidism, sarcoidosis, hyperthyroidism, hypomagnesemia, malignancy with hypercalcemia, non-parathyroid hypercalcemia.	PTH results must always be evaluated in light of concurrent serum calcium levels. PTH tests differ in sensitivity and specificity from assay to assay and from laboratory to laboratory. Carboxyl terminal antibody measures intact, carboxyl terminal and midmolecule fragments. It is 85% sensitive and 95% specific for primary hyperparathyroidism. Amino terminal antibody measures intact and amino terminal fragments. It is about 75% sensitive for hyperparathyroidism. Intact PTH assays are preferred because they detect PTH suppression in nonparathyroid hypercalcemia. Sensitivity of immunometric assays is 85–90% for primary hyperparathyroidism. Endocrinol Metab Clin North Am 1989;18:647. Mayo Clin Proc 1992;67:637. Recent Prog Horm Res 1998;53:283.

Parathyroid hormone-related protein		
Parathyroid hormone-related protein (PTHrP), plasma Assay-specific (pmol/L or undetectable) Tube containing anti-coagulant and protease inhibitors; specimen drawn without a tourniquet. $$	Parathyroid hormone-related protein (PTHrP) is a 139- to 173-amino-acid protein with amino terminal homology to parathyroid hormone (PTH). The homology explains the ability of PTHrP to bind to the PTH receptor and have PTH-like effects on bone and kidney. PTHrP induces increased plasma calcium, decreased plasma phosphorus, and increased urinary cAMP. PTHrP is found in keratinocytes, fibroblasts, placenta, brain, pituitary gland, adrenal gland, stomach, liver, testicular Leydig cells, and mammary glands. Its physiologic role in these diverse sites is unknown. PTHrP is secreted by solid malignant tumors (lung, breast, kidney; other squamous tumors) and produces humoral hypercalcemia of malignancy. PTHrP analysis is by immunoradio-metric assay (IRMA). Assay of choice is amino terminal-specific IRMA. Two-site IRMA assays require sample collection in protease inhibitors because serum proteases destroy immunoreactivity.	**Increased in:** Humoral hypercalcemia of malignancy (80% of solid tumors).	Assays directed at the amino terminal portion of PTHrP are not influenced by renal failure. Increases in PTHrP concentrations are readily detectable with most current assays in the majority of patients with humoral hypercalcemia of malignancy. About 20% of patients with malignancy and hypercalcemia will have low PTHrP levels because their hypercalcemia is caused by local osteolytic processes. N Engl J Med 1990;322:1106. West J Med 1990;153:635. Clin Chem 1992;38:2171. Cancer 1994;73:2223.

Test/Range/Collection	Physiologic Basis	Interpretation	Comments
Partial thromboplastin time, activated, plasma (PTT) 25–35 seconds (range varies) ***Panic:*** ≥60 seconds (off heparin) Blue $$ Fill tube adequately. Do not contaminate specimen with heparin.	Patient's plasma is activated to clot in vitro by mixing it with phospholipid and an activator substance. Test screens the intrinsic coagulation pathway and adequacy of all coagulation factors except XIII and VII. PTT is usually abnormal if any factor level drops below 30–40% of normal.	**Increased in:** Deficiency of any individual coagulation factor except XIII and VII; presence of nonspecific inhibitors (eg, lupus anticoagulant), specific factor inhibitors, von Willebrand's disease (PTT may also be normal), hemophilia A and B), disseminated intravascular coagulation (DIC). Drugs: heparin, warfarin. **Decreased in:** Hypercoagulable states, DIC.	PTT is the best test to monitor adequacy of heparin therapy, but it does not reliably predict the risk of bleeding. Test is not always abnormal in von Willebrand's disease. Test may be normal in chronic DIC. A very common cause of PTT prolongation is the spurious presence of heparin in the plasma sample. Sensitivity and degree of prolongation of PTT depend on particular reagents used. Therapeutic levels of heparin are best achieved using a weight-based dosing nomogram with dose adjustment based on the PTT at 6 hours. JAMA 1989;262:2428. Ann Intern Med 1993;119:874. Thromb Haemost 1995;73:73.

pH

pH, whole blood

Arterial: 7.35–7.45
Venous: 7.31–7.41

Heparinized syringe
$$$

Specimen must be collected in heparinized syringe and immediately transported on ice to lab without exposure to air.

pH assesses the acid-base status of blood, an extremely useful measure of integrated cardiorespiratory function.

The essential relationship between pH, PCO_2 and bicarbonate (HCO_3) is expressed by the Henderson–Hasselbalch equation (at 37 °C):

$$pH = 6.1 + \log\left(\frac{HCO_3^-}{PCO_2 \times 0.03}\right)$$

Arteriovenous pH difference is 0.01–0.03 but is greater in patients with congestive heart failure and shock.

Increased in: *Respiratory alkalosis:* hyperventilation (eg, anxiety), sepsis, liver disease, fever, early salicylate poisoning, and excessive artificial ventilation.

Metabolic alkalosis: Loss of gastric HCl (eg, vomiting), potassium depletion, excessive alkali administration (eg, bicarbonate, antacids), diuretics, volume depletion.

Decreased in: *Respiratory acidosis:* decreased alveolar ventilation (eg, COPD, respiratory depressants), neuromuscular diseases (eg, myasthenia).

Metabolic acidosis (bicarbonate deficit): increased formation of acids (eg, ketosis [diabetes mellitus, alcohol, starvation], lactic acidosis); decreased H^+ excretion (eg, renal failure, renal tubular acidosis, Fanconi's syndrome); increased acid intake (eg, ion-exchange resins, salicylates, ammonium chloride, ethylene glycol, methanol); and increased loss of alkaline body fluids (eg, diarrhea, fistulas, aspiration of gastrointestinal contents, biliary drainage).

The pH of a standing sample decreases because of cellular metabolism.

The correction of pH (measured at 37°C), based on the patient's temperature, is not clinically useful.

Am J Med 1982;72:496.
Crit Care Nurs 1996;16:89.

	Phosphorus

Test/Range/Collection	Physiologic Basis	Interpretation	Comments
Phosphorus, serum 2.5–4.5 mg/dL [0.8–1.45 mmol/L] ***Panic:*** <1.0 mg/dL Marbled $ Avoid hemolysis.	The plasma concentration of inorganic phosphate is determined by parathyroid gland function, action of vitamin D, intestinal absorption, renal function, bone metabolism, and nutrition.	**Increased in:** Renal failure, massive blood transfusion, hypoparathyroidism, sarcoidosis, neoplasms, adrenal insufficiency, acromegaly, hypervitaminosis D, osteolytic metastases to bone, leukemia, milk-alkali syndrome, healing bone fractures, pseudohypoparathyroidism, diabetes mellitus with ketosis, malignant hyperpyrexia, cirrhosis, lactic acidosis, respiratory acidosis. Drugs: phosphate infusions or enemas, anabolic steroids, ergocalciferol, furosemide, hydrochlorothiazide, clonidine, verapamil, potassium supplements, and others. **Decreased in:** Hyperparathyroidism, hypovitaminosis D (rickets, osteomalacia), malabsorption (steatorrhea), malnutrition, starvation or cachexia, GH deficiency, chronic alcoholism, severe diarrhea, vomiting, nasogastric suction, severe hypercalcemia (any cause), acute gout, osteoblastic metastases to bone, severe burns (diuretic phase), respiratory alkalosis, hyperalimentation with inadequate phosphate repletion, carbohydrate administration (eg, intravenous $D_{50}W$ glucose bolus), renal tubular acidosis and other renal tubular defects, diabetic ketoacidosis (during recovery), acid-base disturbances, hypokalemia, pregnancy, hypothyroidism, hemodialysis. Drugs: acetazolamide, phosphate-binding antacids, anticonvulsants, beta-adrenergic agonists, catecholamines, estrogens, isoniazid, oral contraceptives, prolonged use of thiazides, glucose infusion, insulin therapy, salicylates (toxicity).	Thrombocytosis may cause spurious elevation of serum phosphate, but plasma phosphate levels are normal. Clin Lab Med 1993;13:183. Ann Pharmacother 1994;28:626. Am J Med Sci 1994;307:255. J Clin Endocrinol Metab 1998;83:3860.

Platelet aggregation		
Platelet aggregation, whole blood Aggregation by adenosine diphosphate (ADP), collagen, epinephrine, thrombin, ristocetin, and arachidonic acid Drawn by lab $$$$ Whole blood in citrate is drawn into a plastic tube. Platelet-rich plasma (PRP) is obtained by centrifuging at $100 \times g$ for 10–15 minutes.	Platelet aggregometry can provide information concerning possible qualitative platelet defects. Aggregation is measured as an increase in light transmission through stirred platelet-rich plasma (PRP) when a specific agonist is added. Test examines platelet aggregation response to various agonists (eg, ADP, collagen, epinephrine, thrombin, ristocetin, arachidonic acid). Newer lumiaggregation measures aggregation and simultaneous platelet ATP release—the so-called "platelet release reaction."	**Abnormal in:** Acquired defects in the platelet release reaction (eg, drugs, following cardiopulmonary bypass, uremia, paraproteinemias, myeloproliferative disorders), congenital release abnormalities, Glanzmann's thrombasthenia (absent aggregation to ADP, collagen, epinephrine), essential athrombia (similar to Glanzmann's disease except clot retraction is normal), storage pool disease (no secondary wave with ADP, epinephrine, and decreased aggregation with collagen), cyclooxygenase and thromboxane synthetase deficiencies (rare hereditary aspirin-like defects), von Willebrand's disease (normal aggregation with all factors except ristocetin). Drugs: aspirin (absent aggregation curves to ADP and epinephrine, collagen, arachidonate).	Acquired platelet dysfunction is more common than the hereditary form. Hereditary storage pool disease is common enough to be suspected in a child with easy or spontaneous bruising. Test should not be done if the patient has taken aspirin within the previous 10 days. Direct PRP aggregation by ristocetin (1.5 mg/mL) may be normal or abnormal in von Willebrand's disease (vWD). Because this test has limited sensitivity for detection of vWD, it is no longer used for that purpose (see instead Bleeding time, p 59, and von Willebrand factor protein, p 184). Semin Thromb Hemost 1992;18:167. J Clin Invest 1998;101:479. Thromb Haemost 1998;79:211.

		Platelet count	
Test/Range/Collection	**Physiologic Basis**	**Interpretation**	**Comments**
Platelet count, whole blood (Plt) 150–450 × 10³/μL [× 10⁹/L] ***Panic:*** <25 × 10³/μL Lavender $	Platelets are released from mega-karyocytes in bone marrow and are important for normal hemostasis. Platelet counting is done by flow cytometry with size discrimination based on electrical impedance or electro-optical systems.	**Increased in:** Myeloproliferative disorders: polycythemia vera, chronic myeloid leukemia, essential thrombocythemia, myelofibrosis; after bleeding, postsplenectomy, reactive thrombocytosis secondary to inflammatory diseases, iron deficiency, malignancies, alkalosis. **Decreased in:** Decreased production: bone marrow suppression or replacement, chemotherapeutic agents, drugs (eg, ethanol). Increased destruction or removal: splenomegaly, disseminated intravascular coagulation, platelet antibodies (idiopathic thrombocytopenic purpura, posttransfusion purpura, neonatal isoimmune thrombocytopenia, drugs [eg, quinidine, cephalosporins]).	N Engl J Med 1995;332:1132. Am J Med 1995;98:436. Am J Med 1995;98:551. J Clin Pathol 1996;49:664. Ann Intern Med 1998;129:886. Br J Haematol 1998;100:571.

Platelet-associated IgG		
Platelet-associated IgG, whole blood Negative Yellow $$$$ 17 mL of blood is needed.	Antibody screening involves direct testing of a patient's platelets to demonstrate platelet-associated IgG (which may be directed against specific platelet antigens or may represent immune complexes nonspecifically absorbed to the platelet surface) in idiopathic (autoimmune) thrombocytopenic purpura (ITP). It also involves indirect testing of the patient's serum against a panel of reagent platelets to detect circulating antiplatelet antibodies. In alloimmune thrombocytopenia, the patient's direct test is negative and the patient's serum reacts with reagent platelets. Antibody specificity can be identified, and platelets lacking the involved antigen can be transfused.	**Positive in:** Some autoimmune thrombocytopenias (eg, ITP) (90–95%).	In ITP, the direct antiplatelet antibody test may be useful to confirm the diagnosis and monitor subsequent response to therapy. It is also useful in diagnosing posttransfusion purpura and suspected neonatal isoimmune thrombocytopenia. Platelet-associated IgG is also useful for patients with thrombocytopenia or as part of a platelet cross-match prior to transfusion of patients who have repeatedly failed to respond to random donor platelet transfusions. N Engl J Med 1991;324:27. Br J Haematol 1997;96:204.

	Porphobilinogen	

Test/Range/Collection	Physiologic Basis	Interpretation	Comments
Porphobilinogen, urine (PBG) Negative $$ Protect from light.	Porphyrias are characterized clinically by neurologic and cutaneous manifestations and chemically by overproduction of porphyrin and other precursors of heme production. PBG is a water-soluble precursor of heme whose urinary excretion is increased in symptomatic hepatic porphyrias. PBG is detected qualitatively by a color reaction with Ehrlich's reagent and confirmed by extraction into chloroform (Watson-Schwartz test).	**Positive in:** Acute intermittent porphyria, variegate porphyria, coproporphyria, lead poisoning (rare). **Negative in:** 20–30% of patients with hepatic porphyria between attacks.	Positive qualitative urinary PBG tests should be followed up by quantitative measurements. Many labs report frequent false positives with the Watson-Schwartz test. A screening PBG test is insensitive, and a negative test does not rule out porphyria between attacks or the carrier state. Specific porphyrias can be better defined by quantitative measurement of urine PBG and by measurement of erythrocyte uroporphyrinogen-I-synthetase. Mayo Clin Proc 1994;69:289. J Inherit Metab Dis 1997;20:237. Semin Liver Dis 1998;18:57.

	Potassium		
Potassium, serum (K⁺)

3.5–5.0 meq/L [mmol/L]
Panic: <3.0 or >6.0 meq/L

Marbled
$
Avoid hemolysis. | Potassium is predominantly an intracellular cation whose plasma level is regulated by renal excretion. Plasma potassium concentration determines neuromuscular irritability. Elevated or depressed potassium concentrations interfere with muscle contraction. | **Increased in:** Massive hemolysis, severe tissue damage, rhabdomyolysis, acidosis, dehydration, acute or chronic renal failure, Addison's disease, renal tubular acidosis type IV (hyporeninemic hypoaldosteronism), hyperkalemic familial periodic paralysis, exercise (transient). Drugs: potassium salts, potassium-sparing diuretics (eg, spironolactone, triamterene), non-steroidal anti-inflammatory drugs, beta-blockers, ACE inhibitors, high-dose trimethoprim-sulfamethoxazole.

Decreased in: Low potassium intake, prolonged vomiting or diarrhea, renal tubular acidosis types I and II, hyperaldosteronism, Cushing's syndrome, osmotic diuresis (eg, hyperglycemia), alkalosis, familial periodic paralysis, trauma (transient). Drugs: adrenergic agents (isoproterenol), diuretics. | Spurious hyperkalemia can occur with hemolysis of sample, delayed separation of serum from erythrocytes, prolonged fist clenching during blood drawing, and prolonged tourniquet placement. Very high white blood cell or platelet counts may cause spurious elevation of serum potassium, but plasma potassium levels are normal. Crit Care Nurs Q 1990;13:34. Clin Chem 1994;40:1528. Clin Chem 1998;44:849. |

Test/Range/Collection	Physiologic Basis	Interpretation	Comments
Prolactin, serum (PRL) < 20 ng/mL [μg/L] Marbled $$$	Prolactin is a polypeptide hormone secreted by the anterior pituitary. It functions in the initiation and maintenance of lactation in the postpartum period. PRL secretion is inhibited by hypothalamic secretion of dopamine. Prolactin levels increase with renal failure, hypothyroidism, and drugs that are dopamine antagonists.	**Increased in:** Sleep, nursing, nipple stimulation, exercise, hypoglycemia, stress, hypothyroidism, pituitary tumors (prolactinomas and others), hypothalamic/pituitary stalk lesions, renal failure. Drugs: phenothiazines, haloperidol, reserpine, methyldopa, estrogens, opiates, cimetidine. **Decreased in:** Drugs: levodopa.	Serum PRL is used primarily in workup of suspected pituitary tumor (60% of pituitary adenomas secrete PRL). Clinical presentation is usually amenorrhea and galactorrhea in women and impotence in men. (See Amenorrhea algorithm, p 339.) Only 4% of impotence is caused by hyperprolactinemia, and hyperprolactinemia is rare in the absence of low serum testosterone. Clin Endocrinol 1996;44:305. Ann Intern Med 1998;129:472. Clin Endocrinol 1998;48:547.
Prostate-specific antigen, serum (PSA) 0–4 ng/mL [μg/L] Marbled $$$	Prostate-specific antigen is a glycoprotein produced by cells of the prostatic ductal epithelium and is present in the serum of all men. It is absent from the serum of women.	**Increased in:** Prostate carcinoma, benign prostatic hypertrophy (BPH), following prostate examination. **Negative in:** Metastatic prostate carcinoma treated with antiandrogen therapy, postprostatectomy.	PSA is used to monitor recurrence of treated prostate cancer. Decrease in mortality rates resulting from use for cancer screening is unproved, and the risks of early therapy are significant. PSA is often increased in BPH, and the predictive value of a positive test in healthy older men is low. PSA replaces the acid phosphatase test. Hematol Oncol Clin North Am 1996;10:346. Urology 1998;51:789. JAMA 1999;281:1591.

Protein C		
Protein C, plasma 71–176% Blue $$$	Protein C is a vitamin K-dependent proenzyme synthesized in the liver. Following its activation by thrombin, it exerts an anticoagulant effect through inactivation of factors Va and VIIIa using protein S as cofactor. Tests to assay quantitative (antigenic) or functional activity are available. Deficiency is inherited in an autosomal dominant fashion with incomplete penetrance or is acquired. Deficient patients may present with a hypercoagulable state, with recurrent thrombophlebitis or pulmonary emboli.	**Decreased in:** Congenital deficiency, liver disease, cirrhosis (13–25%), warfarin use (28–60%), vitamin K deficiency, disseminated intravascular coagulation (DIC).	Homozygous deficiency of protein C (<1% activity) is associated with fatal neonatal purpura fulminans and massive venous thrombosis. Heterozygous patients (one in 200–300 of the population, with levels 25–50% of normal) may be at risk for venous thrombosis. Interpretation of an abnormally low protein C must be tempered by the clinical setting. Anticoagulant therapy, DIC, and liver disease must not be present. There is overlap between lower limits of normal values and values found in heterozygotes. Kindred with dysfunctional protein C of normal quantity have been identified. N Engl J Med 1986;314:1298. Am J Clin Pathol 1993;99:677. Thromb Haemost 1997;78:344.

	Protein electrophoresis	
Test/Range/Collection	Physiologic Basis	Interpretation	Comments

Test/Range/Collection	Physiologic Basis	Interpretation	Comments
Protein electro-phoresis, serum Adults: Albumin: 3.3–5.7 g/dL α_1: 0.1–0.4 g/dL α_2: 0.3–0.9 g/dL β_2: 0.7–1.5 g/dL γ: 0.5–1.4 g/dL Marbled $$	Electrophoresis of serum will separate serum proteins into albumin, α_1, α_2, β_2, and γ fractions. Albumin is the principal serum protein (see Albumin, p 47). The term "globulin" generally refers to the non-albumin fraction of serum protein. The α_1 fraction contains α_1-antiprotease (90%). α_1-lipoprotein and α_1-acid glycoprotein. The α_2 fraction contains α_2-macroglobulin, haptoglobin, and ceruloplasmin. The β fraction contains transferrin, hemopexin, complement C3, and β-lipoproteins. The γ fraction contains immunoglobulins G, A, D, E, and M.	$\uparrow$ α_1: inflammatory states (α_1-antiprotease), pregnancy. $\uparrow\alpha_2$: nephrotic syndrome, inflammatory states, oral contraceptives, steroid therapy, hyperthyroidism. $\uparrow$ β: hyperlipidemia, hemoglobinemia, iron deficiency anemia. $\uparrow$ γ: polyclonal gammopathies (liver disease, cirrhosis [associated with β–γ "bridging"], chronic infections, autoimmune disease); monoclonal gammopathies (multiple myeloma, Waldenström's macroglobulinemia, lymphoid malignancies, monoclonal gammopathy of undetermined significance). $\downarrow$ α_1: α_1-antiprotease deficiency. $\downarrow$ α_2: in vivo hemolysis, liver disease. $\downarrow$ γ: hypo-β-lipoproteinemias. $\downarrow$ γ: immune deficiency.	Presence of "spikes" in α_2, β_2, or γ regions necessitates the use of immunoelectrophoresis to verify the presence of a monoclonal gammo-pathy (see Immunoelectrophoresis, p 112). If Bence Jones proteins (light chains) are suspected, urine protein electro-phoresis needs to be done. Test is insensitive for detection of decreased levels of immunoglobulins and α_1-antiprotease. Specific quantita-tion is required (see Immunoglobulins, p 113 and α_1-Antiprotease, p 55). If plasma is used, fibrinogen will be detected in the β–γ region. The "acute-phase protein pattern" seen with acute illness, surgery, infarction or trauma is characterized by an $\uparrow\alpha_2$ (haptoglobin) and $\uparrow\alpha_1$ (α_1-antiprotease). Arch Pathol Lab Med 1999;123:114.

	Protein S	Protein, total
Protein S (antigen), plasma 76–178% Blue $$$	Protein S is a vitamin K-dependent glycoprotein, synthesized in the liver. It acts as a cofactor for protein C in producing its anticoagulant effect. Sixty percent of protein S is protein-bound; only free protein S has anti-coagulant function. Deficiency is associated with recurrent venous thrombosis before the age of 40.	**Decreased in:** Congenital protein S deficiency, liver disease, warfarin therapy, disseminated intravascular coagulation, vitamin K deficiency, nephrotic syndrome.	This test measures antigen and not biologic activity. Protein S can also be measured in a functional activity assay. Ann Intern Med 1987;106:677. Thromb Haemost 1997;78:351. Ann Intern Med 1998;128:8. Thromb Haemost 1998;79:802.
Protein, total, plasma or serum 6.0–8.0 g/dL [60–80 g/L] Marbled $ Avoid prolonged venous stasis during collection.	Plasma protein concentration is determined by nutritional state, hepatic function, renal function, hydration, and various disease states. Plasma protein concentration determines the colloidal osmotic pressure.	**Increased in:** Polyclonal or monoclonal gammopathies, marked dehydration. Drugs: anabolic steroids, androgens, corticosteroids, epinephrine. **Decreased in:** Protein-losing enteropathies, acute burns, nephrotic syndrome, severe dietary protein deficiency, chronic liver disease, malabsorption syndrome, agammaglobulinemia.	Serum total protein consists primarily of albumin and globulin. Serum globulin level is calculated as total protein minus albumin. Hypoproteinemia usually indicates hypoalbuminemia, since albumin is the major serum protein. Ann Thorac Surg 1999;67:236.

	Prothrombin time		
Test/Range/Collection	**Physiologic Basis**	**Interpretation**	**Comments**
Prothrombin time, whole blood (PT) 11–15 seconds ***Panic:*** ≥ 30 seconds Blue $ Fill tube completely.	PT screens the extrinsic pathway of the coagulation system. It is performed by adding calcium and tissue thromboplastin to a sample of citrated, platelet-poor plasma and measuring the time required for fibrin clot formation. It is most sensitive to deficiencies in the vitamin K-dependent clotting factors II, VII, IX, and X. It is also sensitive to deficiencies of factor V. It is insensitive to fibrinogen deficiency and not affected by heparin. PT is also used to monitor warfarin therapy. In liver disease, the PT reflects the hepatic capacity for protein synthesis. PT responds rapidly to altered hepatic function because the serum half-lives of factors II and VII are short (hours).	**Increased in:** Liver disease, vitamin K deficiency, intravascular coagulation, circulating anticoagulant, massive transfusion. Drugs: warfarin.	Routine preoperative measurement of PT is unnecessary unless there is clinical history of a bleeding disorder. Efforts to standardize and report the prothrombin time as an INR (International Normalized Ratio) depend on assigning reagents an International Sensitivity Index (ISI) so that: $$INR = \left(\frac{PT\ patient}{PT\ normal} \right)^{ISI}$$ However, assignment of incorrect ISI by reagent manufacturers has caused a greater lack of standardization. Bleeding has been reported to be three times more common in patients with INRs of 3.0–4.5 than in patients with INRs of 2.0–3.0. PT is quite insensitive to individual decreases in factors VII, IX, and X to 50% of normal but is much more sensitive to mild deficiencies in two or more factors. Thus, patients starting warfarin therapy or with liver disease may have elevated prothrombin times with no significant in vivo coagulation defects. JAMA 1989;262:2428. J Lab Clin Med 1996;128:214. J Clin Pathol 1998;51:356.

Q fever antibody		
Q fever antibody, serum <1 : 8 titer Marbled $$$ Submit paired sera, one collected within 1 week of illness and another 2–3 weeks later. Avoid hemolysis.	*Coxiella burnetii* is a rickettsial organism that is the causative organism for Q fever. Most likely mode of transmission is inhalation of aerosols from exposure to common reservoirs, sheep and cattle. Antibodies to the organism can be detected by the presence of agglutinins, by complement fixation (CF), by immunofluorescent antibody testing (IFA), or by ELISA. Agglutinin titers are found 5–8 days after infection. IgM can be detected at 7 days (IFA, ELISA) and may persist for up to 32 weeks (ELISA). IgG (IFA, ELISA) appears after 7 days and peaks at 3–4 weeks. Diagnosis of Q fever is usually confirmed by serologic findings of antiphase II antigen IgM titers of ≥1:50 and IgG titers of ≥ 1 : 200. The finding of elevated levels of both IgM and IgA by ELISA has both high sensitivity and high specificity for acute Q fever. In chronic Q fever, phase 1 antibodies, especially IgG and IgA, are predominant.	**Increased in:** Acute or chronic Q fever (CF antibodies are present by the second week in 65% of cases and by the fourth week in 90%; acute and convalescent titers [IFA or ELISA] detect infection with 89–100% sensitivity and 100% specificity), and recent vaccination for Q fever.	Clinical presentation is similar to that of severe influenza. Typically, there is no rash. Tests are usually performed in large reference labs or public health centers. Occasionally, titers do not rise for 4–6 weeks, especially if antimicrobial therapy has been given. Patients with Q fever have a high prevalence of antiphospholipid antibody (81%), especially as measured by lupus anticoagulant test or measurement of antibodies to cardiolipin. These tests may be useful in diagnosing patients presenting with fever alone. Recent Q fever vaccination causes a rise in antibody titers similar to that seen with acute infection. Antibodies to Q fever do not cross-react with other rickettsial antibodies. Eur J Clin Microbiol Infect Dis 1996;15:749. Clin Diag Lab Immunol 1997;4:384. Chest 1998;114:808. J Clin Microbiol 1998;36:1823. Clin Diag Lab Immunol 1999;6:173.

	Rapid plasma reagin		
Test/Range/Collection	Physiologic Basis	Interpretation	Comments
Rapid plasma reagin, serum (RPR) Nonreactive Marbled $	Measures nontreponemal antibodies that are produced when *Treponema pallidum* interacts with host tissue. The card test is a flocculation test performed by using a cardiolipin-lecithin-cholesterol carbon-containing antigen reagent mixed on a card with the patient's serum. A positive test (presence of antibodies) is indicated when black carbon clumps produced by flocculation are seen by the naked eye.	**Increased in:** Syphilis: primary (78%), secondary (97%), symptomatic late (74%). Biologic false-positives occur in a wide variety of conditions, including leprosy, malaria, intravenous drug abuse, aging, infectious mononucleosis, HIV infection (≤ 15%), autoimmune diseases (SLE, rheumatoid arthritis), pregnancy.	RPR is used as a screening test and in suspected primary and secondary syphilis. Since the test lacks specificity, positive tests should be confirmed with the FTA-ABS or MHA-TP test (see pp 92 and 129, respectively). RPR titers can be used to follow serologic response to treatment. (See Syphilis test table, Table 8-20, p 391.) Ann Intern Med 1991;114:1005. J Clin Microbiol 1995;33:1829. Sex Trans Dis 1998;25:569.

Red cell volume		
Red cell volume, whole blood (RCV) Male: 24-32 Female: 22-28 mL/kg Yellow Lavender (for Hct) $$$ A sample of the patient's whole blood is labeled with radioactive ^{51}Cr (which is taken up into red cells) and reinjected into the patient. Blood is sampled 10 and 60 minutes later to measure radioactivity.	Test measures absolute volume of red cells based on hemodilution of a known quantity of radioactivity in the circulation. Test can distinguish between absolute polycythemia (increased hematocrit [Hct], increased RCV) and relative polycythemia (hemoconcentration) (increased Hct, normal RCV). Alternative techniques can be used to measure RCV without exposing the patient to radiation, including use of biotin-, ^{53}Cr-, and sodium fluorescein-labeled red cells.	**Increased in:** Polycythemia vera, secondary polycythemia due to tissue hypoxemia (pulmonary disease, congenital heart disease, carboxyhemoglobinemia [cigarette smoking], methemoglobinemia, or neoplasms (renal cell carcinoma, hepatoma, large uterine leiomyomas), high altitude, pregnancy.	Test is clinically indicated (but not always required) in the diagnosis of polycythemia vera. Mayo Clin Proc 1991;66:102. Transfusion 1999;39:149. Anesth Analg 1998;87:1234. J Soc Gynecol Investig 1997;4:254.

	Renin activity		
Test/Range/Collection	**Physiologic Basis**	**Interpretation**	**Comments**
Renin activity, plasma (PRA) *High-sodium diet* (75–150 meq Na$^+$/d): supine, 0.2–2.3; standing, 1.3–4.0 ng/mL/h *Low-sodium diet* (30–75 meq Na$^+$/d): standing, 4.0–7.7 ng/mL/h Lavender $$	The renal juxtaglomerular apparatus generates renin, an enzyme that converts angiotensinogen to angiotensin I. The inactive angiotensin I is then converted to angiotensin II, which is a potent vasopressor. Renin activity is measured by the ability of patient's plasma to generate angiotensin I from substrate (angiotensinogen). Normal values depend on the patient's hydration, posture, and salt intake.	**Increased in:** Dehydration, some hypertensive states (eg, renal artery stenosis); edematous states (cirrhosis, nephrotic syndrome, congestive heart failure); hypokalemic states (gastrointestinal sodium and potassium loss, Bartter's syndrome); adrenal insufficiency, chronic renal failure, left ventricular hypertrophy. Drugs: ACE inhibitors, estrogen, hydralazine, nifedipine, minoxidil, oral contraceptives. **Decreased in:** Hyporeninemic hypoaldosteronism, some hypertensive states (eg, primary aldosteronism, severe preeclampsia). Drugs: beta-blockers, aspirin, clonidine, prazosin, reserpine, methyldopa, indomethacin.	PRA alone is not a satisfactory screening test for hyperaldosteronism because suppressed PRA has only 64% sensitivity and 83% specificity for primary hyperaldosteronism. However, when plasma aldosterone and PRA testing are combined, the sensitivity for primary hyperaldosteronism increases to 95% (see Aldosterone, plasma, p 48). Test is also useful in evaluation of hypoaldosteronism (low-sodium diet, patient standing). Measurement of peripheral vein renin activity is not useful in classification of hypertensive patients or in diagnosis of renal artery stenosis. Bilateral renal vein sampling has been used to investigate renal artery stenosis. In general, a renal vein renin (RVR) ratio of 1.5 or more (affected/nonaffected side) is predictive of response to revascularization in >90% of cases, but 60% of cases with RVR ratios <1.5 will also respond. Therefore, the test cannot reliably predict therapeutic response to a surgical procedure. Mayo Clin Proc 1994;69:1172. Acta Obstet Gynecol Scand 1998;77:609. J Hum Hypertens 1998;12:455. Am J Nephrol 1996;16:471.

	Reptilase clotting time	Reticulocyte count
Reptilase clotting time, plasma 13–19 seconds Blue $$	Reptilase is an enzyme derived from the venom of *Bothrops atrox* or *Bothrops jararaca,* South American pit vipers. Reptilase cleaves a fibrinopeptide from fibrinogen directly, bypassing the heparin-antithrombin system, and produces a fibrin clot. The reptilase time will be normal in heparin toxicity, even when the thrombin time is infinite.	**Increased in:** Hypofibrinogenemia, dysfibrinogenemia, afibrinogenemia, and disseminated intravascular coagulation (DIC). **Normal in:** Presence of heparin.	When the thrombin time is prolonged, the reptilase time is useful in distinguishing the presence of an antithrombin (normal reptilase time) from hypo- or dysfibrinogenemia (prolonged reptilase time). The reptilase time is normal when heparin is the cause of a prolonged thrombin time. The reptilase time is only slightly prolonged by fibrin degradation products. Br J Haematol 1971;21:43.
Reticulocyte count, whole blood $33–137 \times 10^3/\mu L$ $[\times 10^9/L]$ Lavender $	Reticulocytes are immature red blood cells that contain cytoplasmic mRNA.	**Increased in:** Hemolytic anemia, blood loss; recovery from iron, B_{12}, or folate deficiency or drug-induced anemia. **Decreased in:** Iron deficiency anemia, aplastic anemia, anemia of chronic disease, megaloblastic anemia, sideroblastic anemia, bone marrow suppression.	This test is indicated in the evaluation of anemia to distinguish hypoproliferative anemia from hemolytic anemia or blood loss. The old method of measuring reticulocytes (manual staining and counting) has poor reproducibility. It has been replaced by automated methods (eg, flow cytometry), which are more precise. Method-specific reference ranges must be used. Am J Hematol 1990;33:13. Am J Clin Pathol 1994;102:623. Clin Lab Haematol 1996;18(Suppl 1):1

	Rh grouping		
Test/Range/Collection	**Physiologic Basis**	**Interpretation**	**Comments**
Rh grouping, red cells (Rh) Red $ Proper identification of specimen is critical.	The Rhesus blood group system is second in importance only to the ABO system. Anti-Rh antibodies are the leading cause of hemolytic disease of the newborn and may also cause hemolytic transfusion reactions. Although there are other Rhesus antigens, only tests for the D antigen are performed routinely in pretransfusion testing, since the D antigen is the most immunogenic. The terms Rh-positive and -negative refer to the presence or absence of the red cell antigen, D, on the cell surface. Persons whose red cells lack D do not regularly have anti-D in their serum. Formation of anti-D almost always results from exposure through transfusion or pregnancy to red cells possessing the D antigen.	Sixty percent of US whites are Rh(D)-positive, 40% negative; 72% of African-Americans are Rh(D)-positive, 28% negative; 95% of Asian-Americans are Rh(D)-positive, 5% negative.	Of D⁻ persons receiving a single D⁺ unit, 50–75% will develop anti-D. The blood of all donors and recipients is therefore routinely tested for D, so that D⁻ recipients can be given D⁻ blood. Donor bloods must also be tested for a weak form of D antigen, called Dᵘ, and must be labeled D⁺ if the Dᵘ test is positive. Recipient blood need not be tested for Dᵘ. *Technical Manual of the American Association of Blood Banks,* 11th ed. American Association of Blood Banks, 1993.

	Rheumatoid factor		**Ribonucleoprotein antibody**
Rheumatoid factor, serum (RF) Negative (<1:16) Marbled $	Rheumatoid factor consists of heterogeneous autoantibodies usually of the IgM class that react against the Fc region of human IgG.	**Positive in:** Rheumatoid arthritis (75–90%), Sjögren's syndrome (80–90%), scleroderma, dermatomyositis, SLE (30%), sarcoidosis, Waldenström's macroglobulinemia. Drugs: methyldopa, others. Low-titer RF can be found in healthy older patients (20%), in 1–4% of normal individuals, and in a variety of acute immune responses (eg, viral infections, including infectious mononucleosis and viral hepatitis), chronic bacterial infections (tuberculosis, leprosy, subacute infective endocarditis), and chronic active hepatitis.	Rheumatoid factor can be useful in differentiating rheumatoid arthritis from other chronic inflammatory arthritides. However, a positive RF test is only one of several criteria needed to make the diagnosis of rheumatoid arthritis. (See also Autoantibodies table, p 367.) RF must be ordered selectively because its predictive value is low (34%) if it is used as a screening test. The test has poor positive predictive value because of its lack of specificity. The subset of patients with seronegative rheumatic disease limits its sensitivity and negative predictive value. *Arch Intern Med* 1992;152:2417.
Ribonucleoprotein antibody, serum (RNP) Negative Marbled $$	This is an antibody to a ribonucleoprotein-extractable nuclear antigen.	**Increased in:** Scleroderma (20–30% sensitivity, low specificity), mixed connective tissue disease (MCTD) (95–100% sensitivity, low specificity), SLE (30%), Sjögren's syndrome, rheumatoid arthritis (10%), discoid lupus (20–30%).	A negative test essentially excludes MCTD. (See also Autoantibodies table, p 367.) *Rheum Dis Clin North Am* 1992;18:283. *Rheum Dis Clin North Am* 1992;18:311. *Rheum Dis Clin North Am* 1994;20:29.

	Rubella antibody		
Test/Range/Collection	**Physiologic Basis**	**Interpretation**	**Comments**
Rubella antibody, serum <1:8 titer Marbled $ For diagnosis of a recent infection, submit paired sera, one collected within 1 week of illness and another 2–4 weeks later.	Rubella (German measles) is a viral infection that causes fever, malaise, coryza, lymphadenopathy, fine maculopapular rash, and congenital birth defects when infection occurs in utero. Antibodies to rubella can be detected by hemagglutination inhibition (HI), complement fixation (CF), indirect hemagglutination (IHA), ELISA, or latex agglutination (LA). Tests can detect IgG and IgM antibody. Titers usually appear as rash fades (1 week) and peak at 10–14 days for HI and 2–3 weeks for other techniques. Baseline titers may remain elevated for life.	**Increased in:** Recent rubella infection, congenital rubella infection, previous rubella infection or vaccination (immunity). Spuriously increased IgM antibody occurs in the presence of rheumatoid factor.	Rubella titers of ≤1:8 indicate susceptibility and need for immunization to prevent infection during pregnancy. Titers of >1:32 indicate immunity from prior infection or vaccination. Definitive diagnosis is based on a four-fold rise in titer or the presence of IgM antibody. To diagnose congenital infection, submit a single specimen for IgM. If positive, submit a second specimen 2–3 months later to rule out maternal antibody transmission across the placenta. The recent resurgence of congenital rubella can largely be prevented with improved rubella testing and vaccination programs. Rev Infect Dis 1985;7(Suppl 1):S108. Am J Clin Pathol 1996;106:170. J Infect Dis 1997;175:749.

Russell's viper venom clotting time		
Russell's viper venom clotting time (dilute), plasma (RVVT) 24–37 seconds Blue $$	Russell viper venom is extracted from a pit viper (*Vipera russelli*), which is common in Southeast Asia (especially Burma) and which causes a rapidly fatal syndrome of consumptive coagulopathy with hemorrhage, shock, rhabdomyolysis, and renal failure. Approximately 70% of the protein content of the venom is phospholipase A₂, which activates factor X in the presence of phospholipid, bypassing factor VII. RVVT is a phospholipid-dependent coagulation test used in detection of antiphospholipid antibodies (so-called lupus anticoagulants). It should be noted that the anticoagulant detected in vitro may be associated with thrombosis (and not bleeding) in vivo.	**Increased in:** Circulating lupus anticoagulants (LAC), severe fibrinogen deficiency (< 50 mg/dL), deficiencies in prothrombin, factor V, factor X, and heparin therapy. **Normal in:** Factor VII deficiency and all intrinsic pathway factor deficiencies.	The lupus anticoagulant may be associated with a prolonged PTT and a positive inhibitor screen (mixing study). If heparin is not present, a dilute Russell viper venom test may be indicated to confirm that the inhibitor is an LAC. Since specific factor inhibitors against factors VIII and IX are associated with clinically significant bleeding and require specific treatment, they must not be missed. The LAC is associated with an increased risk of thrombosis (venous > arterial), recurrent spontaneous abortion, and the primary antiphospholipid syndrome of arterial thrombosis. Haemostasis 1990;20:208. Blood Coagul Fibrinolysis 1990;1:627. Int J Biochem 1994;26:79. Blood Coagul Fibrinolysis 1996;7:31. Thromb Res 1997;85:427.

Test/Range/Collection	Physiologic Basis	Interpretation	Comments
		Salicylate	**Scleroderma-associated antibody**
Salicylate, serum (aspirin) 20–30 mg/dL [200–300 mg/L] *Panic:* >35 mg/dL Marbled $$	At high concentrations, salicylate stimulates hyperventilation, uncouples oxidative phosphorylation, and impairs glucose and fatty acid metabolism. Salicylate toxicity is thus marked by respiratory alkalosis and metabolic acidosis.	**Increased in:** Acute or chronic salicylate intoxication.	The potential toxicity of salicylate levels after acute ingestion can be determined by using the Salicylate nomogram, p 360. Nomograms have become less valid with the increasing popularity of enteric-coated slow-release aspirin preparations. Pediatrics 1960;26:800. Ann Pharmacother 1996;30:935. Am J Emerg Med 1996;14:443.
Scleroderma-associated antibody (Scl-70 antibody), serum Negative Marbled $$	This antibody reacts with a cellular antigen (DNA topoisomerase 1) that is responsible for the relaxation of supercoiled DNA.	**Increased in:** Scleroderma (15–20% sensitivity, high specificity).	Predictive value of a positive test is >95% for scleroderma. Test has prognostic significance for severe digital ischemia in patients with Raynaud's disease and scleroderma. (See also Autoantibodies table, p 367.) Rheum Dis Clin North Am 1990;16:169. J Rheumatol 1991;18:1826. Rheum Dis Clin North Am 1992;18:483. Ann Rheum Dis 1994;53:540. Am J Med 1997;103:242.

Test	Description	Decreased/Positive in	References
Semen analysis, ejaculate Sperm count: >20 × 10^6/mL [10^9/L] Motility score: >60% motile Volume: 2–5 mL Normal morphology: >60% $$ Semen is collected in a urine container after masturbation following 3 days of abstinence from ejaculation. Specimen must be examined promptly.	Sperm are viewed under the microscope for motility and morphology. Infertility can be associated with low counts or with sperm of abnormal morphology or decreased motility.	**Decreased in:** Primary or secondary testicular failure, cryptorchidism, following vasectomy, drugs.	A low sperm count should be confirmed by sending two other appropriately collected semen specimens for evaluation. Functional and computer-assisted sperm analyses increase diagnostic accuracy but are not yet widely available. Endocrinol Metab Clin North Am 1994;23:725. J Androl 1996;17:718. Int J Androl 1997;20:201. Fertil Steril 1997;67:1156.
Smith (anti-Sm) antibody, serum Negative Marbled $$	This antibody to Smith antigen (an extractable nuclear antigen) is a marker antibody for SLE.	**Positive in:** SLE (30–40% sensitivity, high specificity).	A positive test substantially increases posttest probability of SLE. Test rarely needed for the diagnosis of SLE. (See also Autoantibodies table, p 367.) Clin Rheumatol 1990;9:346. Rheum Dis Clin North Am 1992;18:311. Clin Rheumatol 1993;12:350. Arthritis Rheum 1996;39:1055. J Rheumatol 1998;25:1743.

Test/Range/Collection	Physiologic Basis	Interpretation	Comments
Smooth muscle antibodies			**Smooth muscle antibodies**
Smooth muscle antibodies, serum Negative Marbled $$	Antibodies against smooth muscle proteins are found in patients with chronic active hepatitis and primary biliary cirrhosis.	**Positive in:** Autoimmune chronic active hepatitis (40–70%, predominantly IgG antibodies), lower titers in primary biliary cirrhosis (50%, predominantly IgM antibodies), viral hepatitis, infectious mononucleosis, cryptogenic cirrhosis (28%), HIV infection, vitiligo (25%), endometriosis, Behçet's disease (< 2% of normal individuals).	The presence of high titers of smooth muscle antibodies (>1:80) is useful in distinguishing autoimmune chronic active hepatitis from other forms of hepatitis. Gut 1980;21:878. J Clin Pathol 1991;44:64. J Obstet Gynaecol 1991;98:680. Br J Dermatol 1993;20:679.

Sodium		
Sodium, serum (Na⁺) 135—145 meq/L [mmol/L] *Panic:* <125 or >155 meq/L Marbled $	Sodium is the predominant extracellular cation. The serum sodium level is primarily determined by the volume status of the individual. Hyponatremia can be divided into hypovolemia, euvolemia, and hypervolemia categories. (See Hyponatremia algorithm, p 350.)	**Increased in:** Dehydration (excessive sweating, severe vomiting or diarrhea), polyuria (diabetes mellitus, diabetes insipidus), hyperaldosteronism, inadequate water intake (coma, hypothalamic disease). Drugs: steroids, licorice, oral contraceptives. **Decreased in:** Congestive heart failure, cirrhosis, vomiting, diarrhea, excessive sweating (with replacement of water but not salt), salt-losing nephropathy, adrenal insufficiency, nephrotic syndrome, water intoxication, SIADH. Drugs: thiazides, diuretics, ACE inhibitors, chlorpropamide, carbamazepine, antidepressants (selective serotonin reuptake inhibitors), antipsychotics.	Spurious hyponatremia may be produced by severe lipemia or hyperproteinemia if sodium analysis involves a dilution step. The serum sodium falls about 1.6 meq/L for each 100 mg/dL increase in blood glucose. Hyponatremia in a normovolemic patient with urine osmolality higher than plasma osmolality suggests the possibility of SIADH, myxedema, hypopituitarism, or reset osmostat. Treatment of disorders of sodium balance relies on clinical assessment of the patient's extracellular fluid volume rather than the serum sodium. Sodium is commonly measured by ion-selective electrode. Am J Med 1982;72:496. Ann Intern Med 1985;102:164. Postgrad Med 1993;93:227. Med Clin North Am 1997;81:585. Hepatology 1998;28:851. Am J Med 1999;106:399.

	Somatomedin C	
Test/Range/Collection	Physiologic Basis	Interpretation	Comments
Somatomedin C, plasma 123–463 ng/mL (age- and sex-dependent) Lavender $$$$	Somatomedin C is a growth hormone-dependent plasma peptide produced by the liver. It is believed to mediate the growth-promoting effect of growth hormone (GH). It has an anabolic, insulin-like action on fat and muscle and stimulates collagen and protein synthesis. Its level is relatively constant throughout the day.	**Increased in:** Acromegaly (level correlates with disease activity better than GH level). **Decreased in:** Pituitary dwarfism, hypopituitarism, Laron dwarfism (end-organ resistance to GH), fasting for 5–6 days, poor nutrition, hypothyroidism, cirrhosis. Values may be normal in growth hormone-deficient patients with hyperprolactinemia or craniopharyngioma.	A normal somatomedin C level in children is strong evidence that GH deficiency is not present and precludes the need for extensive pituitary function testing. A low level does not prove that GH deficiency is present, since levels may be reduced in malnutrition, malabsorption, chronic systemic illness, and hypothyroidism. Reference range here is for an immunoassay done following displacement of somatomedin C from its binding protein (acid-ethanol extraction). N Engl J Med 1979;301:1138. J Pediatr 1981;99:720. J Clin Endocrinol 1988;66:538. Endocrinol Metab Clin North Am 1992;21:649.

	SS-A/Ro antibody	SS-B/La antibody
SS-A/Ro antibody, serum Negative Marbled $$	Antibodies to Ro (SSA) cellular ribonucleoprotein complexes are found in connective tissue diseases such as Sjögren's syndrome (SS), SLE, rheumatoid arthritis (RA), and vasculitis. **Increased in:** Sjögren's (60–70% sensitivity, low specificity), SLE (30–40%), RA (10%), subacute cutaneous lupus, vasculitis. Useful in counseling women of childbearing age with known connective tissue disease, since a positive test is associated with a small but real risk of neonatal SLE and congenital heart block. The few (< 10%) patients with SLE who do not have a positive ANA commonly have antibodies to SS-A. (See also Autoantibodies table, p 367.) Medicine 1995;74:109. J Rheumatol 1996;23:1897. J Am Acad Dermatol 1996;35 (2 Part 1):147. J Autoimmun 1998;11:29. Br J Dermatol 1998;138:114. Clin Exper Rheumatol 1999;17:63,130.	
SS-B/La antibody, serum Negative Marbled $$	Antibodies to La (SSB) cellular ribonucleoprotein complexes are found in Sjögren's syndrome (SS) and appear to be relatively more specific for SS than are antibodies to SSA. They are quantitated by immunoassay. **Increased in:** Sjögren's (50% sensitivity, higher specificity than anti-SSA), SLE (10%).	Direct pathogenicity and usefulness of autoantibody test in predicting disease exacerbation not proved. (See also Autoantibodies table, p 367.) Arthritis Rheum 1996;39:1055. Ann Rheum Dis 1997;156:272. J Autoimmun 1998;11:29. Clin Exper Rheumatol 1999;17:130.

	T cell receptor gene rearrangement		
Test/Range/Collection	Physiologic Basis	Interpretation	Comments
T cell receptor gene rearrangement Whole blood, bone marrow, or frozen tissue Lavender $$$$	In general, the percentage of T lymphocytes with identical T cell receptors is very low; in malignancies, however, the clonal expansion of one population leads to a large number of cells with identical T cell receptor gene rearrangement. Southern blot is used to identify a monoclonal population.	Positive test results may be seen in T cell neoplasms such as T cell lymphocytic leukemia and cutaneous or nodal T cell lymphomas.	Samples with >10% of cells showing a given T cell rearrangement are considered positive. However, a large monoclonal population is not absolutely diagnostic of malignancy. Am J Hematol 1996;52:171. Mol Pathol 1997;50:77. Arch Dermatol 1998;134:15. J Am Acad Dermatol 1998;39 (4 Part 1):554. Leukemia 1998;12:1081.

	Testosterone	Thrombin time
Testosterone, serum Males: 3.0–10.0 Females: 0.3–0.7 ng/mL [Males: 10–35 Females: 1.0–2.4 nmol/L] Marbled $$$	Testosterone is the principal male sex hormone, produced by the Leydig cells of the testes. Dehydroepiandrosterone (DHEA) is produced in the adrenal cortex, testes and ovaries and is the main precursor for serum testosterone in women. In normal males after puberty, the testosterone level is twice as high as all androgens in females. In serum, it is largely bound to albumin (38%) and to a specific steroid hormone-binding globulin (SHBG) (60%), but it is the free hormone (2%) that is physiologically active. The total testosterone level measures both bound and free testosterone in the serum (by immunoassay).	**Increased in:** Idiopathic sexual precocity (in boys, levels may be in adult range), adrenal hyperplasia (boys), adrenocortical tumors, trophoblastic disease during pregnancy, idiopathic hirsutism, virilizing ovarian tumors, arrhenoblastoma, virilizing luteoma, testicular feminization (normal or moderately elevated), cirrhosis (through increased SHBG), hyperthyroidism. Drugs: anticonvulsants, barbiturates, estrogens, oral contraceptives (through increased SHBG). **Decreased in:** Hypogonadism (primary and secondary, orchidectomy, Klinefelter's, uremia, hemodialysis, hepatic insufficiency, ethanol [men]). Drugs: digoxin, spironolactone, acarbose.	Serum testosterone levels decrease in men after age 50. A free testosterone level is indicated when a normal total testosterone level is thought not to reflect free testosterone levels because of increases in SHBG. In men, there is a small diurnal variation in serum testosterone with a 20% elevation in levels in the evenings. Endocrinol Metab Clin North Am 1992;21:921. Endocrinol Metab Clin North Am 1994;23:709. Fertil Steril 1998;69:286. Arch Androl 1998;40:153. Ann Intern Med 1999;130(4 Part 1):270.
Thrombin time, plasma 24–35 seconds (laboratory-specific) Blue $	Prolongation of the thrombin time indicates a defect in conversion of fibrinogen to fibrin.	**Increased in:** Low fibrinogen (<50 mg/dL), abnormal fibrinogen (dysfibrinogenemia), increased fibrin degradation products (eg, disseminated intravascular coagulation), heparin, fibrinolytic agents (streptokinase, urokinase, tissue plasminogen activator), primary systemic amyloidosis (40%).	Thrombin time can be used to monitor fibrinolytic therapy and to screen for dysfibrinogenemia or circulating anticoagulants. Blood 1991;77:2637.

Test/Range/Collection	Physiologic Basis	Interpretation	Comments
Thyroglobulin, serum 3–42 ng/mL [μg/L] Marbled $$$	Thyroglobulin is a large protein specific to the thyroid gland from which thyroxine is synthesized and cleaved. Highly sensitive immunoradiometric assays (IRMAs) have minimal interference from autoantibodies.	**Increased in:** Hyperthyroidism, subacute thyroiditis, untreated thyroid carcinomas (except medullary carcinoma): follicular cancer (sensitivity 72%, specificity 81%), Hürthle cell cancer (sensitivity 56%, specificity 84%). **Decreased in:** Factitious hyperthyroidism, presence of thyroglobulin autoantibodies, after (>25 days) total thyroidectomy.	Thyroglobulin is useful to follow patients after treatment of non-medullary thyroid carcinomas. Levels fall after successful therapy and rise when metastases develop. Sensitivity of the test is increased if patients are off thyroid replacement for 6 weeks prior to testing or if given T_3 (Cytomel) for the first 4 weeks, then no medication for the last 2 weeks. Athyrotic patients on T_4 (levothyroxine) should have values <5 ng/mL and those off T_4 should have values <10 ng/mL. Clin Chem 1996;42:164. Clin Chem 1996;42:258. Eur J Nucl Med 1997;24:722. Eur J Surg Oncol 1998;24:553. Eur J Endocrinol 1998;138:249.
Thyroglobulin antibody, serum <1:10 (highly method-dependent) Marbled $$	Antibodies against thyroglobulin are produced in autoimmune diseases of the thyroid and other organs. Ten percent of the normal population have slightly elevated titers (especially women and the elderly).	**Increased in:** Hashimoto's thyroiditis (>90%), thyroid carcinoma (45%), thyrotoxicosis, pernicious anemia (50%), SLE (20%), subacute thyroiditis, Graves' disease. **Not Increased in:** Multinodular goiter, thyroid adenomas, and some carcinomas.	The antithyroid peroxidase antibody test is more sensitive than the thyroglobulin antibody test in autoimmune thyroid disease. There is little indication for this test. (See Thyroid Peroxidase Antibody, below.) Am J Med 1983;74:941. Med Clin North Am 1991;75:1. J Clin Endocrinol Metab 1998;83:1121.

Thyroperoxidase antibody		
Thyroperoxidase antibody, serum Negative Marbled $$	Thyroperoxidase (TPO) is a membrane-bound glycoprotein. This enzyme mediates the oxidation of iodide ions and incorporation of iodine into tyrosine residues of thyroglobulin. Its synthesis is stimulated by thyroid-stimulating hormone (TSH). TPO is the major antigen involved in thyroid antibody-dependent cell-mediated cytotoxicity. Antithyroperoxidase antibody assays are performed by ELISA or radioimmunoassay.	**Increased in:** Hashimoto's thyroiditis (>99%), idiopathic myxedema (>99%), Graves' disease (75–85%), Addison's disease (50%), and Riedel's thyroiditis. Low titers are present in approximately 10% of normal individuals and patients with nonimmune thyroid disease.	Thyroperoxidase antibody is an antibody to the main autoantigenic component of microsomes and is a more sensitive and specific test than hemagglutination assays for microsomal antibodies in the diagnosis of autoimmune thyroid disease. Thyroperoxidase antibody testing alone is almost always sufficient to detect autoimmune thyroid disease. J Clin Endocrinol Metab 1990;71:661. Arch Intern Med 1993;153:862. J Clin Endocrinol Metab 1996;81:2595. Thyroid 1997;7:471.

	Thyroid-stimulating hormone		
Test/Range/Collection	**Physiologic Basis**	**Interpretation**	**Comments**
Thyroid-stimulating hormone, serum (TSH; thyrotropin) 0.4–6 μU/mL [mU/L] Marbled $$	TSH is an anterior pituitary hormone that stimulates the thyroid gland to produce thyroid hormones. Secretion is stimulated by thyrotropin-releasing hormone from the hypothalamus. There is negative feedback on TSH secretion by circulating thyroid hormone.	**Increased in:** Hypothyroidism. Mild increases in recovery phase of acute illness. **Decreased in:** Hyperthyroidism, acute medical or surgical illness, pituitary hypothyroidism. Drugs: dopamine, high-dose corticosteroids.	Newer sensitive assays can detect low enough levels of TSH to be useful in the diagnosis of hyperthyroidism as well as hypothyroidism and in distinguishing hyperthyroidism from subnormal TSH values occasionally found in euthyroid sick patients. (See also Thyroid function table, p 393.) Test is useful for following patients taking thyroid medication. Neonatal and cord blood levels are 2–4 times higher than adult levels. J Nucl Med 1985;26:1248. Endocrinol Metab Clin North Am 1992;21:903. Postgrad Med 1993;94:81. Clin Chem 1996;42:140. Clin Chem 1997;43:2428. J R Soc Med 1997;90:547.

	Thyroid-stimulating hormone receptor antibody	Thyroxine, total
Thyroid-stimulating hormone receptor antibody, serum (TSH-R [stim] Ab) < 130% basal activity of adenylyl cyclase Marbled $$$$	Test detects heterogeneous IgG antibodies directed against the TSH receptor on thyroid cells. Frequently, they cause excess release of hormone from the thyroid. Test measures antibodies indirectly by their stimulation of adenylyl cyclase to produce cAMP.	**Increased in:** Graves' disease.	Although TSH-R [stim] Ab is a marker of Graves' disease, the test is not necessary for the diagnosis in most cases. Test is very rarely indicated but may be helpful in (1) pregnant women with a history of Graves' disease, because TSH-R [stim] Ab may have some predictive value for neonatal thyrotoxicosis; (2) patients presenting with exophthalmos who are euthyroid, to confirm Graves' disease. Use of the test to predict relapse of hyperthyroidism at the end of a course of antithyroid drugs is controversial. J Clin Endocrinol Metab 1989;69:1093.
Thyroxine, total, serum (T_4) 5.0–11.0 µg/dL [64–142 nmol/L] Marbled $	Total T_4 is a measure of thyroid gland secretion of T_4, bound and free, and thus is influenced by serum thyroid hormone binding activity.	**Increased in:** Hyperthyroidism, increased thyroid-binding globulin (TBG) (eg, pregnancy, drug). Drugs: amiodarone, high-dose beta-blockers (especially propranolol). **Decreased in:** Hypothyroidism, low TBG due to illness or drugs, congenital absence of TBG. Drugs: phenytoin, carbamazepine, androgens.	Total T_4 should be interpreted with the TBG level or as part of a free thyroxine index. Med Clin North Am 1991;75:1. Med Clin North Am 1991;75:27. Clin Chem 1996;42:146.

Test/Range/Collection	Physiologic Basis	Interpretation	Comments
Thyroxine, free, serum (FT$_4$) Varies with method Marbled $$	FT$_4$ (if done by equilibrium dialysis or ultrafiltration method) is a more direct measure of the free T$_4$ hormone concentration (biologically available hormone) than the free T$_4$ index. FT$_4$, done by a two-step immunoassay is similar to the free thyroxine index. The presence of rheumatoid factor or drug treatment with furosemide, intravenous heparin, and subcutaneous low-molecular-weight heparin may interfere with newer assays for free thyroxine.	**Increased in:** Hyperthyroidism, nonthyroidal illness, especially psychiatric. Drugs: amiodarone, beta-blockers (high dose). **Decreased in:** Hypothyroidism, nonthyroidal illness. Drugs: phenytoin.	FT$_4$I is functionally equivalent to the FT$_4$I (see below). The free thyroxine and sensitive TSH assays have similar sensitivities for detecting clinical hyperthyroidism and hypothyroidism. The TSH assay detects subclinical dysfunction and monitors thyroxine treatment better; the free thyroxine test detects central hypothyroidism and monitors rapidly changing function better. JAMA 1990;263:1529. Arch Intern Med 1996;156:2333. Clin Chem 1996;42:146. Arch Intern Med 1998;158:266.
Thyroxine index, free, serum (FT$_4$I) 6.5–12.5 Marbled $$	Free thyroxine index is expressed as total T$_4$ × T$_3$ (or T$_4$) resin uptake and provides an estimate of the level of free T$_4$, since the T$_3$ (or T$_4$) resin uptake (ie, thyroid hormone binding ratio) is an indirect estimate of the thyroid binding globulin (TBG) concentration. (TBG binds 70% of circulating thyroid hormone.) The unbound form of circulating T$_4$, normally 0.03% of total serum T$_4$, determines the amount of T$_4$ available to cells.	**Increased in:** Hyperthyroidism, nonthyroidal illness, especially psychiatric. Drugs: amiodarone, beta-blockers (high dose). **Decreased in:** Hypothyroidism, nonthyroidal illness. Drugs: phenytoin.	Test is useful in patients with clinically suspected hyper- or hypothyroidism, in elderly patients admitted to geriatric units, or in women over 40 with one or more somatic complaints. (See Thyroid function table, p 393.) Screening for thyroid disease is not indicated in younger women, men, or patients admitted with acute medical or psychiatric illnesses because transient abnormalities are indistinguishable from true thyroid disease. FT$_4$I is functionally equivalent to the FT$_4$ (see above). Ann Intern Med 1990;112:840.

Toxoplasma antibody		
Toxoplasma antibody, serum or CSF (Toxo) IgG: <1:16 IgM: Infant <1:2 Adult <1:8 titer Marbled or CSF $$$ Submit paired sera, one collected within 1 week of illness and another 2–3 weeks later.	_Toxoplasma gondii_ is an obligate intracellular protozoan that causes human infection via ingestion, transplacental transfer, blood products, or organ transplantation. Cats are the definitive hosts of _T gondii_ and pass oocysts in their feces. Human infection occurs through ingestion of sporulated oocysts or via the transplacental route. In the immunodeficient host, acute infection may progress to lethal meningoencephalitis, pneumonitis, or myocarditis. In acute primary infection, IgM antibodies develop 1–2 weeks after onset of illness, peak in 6–8 weeks, and then decline. IgG antibodies develop on a similar time-course but persist for years. In adult infection, the disease usually represents a reactivation, not a primary infection. Therefore, the IgM test is less useful. Approximately 30% of all US adults have antibodies to _T gondii_.	**Increased in:** Acute or congenital toxoplasmosis (IgM), previous toxoplasma exposure (IgG), and false-positive (IgM) reactions (SLE, HIV infection, rheumatoid arthritis).	Single IgG titers of >1:256 are considered diagnostic of active infection; titers of >1:128 are suspicious. Titers of 1:16–1:64 may merely represent past exposure. If titers subsequently rise, they probably represent early disease. IgM titer >1:16 is very important in the diagnosis of congenital toxoplasmosis. High titer IgG antibody results should prompt an IgM test. IgM, however, is generally not found in adult AIDS patients since the disease usually represents a reactivation. Some recommend ordering baseline toxoplasma IgG titers in all asymptomatic HIV-positive patients because a rising toxoplasma titer can help diagnose CNS toxoplasmosis in the future. Culture of the _T gondii_ organism is difficult, and most laboratories are not equipped for the procedure. (See also Brain abscess, p 197.) Ann Intern Med 1984;100:36. N Engl J Med 1988;318:271. Clin Infect Dis 1994;18:14. AIDS 1996;10:1521. J Clin Microbiol 1997;35:174. J Clin Lab Anal 1997;11:214.

Test/Range/Collection	Physiologic Basis	Interpretation	Comments
Triglycerides, serum (TG) <165 mg/dL [<1.65 g/L] Marbled $ Fasting specimen required.	Dietary fat is hydrolyzed in the small intestine, absorbed and resynthesized by mucosal cells, and secreted into lacteals as chylomicrons. Triglycerides in the chylomicrons are cleared from the blood by tissue lipoprotein lipase. Endogenous triglyceride production occurs in the liver. These triglycerides are transported in association with β-lipoproteins in very low density lipoproteins (VLDL).	**Increased in:** Hypothyroidism, diabetes mellitus, nephrotic syndrome, chronic alcoholism (fatty liver), biliary tract obstruction, stress, familial lipoprotein lipase deficiency, familial dysbetalipoproteinemia, familial combined hyperlipidemia, obesity, viral hepatitis, cirrhosis, pancreatitis, chronic renal failure, gout, pregnancy, glycogen storage diseases types I, III, and VI, anorexia nervosa, dietary excess. Drugs: betablockers, cholestyramine, corticosteroids, diazepam, diuretics, estrogens, oral contraceptives. **Decreased in:** Tangier disease (α-lipoprotein deficiency), hypo- and abetalipoproteinemia, malnutrition, malabsorption, parenchymal liver disease, hyperthyroidism, intestinal lymphangiectasia. Drugs: ascorbic acid, clofibrate, nicotinic acid, gemfibrozil.	If serum is clear, the serum triglyceride level is generally <350 mg/dL. Despite extensive research, it remains unclear whether triglycerides are an independent risk factor for coronary artery disease. Triglycerides >1000 mg/dL can be seen when a primary lipid disorder is exacerbated by alcohol or fat intake or by corticosteroid or estrogen therapy. JAMA 1993;269:505. Lancet 1993;342:781. N Engl J Med 1993;328:1220. Med Clin North Am 1994;78:117. Circulation 1997;96:2520. Am J Cardiol 1998;81(4A):70B. Am J Cardiol 1998;82(12A):49U. Am J Med 1998;105(1A):58S. Eur Heart J 1998;19(Suppl A):A36.

Triiodothyronine		
Triiodothyronine, total, serum (T₃) 95–190 ng/dL [1.5–2.9 nmol/L] Marbled $$	T₃ reflects the metabolically active form of thyroid hormone and is influenced by thyroid hormone-binding activity.	**Increased in:** Hyperthyroidism (some), increased thyroid-binding globulin. **Decreased in:** Hypothyroidism, nonthyroidal illness, decreased thyroid-binding globulin. Drugs: amiodarone.	T₃ may be increased in approximately 5% of hyperthyroid patients in whom T₄ is normal (T₃ toxicosis). Therefore, test is indicated when hyperthyroidism is suspected and T₄ value is normal. Test is of no value in the diagnosis of hypothyroidism. Ann Intern Med 1990;112:840. JAMA 1990;263:1529. Am J Med 1994;96:229.

Test/Range/Collection	Physiologic Basis	Interpretation	Comments
Troponin-I, cardiac, serum (cTnI) < 1.5 ng/mL Marbled $$	Troponin is the contractile regulatory protein of striated muscle. It contains three subunits: T, C, and I. Subunit I consists of three forms, which are found in slow-twitch skeletal muscle, fast-twitch skeletal muscle, and cardiac muscle, respectively. Troponin I is predominantly a structural protein and is released into the circulation after cellular necrosis. Cardiac troponin I is expressed only in cardiac muscle, throughout development and despite pathology, and thus its presence in serum can distinguish between myocardial injury and skeletal muscle injury. cTnI is measured by immunoassay using monoclonal antibodies.	**Increased in:** Myocardial infarction (sensitivity 50% at 4 hours, 97% at 6 hours; specificity 95%), cardiac trauma, cardiac surgery, myocardial damage following PTCA, defibrillations, and other cardiac interventions, nonischemic dilated cardiomyopathy. Slight elevations noted in patients with recent aggravated unstable angina, muscular disorders, CNS disorders, HIV infection, chronic renal failure, cirrhosis, sepsis, lung diseases, and endocrine disorders. **Not Increased in:** Skeletal muscle disease (myopathy, myositis, dystrophy), noncardiac trauma or surgery, rhabdomyolysis, severe muscular exertion, chronic renal failure.	Cardiac troponin I is a more specific marker for myocardial infarction than CKMB with roughly equivalent sensitivity early in the course of infarction (4–36 hours). Sensitivity and specificity for peak concentrations of cTnI (100%; 96%) are equivalent to or better than those for CK-MB (88%; 93%) and total CK (73%; 85%). cTnI appears in serum approximately 4 hours after onset of chest pain, peaks at 8–12 hours, and persists for 5–7 days. This prolonged persistence gives it much greater sensitivity than CKMB for diagnosis of myocardial infarction beyond the first 36–48 hours. Minor elevations of cardiac troponin I should be interpreted with caution, particularly in patients suffering from acute illnesses who do not have chest pain or prior myocardial infarction. Clin Chem 1994;40:1291. N Engl J Med 1994;330:670. Clin Chem 1995;41:1266. N Engl J Med 1997;337:1648. Am Heart J 1999;137:332. Am J Emerg Med 1999;17:225.

	Tularemia agglutinins	Type and cross-match
Tularemia agglutinins, serum <1:80 titer Marbled $$	*Francisella tularensis* is an organism of wild rodents (rabbits and hares) that infects humans (eg, trappers and skinners) via contact with animal tissues, by the bite of certain ticks and flies, and by consumption of undercooked meat or contaminated water. Agglutinating antibodies appear in 10–14 days and peak in 5–10 weeks. A four-fold rise in titers is typically needed to prove acute infection. Titers decrease over years.	A type and cross-match is adequate preparation for operative procedures unlikely to require transfusion. Unnecessary type and cross-match orders reduce blood availability and add to costs. In addition, a preordering system should be in place, indicating the number of units of blood likely to be needed for each operative procedure. *Technical Manual of the American Association of Blood Banks,* 11th ed. American Association of Blood Banks, 1993.
	Increased in: Tularemia; cross-reaction with brucella antigens and proteus OX-19 antigen (but at lower titers).	Single titers of >1:160 are indicative of infection. Maximum titers are >1:1280. A history of exposure to rabbits, ticks, dogs, cats, or skunks is suggestive of—but is not a requirement for—the diagnosis. Most common presentation is a single area of painful lymphadenopathy with low-grade fever. Initial treatment should be empiric. Culture of the organism is difficult, requiring special media, and hazardous to laboratory personnel. Serologic tests are the mainstay of diagnosis. Medicine 1985;64:251. N Engl J Med 1993;329:936. Semin Respir Infect 1997;12:61.
Type and cross-match, serum and red cells (Type and cross) Red $$ Specimen label must be signed by the person drawing the blood. A second "check" specimen is needed at some hospitals.	A type and cross-match involves ABO and Rh grouping (see pp 44 and 154, respectively), and antibody screen (see p 53), and cross-match. (Compare with Type and Screen, below.) A major cross-match involves testing recipient serum against donor cells. It uses antihuman globulin to detect recipient's antibodies on donor red cells. If the recipient's serum contains a clinically significant alloantibody by antibody screen, a cross-match is required.	

	Type and screen		
Test/Range/Collection	**Physiologic Basis**	**Interpretation**	**Comments**
Type and screen, serum and red cells Red or lavender $$ Specimen label must be signed by the person drawing the blood. A second "check" specimen is needed at some hospitals.	Type and screen includes ABO and Rh grouping (see pp 44 and 154, respectively) and antibody screen (see p 53). (Compare with Type and Cross-Match, above.)	A negative antibody screen implies that a recipient can receive un-cross-matched type-specific blood with minimal risk. If the recipient's serum contains a clinically significant alloantibody by antibody screen, a cross-match is required.	Type and screen is indicated for patients undergoing operative procedures unlikely to require transfusion. However, in the absence of preoperative indications, routine preoperative blood type and screen testing is not cost-effective and may be eliminated for some procedures, such as laparoscopic cholecystectomy, expected vaginal delivery, and vaginal hysterectomy. *Technical Manual of the American Association of Blood Banks*, 11th ed. American Association of Blood Banks, 1993. Am J Obstet Gynecol 1996;175:1201. Obstet Gynecol 1998;94(4 Part 1):493. Surg Endosc 1999;13:146.

Uric acid			
Uric acid, serum Males: 2.4–7.4 Females 1.4–5.8 mg/dL [Males: 140–440 Females: 80–350 µmol/L] Marbled $	Uric acid is an end product of nucleoprotein metabolism and is excreted by the kidney. An increase in serum uric acid concentration occurs with increased nucleoprotein synthesis or catabolism (blood dyscrasias, therapy of leukemia) or decreased renal uric acid excretion (eg, thiazide diuretic therapy or renal failure).	**Increased in** Renal failure, gout, myeloproliferative disorders (leukemia, lymphoma, myeloma, polycythemia vera), psoriasis, glycogen storage disease (type I), Lesch-Nyhan syndrome (X-linked hypoxanthine-guanine phosphoribosyltransferase deficiency), lead nephropathy, hypertensive diseases of pregnancy, menopause. Drugs: antimetabolite and chemotherapeutic agents, diuretics, ethanol, nicotinic acid, salicylates (low dose), theophylline. **Decreased in:** SIADH, xanthine oxidase deficiency, low-purine diet, Fanconi's syndrome, neoplastic disease (various, causing increased renal excretion), liver disease. Drugs: salicylates (high dose), allopurinol (xanthine oxidase inhibitor).	Sex, age, and renal function affect uric acid levels. The incidence of hyperuricemia is greater in some ethnic groups (eg, Filipinos) than others (whites). Hyperuricemia may be a marker for excess cardiovascular risk. Clin Chem 1992;38:1350. Postgrad Med J 1994;70:486. Metab Clin Experiment 1996;45:1557. Am J Obstet Gynecol 1998;178:1067. Metab Clin Experiment 1998;47:435. J Hum Hypertens 1999;13:153.

Test/Range/Collection	Physiologic Basis	Interpretation	Comments
Vanillylmandelic acid, urine (VMA) 2–7 mg/24 h [10–35 µmol/d] Urine bottle containing hydrochloric acid $$ Collect 24-hour urine.	Catecholamines secreted in excess by pheochromocytomas are metabolized by the enzymes monoamine oxidase and catechol-O-methyltransferase to VMA, which is excreted in urine.	**Increased in:** Pheochromocytoma (96% sensitivity, 100% specificity), neuroblastoma, ganglioneuroma, generalized anxiety. **Decreased in:** Drugs: monoamine oxidase inhibitors.	A 24-hour urine metanephrine test (p 125) is the recommended test for the diagnosis of pheochromocytoma. (See also Pheochromocytoma algorithm, p 355.) A special diet is not needed when VMA test is done by the usual method. <0.1% of hypertensive patients have a pheochromocytoma. Am J Cardiol 1970;26:270. Ann Surg 1974;179:740. Neuropsychobiology 1995;31:6. Psychiatr Res 1995;57:1.
Venereal Disease Research Laboratory test, serum (VDRL) Nonreactive Marbled $	This syphilis test measures nontreponemal antibodies that are produced when *Treponema pallidum* interacts with host tissues. The VDRL usually becomes reactive at a titer of >1:32 within 1–3 weeks after the genital chancre appears.	**Increased in:** Syphilis: primary (59–87%), secondary (100%), late latent (79–91%), tertiary (37–94%); collagen-vascular diseases (rheumatoid arthritis, SLE), infections (mononucleosis, leprosy, malaria), pregnancy, drug abuse.	VDRL is used as a syphilis screening test and in suspected cases of primary and secondary syphilis. Positive tests should be confirmed with an FTA-ABS or MHA-TP test (see pp 92 and 129, respectively). The VDRL has similar sensitivity and specificity to the RPR (see Syphilis test table, p 391). Ann Intern Med 1986;104:368. Ann Intern Med 1991;114:1005. Sex Trans Dis 1998;26:12.

Common Laboratory Tests: Selection and Interpretation

VDRL test, CSF		
Venereal Disease Research Laboratory test, CSF (VDRL) Nonreactive $$ Deliver in a clean plastic or glass tube.	The CSF VDRL test measures nontreponemal antibodies that develop in the CSF when *Treponema pallidum* interacts with the central nervous system.	**Increased in:** Tertiary neurosyphilis (10–27%).

The quantitative VDRL is the test of choice for CNS syphilis.

Since the sensitivity of CSF VDRL is very low, a negative test does not rule out neurosyphilis. Clinical features, CSF white cell count, and CSF protein should be used together to make the diagnosis (see CSF profiles, p 369).

Because the specificity of the CSF VDRL test is high, a positive test confirms the presence of neurosyphilis.

Patients being screened for neurosyphilis with CSF VDRL testing should have a positive serum RPR, VDRL, FTA-ABS, MHA-TP test or other evidence of infection.

Repeat testing may be indicated in HIV-infected patients in whom neurosyphilis is suspected.

When the CSF VDRL is negative but suspicion of CNS syphilis is high, other commonly used laboratory tests (CSF FTA-ABS, serum FTA-ABS, CSF Treponema Pallidum hemagglutination [TPHA], serum TPHA, and CSF cells) can, in combination, identify 87% of patients with neurosyphilis with 94% specificity.

Neurology 1985;35:1368.

West J Med 1988;149:47.

Neurology 1990;40:541.

Am J Clin Pathol 1991;95:397.

Gen Hosp Psychiatry 1995;17:305.

Sex Trans Dis 1996;23:392.

Test/Range/Collection	Physiologic Basis	Interpretation	Comments
Vitamin B₁₂, serum 140–820 pg/mL [100–600 pmol/L] Marbled $$ Serum vitamin B₁₂ specimens should be frozen if not analyzed immediately.	Vitamin B₁₂ is a necessary cofactor for three important biochemical processes: conversion of methyl-malonyl-CoA to succinyl-CoA and methylation of homocysteine to methionine and demethylation of methyltetrahydrofolate to tetrahydrofolate (THF). Consequent deficiency of folate coenzymes derived from THF is probably the crucial lesion caused by B₁₂ deficiency. All vitamin B₁₂ comes from ingestion of foods of animal origin. Vitamin B₁₂ in serum is protein-bound, 70% to transcobalamin I (TC I) and 30% to transcobalamin II (TC II). The B₁₂ bound to TC II is physiologically active; that bound to TC I is not.	**Increased in:** Leukemia (acute myelocytic, chronic myelocytic, chronic lymphocytic, monocytic), marked leukocytosis, polycythemia vera. (Increased B₁₂ levels are not diagnostically useful.) **Decreased in:** Pernicious anemia, gastrectomy, gastric carcinoma, malabsorption (sprue, celiac disease, steatorrhea, regional enteritis, fistulas, bowel resection, *Diphyllobothrium latum* [fish tapeworm] infestation, small bowel bacterial overgrowth), pregnancy, dietary deficiency, HIV infection (with or without malabsorption), chronic high-flux hemodialysis, Alzheimer's disease, drugs (eg, omeprazole, metformin, carbamazepine).	Differentiation among the causes of vitamin B₁₂ deficiency can be accomplished by a vitamin B₁₂ absorption (Schilling's) test (see below). The commonly available competitive protein binding assay measures total B₁₂. It is insensitive to significant decreases in physiologically significant B₁₂ bound to TC II. Specificity of the serum vitamin B₁₂ test (approximately 73%) has not been systematically studied. Neuropsychiatric disorders caused by low serum B₁₂ level can occur in the absence of anemia or macrocytosis. Br J Haematol 1993;83:643. Essays Biochem 1994;28:63. JAMA 1994;272:1233. Ann Intern Med 1994;120:211. Ann Clin Lab Sci 1997;27:249. Nephron 1997;75:259. Am J Med 1998;104:422.

(table header spanning: Vitamin B₁₂)

Vitamin B$_{12}$ absorption test		
Vitamin B$_{12}$ absorption test, 24-hour urine (Schilling's test) Excretion of >8% of administered dose $$$$ Stage I: 0.5–1.0 μCi of ^{57}Co-B$_{12}$ is given orally, followed by 1.0 mg of unlabeled B$_{12}$ IM 2 hours later. A 24-hour urine is collected. Stage II: After 5 days, test is repeated with 60 mg active hog intrinsic factor added to the oral labeled B$_{12}$.	Absorption of vitamin B$_{12}$ is dependent on two factors: adequate intrinsic factor produced by the stomach antrum and normal ileal absorption. Lack of either can lead to B$_{12}$ deficiency.	**Decreased in:** Ileal disease or resection, bacterial overgrowth, B$_{12}$ deficiency (because megaloblastosis of the intestinal wall leads to decreased B$_{12}$ absorption, pernicious anemia (<2.5% excretion of administered dose), postgastrectomy, chronic pancreatitis, cystic fibrosis, giardiasis, Crohn's disease. Previously administered diagnostic and therapeutic radiopharmaceuticals may interfere with performance of the Schilling test for prolonged periods of time. If the patient's creatinine clearance is <60 mL/min, a 48-hour urine should be collected. Pernicious anemia is suggested by an abnormal stage I test, followed by a normal stage II test (ie, addition of intrinsic factor leads to normal intestinal absorption and urinary excretion). Ileal malabsorption gives abnormal results in stages I and II. Low intrinsic factor contributing to B$_{12}$ deficiency is common in AIDS. Egg yolk-bound B$_{12}$ should be used rather than crystalline B$_{12}$ to avoid false negative tests. CRC Crit Rev Clin Lab Sci 1988;26:263. Am J Gastroenterol 1992;87:1781. Mayo Clin Proc 1994;69:144. J Nuclear Med 1995;36:1659. J Nuclear Med 1996;37:1995.

Test/Range/Collection	Physiologic Basis	Interpretation	Comments
Vitamin D₃, 25-hydroxy, serum or plasma (25[OH]D₃) 10–50 ng/mL [25–125 nmol/L] Marbled or green $$$	The vitamin D system functions to maintain serum calcium levels. Vitamin D is a fat-soluble steroid hormone. Two molecular forms exist: D₃ (cholecalciferol), synthesized in the epidermis, and D₂ (ergocalciferol), derived from plant sources. To become active, both need to be further metabolized. Two sequential hydroxylations occur: in the liver to 25(OH)D₃ and then, in the kidney, to 1,25[OH]₂D₃. Plasma levels increase with sun exposure.	**Increased in:** Heavy milk drinkers (up to 64 ng/mL), vitamin D intoxication, sun exposure. **Decreased in:** Dietary deficiency, malabsorption (rickets, osteomalacia), biliary and portal cirrhosis, nephrotic syndrome, lack of sun exposure, osteoarthritis, age. Drugs: phenytoin, phenobarbital.	Measurement of 25(OH)D₃ is the best indicator of both vitamin D deficiency and toxicity. It is indicated in hypocalcemic disorders associated with increased PTH levels, in children with rickets and in adults with osteomalacia. In hypercalcemic disorders, 25(OH)D₃ is useful in disorders associated with decreased PTH levels, or possible vitamin D overdose (hypervitaminosis D). Vitamin D toxicity is manifested by hypercalcemia, hyperphosphatemia, soft tissue calcification and renal failure. Adv Intern Med 1982;27:45. Mayo Clin Proc 1985;60:851. Endocrinol Metab Clin North Am 1989;18:765. Lancet 1995;346:207. Ann Intern Med 1996;125:353. Arthritis Rheum 1999;42:854.

Vitamin D$_3$, 1,25-dihydroxy		
Vitamin D$_3$, 1,25-dihydroxy, serum or plasma (1,25[OH]$_2$D$_3$) 20–76 pg/mL Marbled or green $$$$	1,25-Dihydroxy vitamin D$_3$ is the most potent form of vitamin D. The main actions of vitamin D are the acceleration of calcium and phosphate absorption in the intestine and stimulation of bone resorption.	**Increased in:** Primary hyperparathyroidism, idiopathic hypercalciuria, sarcoidosis, some lymphomas, 1,25(OH)$_2$D$_3$-resistant rickets, normal growth (children), pregnancy, lactation, vitamin D toxicity. **Decreased in:** Chronic renal failure, anephric patients, hypoparathyroidism, 1 α-pseudohypoparathyroidism, post-menopausal osteoporosis.	Test is rarely needed. Measurement of 1.25(OH)$_2$D$_3$ is only useful in distinguishing 1 α-hydroxylase deficiency from 1.25(OH)$_2$D$_3$-resistant rickets or in monitoring vitamin D status of patients with chronic renal failure. Test is not useful for assessment of vitamin D intoxication, because of efficient feedback regulation of 1.25(OH)$_2$D$_3$ synthesis. Adv Intern Med 1982;27:45. N Engl J Med 1989;320:980. Ann Intern Med 1995;122:511.

Test/Range/Collection	Physiologic Basis	Interpretation	Comments
		von Willebrand's factor protein	
von Willebrand's factor protein (immunologic), plasma (vWF) 44–158% units Blue $$$	von Willebrand's factor (vWF) is produced by endothelial cells, circulates in the plasma complexed to factor VIII coagulant protein, and mediates platelet adhesion. vWF is a marker of endothelial injury. Both quantitative and qualitative changes can cause disease. vWF can be measured as protein antigen (immunologic measure) or by ristocetin cofactor activity (functional assay).	**Increased in:** Inflammatory states (acute phase reactant). **Decreased in:** von Willebrand's disease.	In von Willebrand's disease, the platelet count and morphology are generally normal and the bleeding time is usually prolonged (markedly prolonged by aspirin). Variant forms associated with mild thrombocytopenia and angiodysplasia are described. The PTT may not be prolonged if factor VIII coagulant level is >30%. Diagnosis is suggested by bleeding symptoms and family history. Laboratory diagnosis of von Willebrand's disease has become more difficult because of the identification of numerous variant forms. In the classic type I disease, vWF antigen is decreased. Blood 1987;70:895. Mayo Clin Proc 1991;66:832. Thromb Haemost 1998;80:4095.

D-Xylose absorption test		
D-Xylose absorption test, urine >5 g per 5-hour urine (>20% excreted in 5 hours) $$$ Fasting patient is given D-xylose, 25 g in two glasses of water, followed by four glasses of water over the next 2 hours. Urine is collected for 5 hours and refrigerated.	Xylose is normally easily absorbed from the small intestine. Measuring xylose in serum or its excretion in urine after ingestion evaluates the carbohydrate absorption ability of the proximal small intestine.	**Decreased in:** Intestinal malabsorption. small intestinal bacterial overgrowth, renal insufficiency, small intestinal HIV enteropathy, cryptosporidiosis, cytotoxic therapy-related malabsorption.	Test can be helpful in distinguishing intestinal malabsorption (decreased D-xylose absorption) from pancreatic insufficiency (normal D-xylose absorption). Urinary xylose excretion may be spuriously decreased in renal failure, thus limiting the specificity and usefulness of the test. In this case, a serum xylose level (gray top tube) obtained 1 hour after administration of a 25-g dose of D-xylose can be used to evaluate xylose absorption. The normal level should be > 29 mg/dL (1.9 mmol/L). Dig Dis Sci 1991;36:188. J Acquir Immune Defic Syndr 1992;5:1047. Gastroenterology 1995;108:1075. Dig Dis Sci 1997;42:2599. J Clin Oncol 1997;15:2254.

4

Therapeutic Drug Monitoring: Principles and Test Interpretation

Diana Nicoll, MD, PhD, MPA

UNDERLYING ASSUMPTIONS

The basic assumptions underlying therapeutic drug monitoring are that drug metabolism varies from patient to patient and that the plasma level of a drug is more closely related to the drug's therapeutic effect or toxicity than is the dosage.

INDICATIONS FOR DRUG MONITORING

Drugs with a narrow therapeutic index (where therapeutic drug levels do not differ greatly from levels associated with serious toxicity) should be monitored. *Example:* Lithium.

Patients who have impaired clearance of a drug with a narrow therapeutic index are candidates for drug monitoring. The clearance mechanism of the drug involved must be known. *Example:* Patients with renal failure have decreased clearance of gentamicin and therefore are at a higher risk for gentamicin toxicity.

Drugs whose **toxicity is difficult to distinguish from a patient's underlying disease** may require monitoring. *Example:* Theophylline in patients with chronic obstructive pulmonary disease.

Drugs whose efficacy is **difficult to establish clinically** may require monitoring of plasma levels. *Example:* Phenytoin.

SITUATIONS IN WHICH DRUG MONITORING MAY NOT BE USEFUL

Drugs that can be given in extremely high doses before toxicity is apparent are not candidates for monitoring. *Example:* Penicillin.

If there are better means of assessing drug effects, drug level monitoring may not be appropriate. *Example:* Warfarin is monitored by prothrombin time and INR (International Normalized Ratio) determinations, not by serum levels.

Drug level monitoring to assess compliance is limited by the inability to distinguish noncompliance from rapid metabolism without direct inpatient scrutiny of drug administration.

Drug toxicity cannot be diagnosed with drug levels alone; it is a clinical diagnosis. Drug levels within the usual therapeutic range do not rule out drug toxicity in a given patient. *Example:* Digoxin, where other physiologic variables (eg, hypokalemia) affect drug toxicity.

In summary, therapeutic drug monitoring may be useful to guide dosage adjustment of certain drugs in certain patients. Patient compliance is essential if drug monitoring data are to be correctly interpreted.

OTHER INFORMATION REQUIRED FOR EFFECTIVE DRUG MONITORING

Reliability of the Analytic Method

The analytic sensitivity of the drug monitoring method must be adequate. For some drugs, plasma levels are in the nanogram per milliliter range. *Example:* Tricyclic antidepressants, digoxin.

The **specificity** of the method must be known, since the drug's metabolites or other drugs may interfere. Interference by metabolites—which may or may not be pharmacologically active—is of particular concern in immunologic assay methods using antibodies to the parent drug.

The **precision** of the method must be known in order to assess whether changes in levels are caused by method imprecision or by clinical changes.

Reliability of the Therapeutic Range

Establishing the therapeutic range for a drug requires a reliable clinical assessment of its therapeutic and toxic effects, together with plasma drug level measurements by a particular analytic method. In practice, as newer, more specific analytic methods are introduced, the therapeutic ranges for those methods are estimated by comparing the old and new methodologies—without clinical correlation.

Pharmacokinetic Parameters

Five pharmacokinetic parameters that are important in therapeutic drug monitoring include:

1. *Bioavailability.* The bioavailability of a drug depends in part on its formulation. A drug that is significantly metabolized as it first passes through the liver exhibits a marked "first-pass effect," reducing the effective oral absorption of the drug. A reduction in this first-pass effect (eg, because of decreased hepatic blood flow in heart failure) could cause a clinically significant increase in effective oral drug absorption.

2. *Volume of distribution and distribution phases.* The volume of distribution of a drug determines the plasma concentration reached after a loading dose. The distribution phase is the time taken for a drug to distribute from the plasma to the periphery. Drug levels drawn before completion of a long distribution phase may not reflect levels of pharmacologically active drug at sites of action. *Examples:* Digoxin, lithium.

3. *Clearance.* Clearance is either renal or nonrenal (usually hepatic). Whereas changes in renal clearance can be predicted on the basis of serum creatinine or creatinine clearance, there is no routine liver function test for assessment of hepatic drug metabolism. For most therapeutic drugs measured, clearance is independent of plasma drug concentration, so that a change in dose is reflected in a similar change in plasma level. If, however, clearance is dose-dependent, dosage adjustments produce disproportionately large changes in plasma levels and must be made cautiously. *Example:* Phenytoin.

4. *Half-life.* The half-life of a drug depends on its volume of distribution and its clearance and determines the time taken to reach a steady state level. In three or four half-lives, the drug level will be 87.5% to 93.75% of the way to steady state. Patients with decreased drug clearance and therefore increased drug half-lives will take longer to reach a higher steady state level. In general, since non-steady state drug levels are potentially misleading and can be difficult to interpret, it is recommended that most clinical monitoring be done at steady state.

5. *Protein binding of drugs.* All routine drug level analysis involves assessment of both protein-bound and free drug. However, pharmacologic activity depends on only the free drug level. Changes in protein binding (eg, in uremia or hypoalbuminemia) may significantly affect interpretation of reported levels for drugs that are highly protein-bound. *Example:* Phenytoin. In such cases, where the ratio of free to total measured drug level is increased, the usual therapeutic range based on total drug level will not apply.

Drug Interactions

For patients receiving several medications, the possibility of drug interactions affecting drug elimination must be considered. *Example:* Quinidine, verapamil, and amiodarone decrease digoxin clearance.

Time to Draw Levels

In general, the specimen should be drawn after steady state is reached (at least 3 or 4 half-lives after a dosage adjustment) and just before the next dose (trough level).

Peak and trough levels may be indicated to evaluate the dosage of drugs whose half-lives are much shorter than the dosing interval. *Example:* Gentamicin.

Reference

Winter M: *Basic Clinical Pharmacokinetics,* 3rd ed. Applied Therapeutics, 1994.

TABLE 4–1. THERAPEUTIC DRUG MONITORING.

Drug	Effective Concentrations	Half-Life (hours)	Dosage Adjustment	Comments
Amikacin	Peak: 10–25 µg/mL Trough: <10 µg/mL	2–3 ↑ in uremia	↓ in renal dysfunction	Concomitant kanamycin or tobramycin therapy may give falsely elevated amikacin results by immunoassay.
Amitriptyline	160–240 ng/mL	9–46		Drug is highly protein-bound. Patient-specific decrease in protein binding may invalidate quoted range of effective concentration.
Carbamazepine	4–8 µg/mL	10–30		Induces its own metabolism. Metabolite 10,11-epoxide exhibits 13% cross-reactivity by immunoassay. Toxicity: diplopia, drowsiness, nausea, vomiting, and ataxia.
Cyclosporine	150–400 mg/mL (ng/L) whole blood	6–12	Need to know specimen and methodology used	Cyclosporine is lipid-soluble (20% bound to leukocytes; 40% to erythrocytes; 40% in plasma, highly bound to lipoproteins). Binding is temperature-dependent, so whole blood is preferred to plasma or serum as specimen. High-performance liquid chromatography or monoclonal fluorescence polarization immunoassay measures cyclosporine reliably. Polyclonal fluorescence polarization immunoassays cross-react with metabolites, so the therapeutic range used with those assays is higher. Anticonvulsants and rifampin increase metabolism. Erythromycin, ketoconazole, and calcium channel blockers decrease metabolism.
Desipramine	100–250 ng/mL	13–23		Drug is highly protein-bound. Patient-specific decrease in protein binding may invalidate quoted range of effective concentration.

↔= unchanged; ↑ = increased;, ↓ = decreased; **CHF** = congestive heart failure

TABLE 4–1 (CONTINUED).

Drug	Effective Concentrations	Half-Life (hours)	Dosage Adjustment	Comments
Digoxin	0.8–2 ng/mL	42 ↑ in uremia, CHF, hypothyroidism; ↓ in hyperthyroidism	↓ in renal dysfunction, CHF	Bioavailability of digoxin tablets is 50–90%. Specimen must not be drawn within 6 hours of dose. Dialysis does not remove a significant amount. Hypokalemia potentiates toxicity. Digitalis toxicity is a clinical and *not* a laboratory diagnosis. Digibind (digoxin-specific antibody) therapy of digoxin overdose can interfere with measurement of digoxin levels depending on the digoxin assay. Elimination is reduced by quinidine, verapamil, and amiodarone.
Ethosuximide	40–100 mg/L	Child: 30 Adult: 50		Levels used primarily to assess compliance. Toxicity is rare and does not correlate well with plasma concentrations.
Gentamicin	Peak: 4–8 µg/mL Trough: <2 µg/mL	2–5 ↑ in uremia (7.3 on dialysis)	↓ in renal dysfunction	Draw peak specimen 30 minutes after end of infusion. Draw trough just before next dose. In uremic patients, carbenicillin may reduce gentamicin half-life from 46 hours to 22 hours. If a once-daily regimen (5 mg/kg) is used to maximize bacterial killing by optimizing the peak concentration/MIC ratio and to reduce the potential for toxicity, dosage should be reduced if trough concentration is >1 µg/mL (1 mg/L). Measurement of peak concentrations is not recommended with this regimen.
Imipramine	180–350 ng/mL	10–16		Drug is highly protein-bound. Patient-specific decrease in protein binding may invalidate quoted range of effective concentration.
Lidocaine	1–5 µg/mL	1.8 ↔ in uremia, CHF; ↑ in cirrhosis	↓ in CHF, liver disease	Levels increased with cimetidine therapy. CNS toxicity common in the elderly.

↔ = unchanged; ↑ = increased; ↓ = decreased; **CHF** = congestive heart failure

Lithium	0.7–1.5 meq/L	22 ↑ in uremia	↓ in renal dysfunction	Thiazides and loop diuretics may increase serum lithium levels.
Methotrexate		8.4 ↑ in uremia	↓ in renal dysfunction	7-Hydroxymethotrexate cross-reacts 1.5% in immunoassay. To minimize toxicity, leucovorin should be continued if methotrexate level is >0.1 µmol/L at 48 hours after start of therapy. Methotrexate > 1 µmol/L at >48 hours requires an increase in leucovorin rescue therapy.
Nortriptyline	50–40 ng/mL	18–44		Drug is highly protein-bound. Patient-specific decrease in protein binding may invalidate quoted range of effective concentration.
Phenobarbital	10–30 µg/mL	86 ↑ in cirrhosis	↓ in liver disease.	Metabolized principally by the hepatic microsomal enzyme system. Many drug-drug interactions.
Phenytoin	10–20 µg/mL ↓ in uremia, hypoalbuminemia	Dose-dependent		Metabolite cross-reacts 10% in immunoassay. Metabolism is capacity-limited. Increase dose cautiously when level approaches therapeutic range, since new steady state level may be disproportionately higher. Drug is very highly protein-bound, and when protein-binding is decreased in uremia and hypoalbuminemia, the usual therapeutic range does not apply. In this situation, use a reference range of 5–10 µg/mL.
Primidone	5–10 µg/mL	8		Phenobarbital cross-reacts 0.5%. Metabolized to phenobarbital. Primidone/phenobarbital ratio >1:2 suggests poor compliance.
Procainamide	4–8 µg/mL	3 ↑ in uremia	↓ in renal dysfunction	Thirty percent of patients with plasma levels of 12–16 µg/mL have ECG changes; 40% of patients with plasma levels of 16 µg/mL have severe toxicity. Metabolite N-acetylprocainamide is active.

↔ = unchanged; ↑ = increased; ↓ = decreased; **CHF** = congestive heart failure

TABLE 4–1 (CONTINUED).

Drug	Effective Concentrations	Half-Life (hours)	Dosage Adjustment	Comments
Quinidine	1–5 µg/L	7 ↔ in CHF ↑ in liver disease	↓ in liver disease, CHF	Effective concentration is lower in chronic liver disease and nephrosis where binding is decreased.
Salicylate	150–300 µg/mL (15–30 mg/dL)	Dose-dependent		See Figure 8–23, p 360, for nomogram of salicylate toxicity.
Theophylline	5–20 µg/mL	9	↓ in CHF, cirrhosis, and with cimetidine	Caffeine cross-reacts 10%. Elimination is increased 1.5–2 times in smokers. 1,3-Dimethyl uric acid metabolite increased in uremia and because of cross-reactivity may cause an apparent slight increase in serum theophylline.
Tobramycin	Peak: 5–10 µg/mL Trough: <2 µg/mL	2–3 ↑ in uremia	↓ in renal dysfunction	Tobramycin, kanamycin, and amikacin may cross-react in immunoassay. If a once-daily regimen is used to maximize bacterial killing by optimizing the peak concentration/MIC ratio and to reduce the potential for toxicity, dosage should be reduced if trough concentration is >1 µg/mL (1 mg/L). Measurement of peak concentrations is not recommended with this regimen.
Valproic acid	55–100 µg/mL	13–19		Ninety-five percent protein-bound. Reduced binding in uremia and cirrhosis.
Vancomycin	Trough: 5–15 µg/mL	6 ↑ in uremia	↓ in renal dysfunction	Toxicity in uremic patients leads to irreversible deafness. Keep peak level <30–40 µg/mL to avoid toxicity.

↔ = unchanged; ↑ = increased; ↓ = decreased; **CHF** = congestive heart failure

5

Microbiology: Test Selection

Mary K. York, PhD

HOW TO USE THIS SECTION

This section displays information about clinically important infectious diseases in tabular form. Included in these tables are the *Organisms* involved in the disease/syndrome listed; *Specimens/Diagnostic Tests* that are useful in the evaluation; and *Comments* regarding the tests and diagnoses discussed. Topics are listed by body area/organ system: Central Nervous System, Eye, Ear, Sinus, Upper Airway, Lung, Heart and Vessels, Abdomen, Genitourinary, Bone, Joint, Muscle, Skin, and Blood.

Organisms

This column lists organisms that are known to cause the stated illness. Scientific names are abbreviated according to common usage (eg, *Streptococcus pneumoniae* as *S pneumoniae* or pneumococcus). Specific age or risk groups are listed in order of increasing age or frequency (eg, Infant, Child, Adult, HIV).

When bacteria are listed, Gram stain characteristics follow the organism name in parentheses—eg, "*S pneumoniae* (GPDC)." The following abbreviations are used:

GPC	Gram-positive cocci	**GNC**	Gram-negative cocci
GPDC	Gram-positive diplococci	**GNDC**	Gram-negative diplococci
GPCB	Gram-positive coccobacilli	**GNCB**	Gram-negative coccobacilli
GPR	Gram-positive rods	**GNR**	Gram-negative rods
GVCB	Gram-variable coccobacilli	**AFB**	Acid-fast bacilli

When known, the frequency of the specific organism's involvement in the disease process is also provided in parentheses—eg, "*S pneumoniae* (GPDC) (50%)."

Specimen Collection/Diagnostic Tests

This column describes the collection of specimens, laboratory processing, useful radiographic procedures, and other diagnostic tests. Culture or test sensitivities with respect to the diagnosis in question are placed in parentheses immediately following the test when known—eg, "Gram stain (60%)." Pertinent serologic tests are also listed. Keep in mind that few infections can be identified by definitive diagnostic tests and that clinical judgment is critical to making difficult diagnoses when test results are equivocal.

Comments

This column includes general information about the utility of the tests and may include information about patient management. Appropriate general references are also listed.

Syndrome Name/Body Area

In the last two columns the syndrome name and body area are placed perpendicular to the rest of the table to allow for quick referencing.

CENTRAL NERVOUS SYSTEM		
Brain Abscess		
Organism	**Specimen/Diagnostic Tests**	**Comments**
Brain Abscess Usually polymicrobial Child: anaerobes (40%), *S aureus* (GPC), *S pneumoniae* (GPDC), *S pyogenes* (GPC in chains), viridans streptococci (GPC in chains), less common, Enterobacteriaceae (GNR), *P aeruginosa* (GNR), *H influenzae* (GNCB), *N meningitidis* (GNDC) Adults: Viridans and anaerobic streptococci (GPC in chains) (60–70%), bacteroides (GNR) (20–40%), Enterobacteriaceae (GNR) (23–33%), *S aureus* (GPC) (10–15%), other anaerobes, including fusobacterium (GNR) and actinomyces (GPR), *T solium* (cysticerci) Immunocompromised : *T gondii*, *C neoformans*, nocardia (GPR), mycobacteria (AFB), fungi, *E histolytica*. Posttraumatic: *S aureus* (GPC), Enterobacteriaceae (GNR), coagulase-negative staphylococci (GPC), *P acnes* (GPR)	Blood for bacterial cultures. Brain abscess aspirate for Gram stain (82%), bacterial (88%), AFB, fungal cultures, and cytology. Lumbar puncture is dangerous and contraindicated. Sources of infection in the ears, sinuses, lungs or bloodstream should be sought for culture when abscess is found. CT scan and MRI are the most valuable imaging procedures and can guide biopsy if a specimen is needed. (See CT scan, MRI of head, p 245.) Serum toxoplasma antibody in HIV-infected patients may not be positive at outset of presumptive therapy. If negative or if no response to empiric therapy, biopsy may be needed to rule out lymphoma, fungal infection, or tuberculosis. Biopsy material should be sent for toxoplasma antigen (DFA). Detection of toxoplasma DNA in blood or CSF samples by PCR techniques is now available from specialized or reference laboratories. A positive PCR result must be interpreted in the context of the clinical presentation. Active or recent infection is indicated by a positive IgM antibody test. (See also toxoplasma antibody, p 171.)	Occurs in patients with otitis media and sinusitis. Also seen in patients with cyanotic congenital heart disease and right-to-left shunting (eg, tetralogy of Fallot) or arteriovenous vascular abnormalities of the lung (eg, Osler-Weber-Rendu). Majority of toxoplasmosis abscesses are multiple and are seen on MRI in the basal ganglia, parietal and frontal lobes. 99mTechnetium brain scan is a very sensitive test for abscess and the test of choice where CT and MRI are unavailable. J Child Neurol 1995;10:283. Clin Infect Dis 1996;23:1061. Clin Infect Dis 1997;25:763. Neurol Clin 1998;16:419.

	CENTRAL NERVOUS SYSTEM	
	Encephalitis	
Organism	**Specimen / Diagnostic Tests**	**Comments**
Encephalitis Arboviruses (California group, St. Louis, western equine), enteroviruses (coxsackie, echo, polio), herpes simplex (HSV). *B henselae*, lymphocytic choriomeningitis, mumps, tick-borne encephalitis virus, post-infectious (following influenza, human herpes virus 6 [HHV-6], measles, mumps, rubella, varicella-zoster [VZV]), rabies, Creutzfeldt-Jakob Postvaccination: Rabies, pertussis. Immunocompromised: Cytomegalovirus (CMV), toxoplasmosis, papovavirus (PML)	CSF for pressure (elevated), cell count (WBCs elevated but variable [10–2000/µL], mostly lymphocytes), protein (elevated, especially IgG fraction), glucose (normal), RBCs (especially in herpesvirus). Repeat examination of CSF after 24 hours often useful. (See CSF profiles, p 369.) CSF cultures for viruses and bacteria (low yield). CSF PCR in reference laboratories for CMV (33%), HSV (98%), VZV, and enterovirus. Identification of HSV DNA in CSF by PCR techniques is now the definitive diagnostic test. Throat swab for enterovirus, mumps. Stool culture for enterovirus, which is frequently shed for weeks (especially in children). Urine culture for mumps. Culture of both skin biopsy from hairline and saliva for rabies. Single serum for bartonella (cat-scratch disease) IgM and IgG. Paired sera for arboviruses, mumps, or rabies should be drawn acutely and after 1–3 weeks of illness. Serologic tests are often of academic interest only. Not indicated for herpes simplex.	CT scan with contrast or MRI with gadolinium showing temporal lobe lesions suggests herpes simplex. Polyradiculopathy is highly suggestive of CMV in AIDS. Clin Neuropathol 1995;14:187. Ann Intern Med 1996;125:577. Clin Infect Dis 1996;23:219. Postgrad Med 1998;103:123. Ann Intern Med 1998;128:922. J Neurosurg 1998;89:640. J Child Neurol 1999;14:1. J Clin Microbiol 1999;37:2127.

CENTRAL NERVOUS SYSTEM		
Aseptic Meningitis		
Aseptic Meningitis Acute: Enteroviruses (coxsackie, echo, polio) (90%), mumps, herpes simplex (HSV), HIV (primary HIV seroconversion), varicella-zoster (VZV), lymphocytic choriomeningitis virus (rare). Recurrent: Herpes simplex type 2 (Mollaret's syndrome)	CSF for pressure (elevated), cell count (WBCs 10–100/µL, PMNs early, lymphocytes later), protein (normal or slightly elevated), and glucose (normal). (See CSF profiles, p 369.) CSF viral culture can be negative despite active viral infection. Enteroviruses can be isolated from the CSF in the first few days after onset but only rarely after the first week. Detection of enteroviral RNA in CSF by PCR from specialized or reference laboratories. Urine viral culture for mumps. Vesicle direct fluorescent antibody (DFA) or culture for HSV or VZV. Paired sera for viral titers: poliovirus, mumps, and VZV. Not practical for other organisms unless actual isolate known and then only useful epidemiologically. Detection of VZV or HSV in CSF by PCR.	Aseptic meningitis is acute meningeal irritation in the absence of pyogenic bacteria or fungi. Diagnosis is usually made by the examination of the CSF and by ruling out other infectious causes (eg, syphilis, tuberculosis). Consider nonsteroidal anti-inflammatory drugs as a noninfectious cause. Enteroviral aseptic meningitis is rare after age 40. Patients with deficiency of the complement regulatory protein factor I may have recurrent aseptic meningitis. J Clin Microbiol 1997;35:691. Clin Microbiol Rev 1998;11:202. Acta Neurol Scand 1998;98:209.

	CENTRAL NERVOUS SYSTEM	
	Bacterial Meningitis	
Organism	**Specimen/Diagnostic Tests**	**Comments**
Bacterial Meningitis Neonate: *E coli* (GNR), group B or D streptococci (GPC), *L monocytogenes* (GPR). Infant: Group B streptococci, *S pneumoniae* (GPC), *N meningitidis* (GNDC), *Listeria monocytogenes* (GPR), *H influenzae* (GNCB). Child: *S pneumoniae*, *N meningitidis*, *H influenzae*. Adult: *S pneumoniae*, *N meningitidis*, *L monocytogenes*. Postneurosurgical: *S aureus* (GPC), *S pneumoniae*, *P acnes* (GPR), coagulase-negative staphylococci (GPC), pseudomonas (GNR), *E coli* (GNR), other Enterobacteriaceae. Alcoholic patients and the elderly: In addition to the adult organisms, Enterobacteriaceae, pseudomonas, *H influenzae*.	CSF for pressure (> 180 mm H_2O), cell count (WBCs 1000–100,000/μL, >50% PMNs), protein (150–500 mg/dL), glucose (<40% of serum). (See CSF profiles, p 369.) CSF for Gram stain of cytocentrifuged material (positive in 70–80%). CSF culture for bacteria. Blood culture positive in 40–60% of patients with pneumococcal, meningococcal, and *H influenzae* meningitis. CSF antigen tests are no longer considered useful because of their low sensitivity and false-positive results.	The first priority in the care of the patient with suspected acute meningitis is therapy, then diagnosis. Antibiotics should be started within 30 minutes of presentation. The death rate for meningitis is about 50% for pneumococcal, less for others. With recurrent *N meningitidis* meningitis, suspect a terminal complement component deficiency. With other recurrent bacterial meningitides, suspect a CSF leak. Postgrad Med 1998;103:102. Medicine (Baltimore) 1998;77:313. Infect Dis Clin North Am 1999;13:711. Infect Dis Clin North Am 1999;13:579.

CENTRAL NERVOUS SYSTEM		
Fungal Meningitis		
Fungal Meningitis *C neoformans* (spherical, budding yeast), *C immitis* (spherules), *H capsulatum*. Immunocompromised: Aspergillus sp, *P boydii*, candida sp.	CSF for pressure (normal or elevated), cell count (WBCs 50–1000/µL, mostly lymphocytes), protein (elevated), and glucose (decreased). Serum cryptococcal antigen (CrAg) for *C neoformans* (99%). For other fungi, collect at least 5 mL of CSF for fungal culture. Initial cultures are positive in 40% of coccidioides cases and 27–65% of histoplasma cases. Repeat cultures are frequently needed. Culture of bone marrow, skin lesions, or other involved organs should also be performed if clinically indicated. CSF India ink preparation for cryptococcus is not recommended because it is positive in only 50% of cases. Serum coccidioidal serology is a concentrated serum immunodiffusion test for the organism (75–95%). CSF serologic testing is rarely necessary. (See coccidioides serology: p 74.) Complement fixation test for histoplasma is available from public health department laboratories (see p 109). Histoplasma antigen can be detected in urine, blood, or CSF in 61% of cases of histoplasma meningitis.	The clinical presentation of fungal meningitis in immunocompromised patients is that of an indolent chronic meningitis. Prior to AIDS, cryptococcal meningitis was seen both in patients with cellular immunologic deficiencies and in patients who lacked obvious defects (about 50% of cases). Cryptococcus is the most common cause of meningitis in AIDS patients and may present with normal CSF findings. Titer of CSF CrAg can be used to monitor therapeutic success (falling titer) or failure (unchanged or rising titer) or to predict relapse during suppressive therapy (rising titer). Clin Microbiol Rev 1995;8:515. Emerg Infect Dis 1996;2:109. Clin Infect Dis 1996;22:240. Scand J Infect Dis 1998;30:485.

	CENTRAL NERVOUS SYSTEM
	Spirochetal Meningitis

Organism	Specimen/Diagnostic Tests	Comments
Spirochetal Meningitis/ Neurologic diseases *B burgdorferi* (neuroborreliosis), *T pallidum* (neurosyphilis), leptospira, other borreliae	**Neuroborreliosis:** CSF for pressure (normal or elevated), cell count (WBCs elevated, mostly lymphocytes), protein (may be elevated), and glucose (normal). Serum and CSF for serologic testing. False-positive serologic tests may occur. Western blots should be used to confirm borderline or positive results. CSF serology for anti-*B burgdorferi* IgM (90%). Culture and PCR less specific. For Lyme disease serologies, see p 122. **Acute syphilitic meningitis:** CSF for pressure (elevated), cell count (WBCs 25–2000/μL, mostly lymphocytes), protein (elevated), and glucose (normal or low). (See CSF profiles, p 369.) Serum VDRL. (See VDRL, serum, p 178.) CSF VDRL is the preferred test (see p 179), but is only 66% sensitive for acute syphilitic meningitis. **Neurosyphilis:** CSF for pressure (normal), cell count (WBCs normal or slightly increased, mostly lymphocytes), protein (normal or elevated), glucose (normal), and CSF VDRL. Serum VDRL, FTA-ABS, or MHA-TP should be done. **Leptospirosis:** CSF cell count (WBCs <500/μL, mostly monocytes), protein (slightly elevated), and glucose (normal). Urine for dark-field examination of sediment. Blood and CSF dark-field examination only positive in acute phase prior to meningitis. Serum for serology for IgM.	Neurosyphilis is a late stage of infection and can present with meningovascular (hemiparesis, seizures, aphasia), parenchymal (general paresis, tabes dorsalis), or asymptomatic (latent) disease. Because there is no single highly sensitive or specific test for neurosyphilis, the diagnosis must depend on a combination of clinical and laboratory data. Therapy of suspected neurosyphilis should not be withheld on the basis of a negative CSF VDRL if clinical suspicion is high. In HIV neurosyphilis, treatment failures may be common. Lyme disease can present as a lymphocytic meningitis, facial palsy, or painful radiculitis. Leptospirosis follows exposure to rats. Semin Neurol 1998;18:185. J Neurol Sci 1998;153:182. Clin Infect Dis 1998;26:151. J Clin Microbiol 1998;36:3138. J Emerg Med 1998;16:851.

CENTRAL NERVOUS SYSTEM	
Parasitic Meningoencephalitis	**Tuberculous Meningitis**

Parasitic Meningoencephalitis

T gondii, E chaffeensis (human monocytic ehrlichiosis) (HME) and other species of human granulocytic ehrlichiosis (HGE), *E histolytica, N fowleri, T solium* (cysticerci).

CSF for pressure (normal or elevated), cell count (WBCs 100–1000/μL, chiefly monocytes, lymphocytes), protein (elevated), glucose (normal).
Serology as for brain abscess.

Ehrlichiosis: White blood cell count low (1300–4000/μL), platelets low (50,000–140,000/μL), hepatic aminotransferases (tenfold above normal). Buffy coat for Giemsa (1% in HME, 18–80% in HGE), PCR of blood available (50–90% depending on prior therapy). Serum IgG and IgM usually not positive until the third week.

Naegleria: CSF wet mount, culture, and Giemsa stain.

Cysticercosis: Characteristic findings on CT and MRI are diagnostic. Serology is less sensitive.

Naegleria follows exposure to warm fresh water. Ehrlichia follows exposure to horses and ticks.
Pediatr Neurol 1996;15:230.
J Neuroophthalmol 1997;17:47.
Infect Dis Clin North Am 1998;12:123.

Tuberculous Meningitis

M tuberculosis (MTb) (acid-fast bacilli [AFB])

CSF for pressure (elevated), cell count (WBCs 100–500/μL, PMNs early, lymphocytes later), protein (elevated), glucose (decreased). (See CSF culture, p 369.)
CSF for AFB stain. Stain is positive in only 30%. Cytocentrifugation and repeat smears increase yield.
CSF for AFB culture (positive in <70%). Repeated sampling of the CSF during the first week of therapy is recommended; ideally, 3 or 4 specimens of 5–10 mL each should be obtained (87% yield with 4 specimens). PCR available but not yet validated. DNA probes are available for rapid confirmation from mycobacterial growth.

Tuberculous meningitis is usually secondary to rupture of a subependymal tubercle rather than blood-borne invasion.
Since CSF stain and culture are not sensitive for tuberculosis, diagnosis and treatment should be based on a combination of clinical and micro-biologic data.
Evidence of inactive or active extrameningeal tuberculosis, especially pulmonary, is seen in 75% of patients.
Radiol Clin North Am 1995;33:733.
Surg Neurol 1995;44:378.
Acta Neurol Belg 1995;95:80.

	EYE	
	Conjunctivitis	
Organism	**Specimen / Diagnostic Tests**	**Comments**
Conjunctivitis Neonate (ophthalmia neonatorum): *C trachomatis, N gonorrhoeae* (GNDC), herpes simplex (HSV) Children and adults: adenovirus, staphylococci (GPC), herpes simplex (HSV), *H influenzae* (GNCB), *S pneumoniae* (GPDC), *S pyogenes* (GPC), varicella-zoster (VZV), *N gonorrhoeae* (GNDC), *M lacunata* (GNCB), bartonella sp (Parinaud's oculoglandular syndrome). Adult inclusion conjunctivitis/trachoma: *C trachomatis.* Acute hemorrhagic conjunctivitis (acute epidemic keratoconjunctivitis): enterovirus, coxsackievirus.	Conjunctival Gram stain is especially useful if gonococcal infection is suspected. Bacterial culture for severe cases (routine bacterial culture) or suspected gonococcal infection. Conjunctival scrapings or smears by direct immunofluorescent monoclonal antibody staining for *C trachomatis.* Cell culture for chlamydia. Detection of chlamydial DNA on ocular swabs by PCR techniques is available but not yet validated. Ocular HSV and VZV PCR available in reference laboratories.	The causes of conjunctivitis change with the season. Adenovirus occurs mainly in the fall, *H influenzae* in the winter. Gonococcal conjunctivitis is an ophthalmologic emergency. Cultures are usually unnecessary unless chlamydia or gonorrhea is suspected or the case is severe. Consider noninfectious causes (eg, allergy, contact lens deposits, trauma) Clin Ther 1995:17:800. Clin Infect Dis 1995;21:479. Postgrad Med 1997:101:185. Am Fam Physician 1998;57:735.

EYE		
Keratitis		
Endophthalmitis		

Keratitis

Bacteria: *P aeruginosa* (GNR), staphylococci (GPC), *S pneumoniae* (GPDC), moraxella sp.
Virus: Herpes simplex (HSV) (dendritic pattern on fluorescein slitlamp examination), varicella-zoster virus (VZV)
Contact lens: Acanthamoeba, Enterobacteriaceae (GNR).
Fungus: Candida, fusarium, aspergillus, rhodotorula, and other filamentous fungi.
Parasite: *O volvulus* (river blindness), microsporidia (HIV)

Corneal scrapings for Gram stain, KOH, and culture. Routine bacterial culture is used for most bacterial causes, viral culture for herpes, and special media for acanthamoeba (can be detected with trichrome or Giemsa stain of smears).
Treatment depends on Gram stain appearance and culture.
Corneal biopsy may be needed if initial cultures are negative.

Prompt ophthalmologic consultation is mandatory. Acanthamoeba infection occurs in soft contact (extended-wear) lens wearers and may resemble HSV infection on fluorescein examination (dendritic ["branching"] ulcer).
Bacterial keratitis is usually caused by contact lens use or trauma. Fungal keratitis is usually caused by trauma.
Int Ophthalmol Clin 1998;38:115.
Int Ophthalmol Clin 1998;38:107.
CLAO J 1998;24:52.
Cornea 1998;17:3.
Clin Microbiol Rev 1999;12:445.
Cornea 1999;18:144.

Endophthalmitis

Spontaneous or postoperative: *S aureus* (GPC), coagulase-negative staphylococci (GPC), *S pneumoniae* (GPDC), candida sp; streptococci, non-group B (GPC in chains).
Trauma: Bacillus sp (GPR), fungi.
Post-filtering bleb: Viridans group streptococcus (57%), *S pneumoniae* (GPDC), *H influenzae* (GNCB).
IV drug abuse: Add *B cereus*.

Culture material from anterior chamber, vitreous cavity, and wound abscess for bacteria, mycobacteria, and fungi. Traumatic and postoperative cases should have aqueous and vitreous aspiration for culture and smear (56%).
Conjunctival cultures are inadequate and misleading.

Endophthalmitis is an inflammatory process of the ocular cavity and adjacent structures. Rapid diagnosis is critical, since vision may be compromised. Bacterial endophthalmitis usually occurs as a consequence of ocular surgery. Prophylactic antibiotic use is of unproved benefit, though topical antibiotics are widely used.
Also consider retinitis in immunocompromised patients, caused by CMV, HSV, VZV, and toxoplasma (retinochoroiditis), which is diagnosed by retinal examination.
Int Ophthalmol Clin 1996;36:163.
Ophthalmology 1996;103:757.
Clin Infect Dis 1997;24:1172.
Curr Opin Ophthalmol 1998;9:66.
Surv Ophthalmol 1998;43:193.

	EAR	
	Otitis Media	

Organism	Specimen/Diagnostic Tests	Comments
Otitis Media Infant, child, and adult: *S pneumoniae* (30%) (GPDC), *H influenzae* (30%) (GNCB), *M catarrhalis* (10%) (GNDC), *S aureus* (GPC), *S pyogenes* (GPC in chains), *M pneumoniae*, *C pneumoniae*, "sterile." Neonate: Same as above plus Enterobacteriaceae (GNR), group B streptococcus (GPC). Endotracheal intubation: Pseudomonas sp (GNR), klebsiella (GNR), Enterobacteriaceae (GNR). Chronic: *S aureus* (GPC), *P aeruginosa* (GNR), anaerobes, *M tuberculosis* (AFB).	Tympanocentesis aspirate for Gram stain and bacterial culture in the patient who has a toxic appearance. Otherwise, microbiologic studies of effusions are so consistent that empiric treatment is acceptable. CSF examination if clinically indicated. Nasopharyngeal swab may be substituted for tympanocentesis. Blood culture in the toxic patient.	Peak incidence of otitis media occurs in the first 3 years of life, especially between 6 and 24 months of age. In neonates, predisposing factors include cleft palate, hypotonia, mental retardation (Down's syndrome). Tympanocentesis is indicated if the patient fails to improve after 48 hours or develops fever. It may hasten resolution and decrease sterile effusion. Persistent middle ear effusion may require placement of ventilating or tympanostomy tubes. Bullous myringitis suggests mycoplasma. Emerging antibiotic resistance should be considered in choice of empiric antibiotic therapy. Int J Pediatr Otorhinolaryngol 1995;31:153. Pediatr Clin North Am 1996;43:1165. Pediatr Infect Dis J 1997;16:449. Pediatr Infect Dis J 1998;17:1105. Pediatr Infect Dis J 1999;18:1.

EAR		
Otitis Externa		
Otitis Externa Acute localized: *S aureus* (GPC), anaerobes (32%), *S pyogenes* (GPC in chains). "Swimmer's ear": Pseudomonas sp (GNR), Enterobacteriaceae (GNR), vibrio (GNR), fungi (rare). Chronic: Usually secondary to seborrhea or eczema. Diabetes mellitus, AIDS ("malignant otitis externa"): *P aeruginosa* (GNR), aspergillus sp. Furuncle of external canal: *S aureus*.	Ear drainage for Gram stain and bacterial culture, especially in malignant otitis externa. CT or MRI can aid in diagnosis by demonstrating cortical bone erosion or meningeal enhancement.	Infection of the external auditory canal is similar to infection of skin and soft tissue elsewhere. If malignant otitis externa is present, exclusion of associated osteomyelitis and surgical drainage may be required. Clin Infect Dis 1992;15:955. Otolaryngol Clin North Am 1996;29:761. Nurse Pract 1998;23:125. Aust Fam Physician 1999;28:217.

	SINUS	
	Sinusitis	
Organism	**Specimen/Diagnostic Tests**	**Comments**
Sinusitis	Nasal aspirate for bacterial culture is not usually helpful.	Diagnosis and treatment of sinusitis is usually based on clinical and radiologic features. Microbiologic studies can be helpful in severe or atypical cases.
Acute: *S pneumoniae* (GPC) (31%), *H influenzae* (GNCB) (21%), *M catarrhalis* (GNDC), *S pyogenes* (2–5%) (GPC), anaerobes (2–5%), viruses (adenovirus, influenza, parainfluenza), *S aureus* (GPC) (rare).	Maxillary sinus aspirate for bacterial culture may be helpful in severe or atypical cases.	Sinus CT scan (or MRI) is better than plain x-ray for diagnosing sinusitis, particularly if sphenoid sinusitis is suspected. However, sinus CT scans should be interpreted cautiously, since abnormalities are also seen in patients with the common cold.
Chronic (child): Viridans and anaerobic streptococci (GPC in chains) (23%), *S aureus* (19%), *S pneumoniae*, *H influenzae*, *M catarrhalis*, *P aeruginosa* (GNR) in cystic fibrosis.		Acute and chronic sinusitis occur frequently in HIV-infected patients, may be recurrent or refractory, and may involve multiple sinuses (especially when the CD4 cell count is <200/μL).
Chronic (adult): Coagulase-negative staphylococci (GPC) (36%), *S aureus* (GPC in chains) (25%), viridans streptococci (GPC) (8%), corynebacteria (GPR) (5%), anaerobes (6%), including bacteroides sp, prevotella sp (GNR), peptostreptococcus (GPC), fusobacterium sp (GNR).		Acute sinusitis often results from bacterial superinfection following viral upper respiratory infection. Pediatr Clin North Am 1996;43:1297. J Otolaryngol 1996;25:249. Acta Otorhinolaryngol Belg 1997;51:305. CMAJ 1997;15:156(Suppl 6):S1. Clin Infect Dis 1997;25:267. Ann Otol Rhinol Laryngol 1998;107:942.
Hospitalized with nasogastric tube or nasotracheal intubation: Enterobacteriaceae (GNR), pseudomonas sp (GNR).		
Fungal: Zygomycetes (rhizopus), aspergillus, *P boydii*.		
Immunocompromised: *P aeruginosa* (GNR), cytomegalovirus (CMV), aspergillus sp. and other filamentous fungi plus microsporidia, *Cryptosporidium parvum*, acanthamoeba in HIV-infected patients.		

UPPER AIRWAY		
Pharyngitis		**Laryngitis**

Pharyngitis

Exudative: *S pyogenes* (GPC) (15–30%), viruses (rhinovirus, coronavirus, adenovirus) (25%), group C streptococcus (GPC), Epstein-Barr virus (mononucleosis), *N gonorrhoeae* (GNDC), *Arcanobacterium hemolyticum* (GPR). Membranous: *C diphtheriae* (GPR), *C pseudodiphtheriicum* (GPR), Epstein-Barr virus.

Throat swab for culture. Place in sterile tube or transport medium. If *N gonorrhoeae* suspected, use chocolate agar or Thayer-Martin media. If *C diphtheriae* suspected, use Tinsdale or blood agar. Throat swabs are routinely cultured for group A streptococcus only. If other organisms are suspected, this must be stated. Throat culture is about 70% sensitive for group A streptococcus. "Rapid" tests for group A streptococcus can speed diagnosis and aid in the treatment of family members. However, false-negative results may lead to underdiagnosis and failure to treat.

Controversy exists over how to evaluate patients with sore throat. Some authors suggest culturing all patients and then treating only those with positive cultures. In patients with compatible histories, be sure to consider pharyngeal abscess or epiglottitis, both of which may be life-threatening. Complications include pharyngeal abscess and Lemierre's syndrome (infection with fusobacterium sp.), which can progress to sepsis and multi-organ failure.
Clin Infect Dis 1995;20:1512.
Nurse Pract 1996;21:38.
Clin Infect Dis 1997;25:574.
J Clin Microbiol 1998;36:3468.
Int J Pediatr Otorhinolaryngol 1998;45:51.

Laryngitis

Virus (90%) (influenza, rhinovirus, adenovirus, parainfluenza, Epstein-Barr virus), *S pyogenes* (GPC) (10%), *M catarrhalis* (GNDC) (55% of adults), *M tuberculosis*, fungus (cryptococcosis, histoplasmosis). Immunocompromised: *Candida* sp, cytomegalovirus, herpes simplex (HSV).

Diagnosis is made by clinical picture of upper respiratory infection with hoarseness.

Laryngitis usually occurs with common cold or influenzal syndromes. Fungal laryngeal infections occur most commonly in immunocompromised patients (AIDS, cancer, organ transplants, corticosteroid therapy, diabetes mellitus). Consider acid reflux for chronic cases.
Am Otol Rhinol Laryngol 1993;102:209.
J Infect Dis 1996;174:636.
Head Neck 1996;18:455.
J Voice 1998;12:9:1.

	UPPER AIRWAY
	Laryngotracheobronchitis

Organism	Specimen / Diagnostic Tests	Comments
Laryngotracheobronchitis Infant/child: Respiratory syncytial virus (RSV) (50–75%) (bronchiolitis), adenovirus, parainfluenza virus (croup), *B pertussis* (GNCB) (whooping cough), other viruses, including rhinovirus, coronavirus, influenza. Adolescent/adult: Usually viruses, *M pneumoniae*, *C pneumoniae*, *B pertussis*. Chronic adult: *S pneumoniae* (GPDC), *H influenzae* (GNCB), *M catarrhalis* (GNDC), klebsiella (GNR), other Enterobacteriaceae (GNR), viruses (eg, influenza), aspergillus (allergic bronchopulmonary aspergillosis). Chronic obstructive airway disease: Viral (25–50%) *S pneumoniae* (GPC), *H influenzae* (GNCB), *S aureus* (GPC), Enterobacteriaceae (GNR), anaerobes (<10%).	Nasopharyngeal aspirate for respiratory virus direct fluorescent antigen (DFA), for viral culture (rarely indicated), and for PCR for *B pertussis*. PCR for pertussis is test of choice; culture and DFA are less sensitive. Cellular examination of early morning sputum will show many PMNs in chronic bronchitis. Sputum Gram stain and culture for ill adults. In chronic bronchitis, mixed flora are usually seen with oral flora or colonized *H influenzae* or *S pneumoniae* on culture. Paired sera for viral, mycoplasmal, and chlamydial titers can help make a diagnosis retrospectively in infants and children but are not clinically useful except for seriously ill patients.	Chronic bronchitis is diagnosed when sputum is coughed up on most days for at least 3 consecutive months for more than 2 successive years. Bacterial infections are usually secondary infections of initial viral or mycoplasma-induced inflammation. Airway endoscopy can aid in the diagnosis of bacterial tracheitis in children. J Infect 1997;35:189. Wien Klin Wochenschr 1997;109:574. J Clin Microbiol 1997;35:2435. Nurse Pract 1997;22:104. Infect Dis Clin North Am 1998;12:671. Monaldi Arch Chest Dis 1999;54:43. Can Respir J 1999;6:40A.

UPPER AIRWAY		
Epiglottitis		
Epiglottitis Child: *H influenzae* type B (GNCB). Adult: *S pyogenes* (GPC), *H influenzae*. HIV: Candida	Blood for bacterial culture: positive in 50–100% of children with *H influenzae*. Lateral neck x-ray may show an enlarged epiglottis but has a low sensitivity (31%).	Acute epiglottitis is a rapidly moving cellulitis of the epiglottis and represents an airway emergency. Epiglottitis can be confused with croup, a viral infection of gradual onset that affects infants and causes inspiratory and expiratory stridor. Airway management is the primary concern, and an endo-tracheal tube should be placed or tracheostomy performed as soon as the diagnosis of epiglottitis is made in children. A tracheostomy set should be at the bedside for adults. Am J Emerg Med 1996;14:421. Mayo Clin Proc 1998;73:1102. J Otolaryngol 1998;27:332. Pediatr Infect Dis J 1999;18:490.

	LUNG
	Community-Acquired Pneumonia

Organism	Specimen/Diagnostic Tests	Comments
Community-Acquired Pneumonia	Sputum for Gram stain desirable; culture, if empiric therapy fails or patient is seriously ill. An adequate specimen should have <10 epithelial cells and >25 PMNs per low-power field. Special sputum cultures for legionella are available. DFA for legionella sp has a sensitivity of 25–70% and a specificity of 95%. (Positive predictive value is low in areas of low disease prevalence.)	About 60% of cases of community-acquired pneumonia have an identifiable microbial cause. Pneumatoceles suggest *S aureus* but are also reported with pneumococcus, group A streptococcus, *H influenzae*, and Enterobacteriaceae (in neonates).
Neonate: *E coli* (GNR), group A or B streptococcus (GPC), *S aureus* (GPC), pseudomonas sp (GNR), *C trachomatis*.		
Infant/child (<5 years): Virus, *S pneumoniae* (GPC), *H influenzae* (GNCB), *S aureus*.	Blood for bacterial cultures, especially in ill patients.	An "atypical pneumonia" presentation (diffuse pattern on chest x-ray with lack of organisms on Gram stain of sputum) should raise suspicion of mycoplasma, legionella, or chlamydial infection. Consider hantavirus pulmonary syndrome if pulmonary symptoms follow afebrile illness.
Age 5–40 years: Virus, *M pneumoniae*, *C pneumoniae* (formerly known as TWAR strain), *C psittaci*, *S pneumoniae*, legionella sp.	Pleural fluid for bacterial culture if significant effusion is present.	
Age >40 without other disease: *S pneumoniae* (GPDC), *H influenzae* (GNCB), *S aureus* (GPC), *M catarrhalis* (GNDC), *C pneumoniae*, legionella sp (GNR), *C pseudodiphtheriticum* (GPR), *S pyogenes* (GPC), *K pneumoniae* (GNR), Enterobacteriaceae (GNR), *N meningitidis* (GNDC), viruses (eg. influenza)	Bronchoalveolar lavage or brushings for bacterial, fungal, and viral antigen tests and AFB culture in immunocompromised patients and atypical cases.	Aspirations are most commonly associated with stroke, alcoholism, drug abuse, sedation, and periodontal disease.
	Paired sera for *M pneumoniae* complement fixation testing can diagnose infection retrospectively.	Am Rev Resp Dis 1993;148:1418. Clin Infect Dis 1998;27:566. Clin Infect Dis 1998;26:811.
Cystic fibrosis: *P aeruginosa* (GNR), *Burkholderia cepacia*.	Serologic tests for *C pneumoniae*, *C psittaci* strains, and Q fever are available. Serologic tests and PCR for hantavirus (IgM and IgG) are available.	Lancet 1998;352:1295. Infect Dis Clin North Am 1998;12:689. Can Respir J 1999;6(Suppl A):15.
Elderly: *S pneumoniae* (GPDC), *H influenzae* (GNCB), *S aureus* (GPC), Enterobacteriaceae (GNR), *M catarrhalis* (GNDC), group B streptococcus (GPC), legionella (GNR), nocardia (GPR), influenza.	Other special techniques (bronchoscopy with telescoping plugged catheter on protected brush, transtracheal aspiration, transthoracic fine-needle aspiration, or, rarely, open lung biopsy) can be used to obtain specimens for culture in severe cases, in immunocompromised patients, or in cases with negative conventional cultures and progression despite empiric antibiotic therapy.	
Aspiration: *S pneumoniae* (GPDC), *K pneumoniae* (GNR), Enterobacteriaceae (GNR), bacteroides sp and other oral anaerobes.		
Fungal: *H capsulatum*, *C immitis*, *B dermatitidis*		
Exposure to birthing animals, sheep: *C burnetii* (Q fever), rabbits: *F tularensis* (tularemia), deer mice: hantavirus, birds: *C psittaci*.		

	LUNG	
	Anaerobic Pneumonia	**Hospital-Acquired Pneumonia**
Anaerobic Pneumonia/Lung Abscess Usually polymicrobial: bacteroides sp (15% *B fragilis*), peptostreptococcus, micro-aerophilic streptococcus, veillonella, *S aureus*, *P aeruginosa*, type 3 *S pneumoniae* (rare), klebsiella (rare).	Sputum Gram stain and culture for anaerobes are of little value because of contaminating oral flora. Bronchoalveolar sampling (brush or aspirate) for Gram stain will usually make an accurate diagnosis. As contamination is likely with a bronchoscope alone, a Bartlett tube should be used. Percutaneous transthoracic needle aspiration may be useful for culture and for cytology to demonstrate coexistence of an underlying carcinoma. Blood cultures are usually negative.	Aspiration is the most important background feature of lung abscess. Without clear-cut risk factors such as alcoholism, coma, or seizures, bronchoscopy is often performed to rule out neoplasm. Am J Ment Retard 1995;99:579. J Periodontol 1996;67:1114. Curr Opin Pulm Med 1997;3:120.
Hospital-Acquired Pneumonia *P aeruginosa* (GNR), klebsiella (GNR), *S aureus* (GPC), acinetobacter (GNR), Enterobacteriaceae (GNR), *S pneumoniae* (GPDC), *H influenzae* (GNCB), influenza virus, respiratory syncytial virus (RSV), legionella (GNR), oral anaerobes. Mendelson's syndrome (see comments): No organisms initially, then pseudomonas, Enterobacteriaceae, *S aureus*, *S pneumoniae*.	Sputum Gram stain and culture for bacteria (aerobic and anaerobic) and fungus (if suspected). Blood cultures for bacteria are often negative. Endotracheal aspirate or bronchoalveolar sample for bacterial and fungal culture in selected patients.	Most cases are related to aspiration. Hospital-acquired aspiration pneumonia is associated with intubation and the use of broad-spectrum antibiotics. A strong association between aspiration pneumonia and swallowing dysfunction is demonstrable by videofluoroscopy. Mendelson's syndrome is due to acute aspiration of gastric contents (eg, during anesthesia or drowning). Infect Dis Clin North Am 1997;11:427. Infect Dis Clin North Am 1998;12:761. Am J Med 1998;105:319. Chest 1999;115:28S.

	LUNG	
	Pneumonia in Immunocompromised Host	
Organism	**Specimen/Diagnostic Tests**	**Comments**
Pneumonia in the Immuno-compromised Host Child with HIV infection: Lymphoid interstitial pneumonia (LIP). AIDS: *M avium* (31%), *P carinii* (13%), cytomegalovirus (CMV) (11%), *H capsulatum* (7%), *S pneumoniae* (GPDC), *H influenzae* (GNCB), *P aeruginosa* (GNR), Enterobacteriaceae (GNR), *C neoformans*, *C pseudo-diphtheriticum* (GPR), *M tuberculosis* (AFB), *C immitis*, *P marneffei*, *Rhodococcus equi* (GPR). Neutropenic: Pseudomonas sp (GNR), klebsiella, enterobacter (GNR), bacteroides sp and other oral anaerobes, legionella, candida, aspergillus, mucor. Transplant recipients: Cytomegalovirus (CMV) (60–70%), *P aeruginosa* (GNR), *S aureus* (GPC), *S pneumoniae* (GPDC), legionella (GNR), respiratory syncytial virus (RSV), influenza virus, *P carinii*, aspergillus, *P boydii*, nocardia sp, strongyloides.	Expectorated sputum for Gram stain and bacterial culture, if purulent. Sputum induction or bronchiolar lavage for Giemsa or methenamine silver staining or direct fluorescent antibody (DFA) for *P carinii* trophozoites or cysts; for mycobacterial, fungal staining and culture, for legionella culture, and for CMV culture. Blood for CMV antigenemia or PCR from transplant patients. Blood or bone marrow fungal culture for histoplasmosis (positive in 50%), coccidioidomycosis (positive in 30%). Blood culture for bacteria. Blood cultures are more frequently positive in HIV-infected patients with bacterial pneumonia and often are the only source where a specific organism is identified; bacteremic patients have higher mortality rates. Histoplasma polysaccharide antigen positive in 90% of AIDS patients with disseminated histoplasmosis; antigen increases ≥ 2 RIA units with relapse. Immunodiffusion or CIE is useful for screening for, and CF for confirmation of, suspected histoplasmosis or coccidioidomycosis. Serum cryptococcal antigen when pulmonary cryptococcosis is suspected. Serum lactate dehydrogenase (LDH) levels are elevated in 63% and hypoxemia with exercise (Pao$_2$ < 75 mm Hg) occurs in 57% of PCP cases.	In PCP, the sensitivities of the various diagnostic tests are: sputum induction 80% (in experienced labs), bronchoscopy with lavage 90–97%, trans-bronchial biopsy 94–97%. In PCP, chest x-ray may show interstitial (36%) or alveolar (25%) infiltrates or may be normal (39%), particularly if leukopenia is present. Recurrent episodes of bacterial pneumonia are common. Kaposi's sarcoma of the lung is a common neoplastic process that can imitate infection in homosexual and African HIV-infected patients. J Antimicrob Chemother 1995;36(Suppl B):59. Semin Respir Infect 1996;11:119. Infect Dis Clin North Am 1998;12:781. J Thorac Imaging 1998;13:247. Haematologica 1999;84:71. Clin Infect Dis 1999;28:341.

LUNG		
Mycobacterial Pneumonia		
Mycobacterial Pneumonia *M tuberculosis* (MTb), *M kansasii*, *M avium-intracellulare* complex (AFB, acid-fast beaded rods).	Sputum for AFB stain and culture. First morning samples are best, and at least three samples are required. Culture systems detect mycobacterial growth in as little as several days to 6 weeks. Bronchoalveolar lavage for AFB stain and culture or gastric washings for AFB culture can be used if sputum tests are negative. Sputum or bronchoalveolar lavage for PCR to MTb available for confirmation of smear positive (99%), less sensitive for smear negative (75%). CT- or ultrasound-guided transthoracic fine-needle aspiration cytology can be used if clinical or radiographic features are nonspecific or if malignancy is suspected.	AFB found on sputum stain do not necessarily make the diagnosis of tuberculosis, because *M kansasii* and *M avium-intracellulare* look identical. Tuberculosis is very common in HIV-infected patients, in whom the chest x-ray appearance may be atypical and occasionally (4%) may mimic PCP (especially in patients with CD4 cell counts <200/µL). In one study, only 2% of patients sent for sputum induction for PCP had tuberculosis. Consider HIV testing if MTb is diagnosed. Delayed diagnosis of pulmonary tuberculosis is common (up to 20% of cases), especially among patients who are older or who do not have respiratory symptoms. In any patient with suspected tuberculosis, respiratory isolation is required. Chest 1998;114:317. Respiration 1998;65:163. CMAJ 1999;160:1725. Chest Surg Clin North Am 1999;9:227.

	LUNG	
	Empyema	
Organism	**Specimen/Diagnostic Tests**	**Comments**
Empyema Neonate: *E coli* (GNR), group A or B streptococcus (GPC), *S aureus* (GPC), pseudomonas sp (GNR). Infant/child (<5 years): *S aureus* (GPC), *S pneumoniae* (GPC), *H influenzae* (GNCB), anaerobes. Child (>5 years)/adult, Acute: *S pneumoniae* (GPC), group A streptococcus (GPC), *S aureus* (GPC), *H influenzae* (GNCB), legionella. Child (>5 years)/adult, chronic: Anaerobic streptococci, bacteroides sp, prevotella sp. porphyromonas sp. fusobacterium sp. Enterobacteriaceae, *E coli*, *Klebsiella pneumoniae*, *M tuberculosis*.	Pleural fluid for cell count (WBCs 25,000–100,000/μL, mostly PMNs), protein (>50% of serum), glucose (< serum, often very low), pH (<7.20), LDH (>60% of serum). (See Pleural fluid profiles, p 382.) Blood cultures for bacteria. Sputum for Gram stain and bacterial culture. Special culture can also be performed for legionella when suspected. Pleural fluid for Gram stain and bacterial culture (aerobic and anaerobic).	Chest tube drainage is paramount. The clinical presentation of empyema is nonspecific. Chest CT with contrast is helpful in demonstrating pleural fluid accumulations due to mediastinal or subdiaphragmatic processes and can identify loculated effusions, bronchopleural fistulae, and lung abscesses. About 25% of cases result from trauma or surgery. Bronchoscopy is indicated when the infection is unexplained. Occasionally, multiple thoracenteses may be needed to diagnose empyema. Curr Opin Pulm Med 1998;4:185. Clin Chest Med 1998;19:363. Semin Respir Infect 1999;14:18. Semin Respir Infect 1999;14:82.

HEART AND VESSELS		
Pericarditis		**Tuberculous Pericarditis**
Pericarditis Viruses: Enteroviruses (coxsackie, echo), influenza, Epstein-Barr, herpes zoster, mumps, HIV, CMV. Bacteria: *S aureus* (GPC), *S pneumoniae* (GPC), mycoplasma, *S pyogenes* (GPC), Enterobacteriaceae (GNR), *N meningitidis* (GNDC). Fungi: Candida (immunocompromised)	In acute pericarditis, specific bacterial diagnosis is made in only 19%. Pericardial fluid aspirate for Gram stain and bacterial culture (aerobic and anaerobic). In acute pericarditis, only 54% have pericardial effusions. Blood for buffy coat, stool or throat for enteroviral culture. PCR available in reference laboratories. Surgical pericardial drainage with biopsy of pericardium for culture (22%) and histologic examination. Paired sera for enterovirus (coxsackie) and mycoplasma.	Viral pericarditis is usually diagnosed clinically (precordial pain, muffled heart sounds, pericardial friction rub, cardiomegaly). The diagnosis is rarely aided by microbiologic tests. CT and MRI may demonstrate pericardial thickening. Bacterial pericarditis is usually secondary to surgery, immunosuppression (including HIV), esophageal rupture, endocarditis with ruptured ring abscess, extension from lung abscess, aspiration pneumonia or empyema, or sepsis with pericarditis. Ann Thorac Surg 1997;63:1200. Emerg Med Clin North Am 1998;16:665. Am Heart J 1999;137:516. Clin Cardiol 1999;22:334.
Tuberculous Pericarditis *Mycobacterium tuberculosis* (MTb, AFB, acid-fast beaded rods)	PPD skin testing should be performed (negative in a sizable minority). Pericardial fluid obtained by needle aspiration can show AFB by smear (rare) or culture (low yield). The yield is improved by obtaining three or four repeated specimens for smear and culture. Pericardial biopsy for culture and histologic examination has highest diagnostic yield. Other sources of culture for MTb besides pericardium are available in 50% of patients. Pericardial fluid may show markedly elevated levels of adenosine deaminase.	Spread from nearby caseous mediastinal lymph nodes or pleurisy is the most common route of infection. Acutely, serofibrinous pericardial effusion develops with substernal pain, fever, and friction rub. Tamponade may occur. Tuberculosis accounts for 4% of cases of acute pericarditis, 7% of cases of cardiac tamponade, and 6% of cases of constrictive pericarditis. One-third to one-half of patients develop constrictive pericarditis despite drug therapy. Constrictive pericarditis occurs 2–4 years after acute infection. JAMA 1991;266:91. Intern Med 1993;32:675. Am Heart J 1993;126:249. J Infect 1997;35:215.

	HEART AND VESSELS
	Infectious Myocarditis

Organism	Specimen/Diagnostic Tests	Comments
Infectious Myocarditis Enteroviruses (especially coxsackie B), adenovirus, influenza virus, HIV, *Borrelia burgdorferi* (Lyme disease), scrub typhus, *Rickettsia rickettsii* (Rocky Mountain spotted fever), *Coxiella burnetii* (Q fever), *Mycoplasma pneumoniae, Chlamydia pneumoniae, C diphtheriae* (GPR), *Trichinella spiralis* (trichinosis), *Trypanosoma cruzi* (Chagas' disease), toxoplasma.	Endomyocardial biopsy for pathologic examination, PCR, and culture in selected cases. Indium-111 antimyosin antibody imaging is more sensitive than endomyocardial biopsy. Stool or throat swab for enterovirus culture. Blood for enterovirus PCR (reference labs) and culture of white cells. Paired sera for coxsackie B, *Mycoplasma pneumoniae, Chlamydia pneumoniae*, scrub typhus, *Rickettsia rickettsii, Coxiella burnetii*, trichinella, toxoplasma. Single serum for HIV, *Borrelia burgdorferi, Trypanosoma cruzi.* Gallium scanning is sensitive but not specific for myocardial inflammation. Antimyosin antibody scintigraphy has a high specificity but a lower sensitivity for the detection of myocarditis.	Acute infectious myocarditis should be suspected in a patient with dynamically evolving changes in ECG, echocardiography, and serum CK levels and symptoms of an infection. The value of endomyocardial biopsy in such cases has not been established. In contrast, an endomyocardial biopsy is needed to diagnose lymphocytic or giant cell myocarditis. The incidence of myocarditis in AIDS may be as high as 46%. Many patients with acute myocarditis progress to dilated cardiomyopathy. Adv Pediatr 1997;44:141. J Infect 1998;37:99. J Am Coll Cardiol 1998;32:1371. Emerg Med Clin North Am 1998;16:665. Adv Intern Med 1999;44:293. Circulation 1999;99:2011.

HEART AND VESSELS
Infective Endocarditis

Infective Endocarditis		
Viridans group streptococci (GPC), enterococcus (GPC), nutritionally deficient streptococcus (GPC), *S aureus* (GPC), *S pneumoniae* (GPC), *Erysipelothrix rhusiopathiae* (GPR), brucella (GNR), *Coxiella burnetii, C pneumoniae*. Slow-growing fastidious GNRs: *H parainfluenzae, H aphrophilus,* actinobacillus, cardiobacterium, capnocytophaga, eikenella, kingella (HACEK).	Blood cultures for bacteria. Three blood cultures are sufficient in 97% of cases. Blood cultures are frequently positive with gram-positive organisms but can be negative with gram-negative or anaerobic organisms. If the patient is not acutely ill, therapy can begin after cultures identify an organism. Transesophageal echocardiography (TEE) can help in diagnosis by demonstrating the presence of valvular vegetations (sensitivity > 90%), prosthetic valve dysfunction, valvular regurgitation, secondary "jet" or "kissing" lesions, and paravalvular abscess. SPECT immunoscintigraphy with antigranulocyte antibody can be used in cases of suspected infective endocarditis if echocardiography is non-diagnostic.	Patients with congenital or valvular heart disease should receive prophylaxis before dental procedures or surgery of the upper respiratory, genitourinary, or gastrointestinal tract. In left-sided endocarditis, patients should be watched carefully for development of valvular regurgitation or ring abscess. The size and mobility of valvular vegetations on TEE can help to predict the risk of arterial embolization. Clin Infect Dis 1997;25:1448. Infect Dis Clin North Am 1999;13:833. Clin Infect Dis 1999;29:1. Clin Infect Dis 1999;46:275. J Infection 1999;39:27. Am J Med 1999;107:198. J Infection 1999;38:87. Postgrad Med J 1999;75:540. Clin Infect Dis 1999;28:106.

HEART AND VESSELS
Prosthetic Valve Infective Endocarditis

Organism	Specimen/Diagnostic Tests	Comments
Prosthetic Valve Infective Endocarditis (PVE) Early (<2 months): Coagulase-negative staphylococci (usually *S epidermidis* with 80% methicillin-resistant) (GPC) (27%), *S aureus* (GPC) (20%), Enterobacteriaceae (GNR), diphtheroids (GPR), candida (yeast). Late (>2 months): Viridans group streptococci (GPC) (42%), coagulase-negative staphylococci (21%), *S aureus* (11%), enterococcus (GPC), Enterobacteriaceae.	Blood cultures for bacteria and yeast. Three sets of blood cultures are sufficient in 97% of cases. Draw blood cultures before temperature spike. While more invasive, transesophageal echocardiography is superior in predicting which patients with infective endocarditis have perivalvular abscess or prosthetic valve dysfunction and which are most susceptible to systemic embolism.	In a large series using perioperative prophylaxis, the incidences of early-onset and late-onset prosthetic valve endocarditis were 0.78% and 1.1%, respectively. The portals of entry of early-onset PVE are intraoperative contamination and postoperative wound infections. The portals of entry of late-onset PVE appear to be the same as those of native valve endocarditis, and the microbiologic profiles are also similar. Clinically, patients with late-onset PVE resemble those with native valve disease. However, those with early-onset infection are often critically ill, more often have other complicating problems, are more likely to go into shock and are more likely to have conduction abnormalities due to ring abscess. Medicine (Baltimore) 1997;76:94. Clin Infect Dis 1997;24:884. J Infect 1999;39:27.

HEART AND VESSELS		
Infectious Thrombophlebitis		
Infectious Thrombophlebitis Associated with venous catheters: *S aureus* (GPC) (65–78%), coagulase-negative staphylococci (GPC), candida sp (yeast), pseudomonas sp (GNR), Entero-bacteriaceae (GNR). Hyperalimentation with catheter: Candida sp, *Malassezia furfur* (yeast). Indwelling venous catheter (eg, Broviac, Hickman, Gershorn): *S aureus*, coagulase-negative staphylococci, diphtheroids (GPR), pseudomonas sp, Entero-bacteriaceae, candida sp. Postpartum or post-abortion pelvic thrombophlebitis: Bacteroides (GNR), Enterobacteriaceae, clos-tridium (GPR), streptococcus (GPC).	Blood cultures for bacteria (positive in 80–90%). Catheter tip for bacterial culture to document etiol-ogy. More than 15 colonies (CFUs) suggests colonization or infection. CT and MRI are the studies of choice in the evalua-tion of puerperal septic pelvic thrombophlebitis.	Thrombophlebitis is an inflammation of the vein wall. Infectious thrombophlebitis is associated with microbial invasion of the vessel and is associated with bacteremia and thrombosis. Risk of infection from an indwelling peripheral venous catheter goes up significantly after 4 days. Arch Surg 1996;131:95. AJR Am J Roentgenol 1997;169:1039. Pediatr Infect Dis J 1997;16:63. World J Surg 1999;23:589. Support Care Cancer 1999;7:386. Infection 1999;27(Suppl 1):S11.

ABDOMEN		
	Gastritis	Infectious Esophagitis

Organism	Specimen/Diagnostic Tests	Comments
Gastritis *Helicobacter pylori*	Serum for antibody test (76–90% sensitivity but low specificity) (see p 100). Stool for antigen detection test and [^{13}C]urea breath test (99%) are specific noninvasive tests. Gastric mucosal biopsy for rapid urea test (89%), culture (89%), histology (92%), and PCR (99%) (reference laboratories).	Also associated with duodenal ulcer, gastric carcinoma, and gastroesophageal reflux disease. Clin Microbiol Rev 1997;10:720. Aliment Pharmacol Ther 1998;12 (Suppl 1):61.] J Clin Microbiol 1999;37:3328. J Gastroenterol 1999;34(Suppl 11):67. J Clin Microbiol 2000;38:13. Am J Gastroenterol 2000;95:72.
Infectious Esophagitis Candida sp (yeast), herpes simplex (HSV), cytomegalovirus (CMV), varicella-zoster (VZV), *Helicobacter pylori* (GNR), cryptosporidium. (Rare causes: *Mycobacterium tuberculosis* [AFB], aspergillus, histoplasma, blastomyces, HIV).	Barium esophagram reveals abnormalities in the majority of cases of candidal esophagitis. Endoscopy with biopsy and brushings for culture and cytology has the highest diagnostic yield (57%) and should be performed if clinically indicated or if empiric antifungal therapy is unsuccessful.	Thrush and odynophagia in an immunocompromised patient warrants empiric therapy for candida. Factors predisposing to infectious esophagitis include HIV infection, exposure to radiation, cytotoxic chemotherapy, recent antibiotic therapy, corticosteroid therapy, and neutropenia. Gastrointest Endosc 1996;44:587. Med Pediatr Oncol 1997;28:299. Am J Gastroenterol 1998;93:394, 2239. Am J Gastroenterol 1999;94:339.

ABDOMEN

Infectious Colitis/Dysentery

Infectious Colitis/Dysentery		
Infant: *E coli* (enteropathogenic). Child/Adult without travel, afebrile, no gross blood or WBCs in stool: Rotaviruses, caliciviruses (eg, Norwalk agent), *E coli* (GNR). Child/Adult with fever, bloody stool or history of travel to subtropics/tropics (varies with epidemiology): *Campylobacter jejuni* (GNR), *E coli* (GNR). (enterotoxigenic, enteroinvasive, enterohemorrhagic O157:H7), shigella (GNR), salmonella (GNR), *Yersinia enterocolitica* (GNR), *Clostridium difficile* (GPR), aeromonas (GNR), vibrio (GNR), cryptosporidium, *Entamoeba histolytica, Giardia lamblia*, cyclospora, strongyloides, edwardsiella (GNR). Child/Adult with vomiting and no fever: *S aureus* (GPC), *Bacillus cereus* (GPR).	Stool for occult blood helpful to diagnosis of *E coli* O157:H7, salmonella, *E histolytica*. Stool collected culture, ova and parasites examination. Two samples are often needed. The sensitivity of the stool culture is only 72%, but its specificity is 100% (using PCR as standard). One repeat culture may increase sensitivity. Special culture technique is needed for yersinia, *E coli*, and vibrio. Cultures for salmonella or shigella are not helpful in patients hospitalized more than 72 hours. Proctosigmoidoscopy is indicated in patients with chronic or recurrent diarrhea or in diarrhea of unknown cause for smears of aspirates (may show organisms) and biopsy. Cultures of biopsy specimens have somewhat higher sensitivities than stool cultures. Rectal and jejunal biopsies may be necessary in HIV-infected patients. Need modified acid-fast stain for cryptosporidium. Immunodiagnosis of *G lamblia*, cryptosporidium, or *E histolytica* cysts in stool is highly sensitive and specific.	Acute dysentery is diarrhea with bloody, mucoid stools, tenesmus, and pain on defecation and implies an inflammatory invasion of the colonic mucosa. BUN and serum electrolytes may be indicated for supportive care. Severe dehydration is a medical emergency. Necrotizing enterocolitis is a fulminant disease of premature newborns; cause is unknown but human breast milk is protective. Air in the intestinal wall (pneumatosis intestinalis), in the portal venous system, or in the peritoneal cavity seen on plain x-ray can confirm diagnosis. 30–50% of these infants will have bacteremia or peritonitis. Risk factors for infectious colitis include poor hygiene and immune compromise (infancy, advanced age, corticosteroid or immunosuppressive therapy, HIV infection). J Infect 1996 Nov;33:143. Arch Virol Suppl 1997;13:153. J Infect Dis. 1997 Dec;176 (Suppl 2):S103. Am Fam Physician 1998;58:1769. J Diarrhoeal Dis Res. 1998;16:248. Adv Pediatr 1999;46:353. Emerg Infect Dis 1999;5:607. Annu Rev Med 1999;50:355. Clin Lab Med 1999;19:553, 691. Clin Infect Dis 1999;29:356.

	ABDOMEN
	Antibiotic-Associated Colitis

Organism	Specimen / Diagnostic Tests	Comments
Antibiotic-Associated Pseudomembranous Colitis *Clostridium difficile* (GPR) toxin, *Clostridium perfringens* (GPR), *Staphylococcus aureus* (GPC), *Klebsiella oxytoca* (GNR).	Send stool for *C difficile*, cytotoxin A by tissue culture or toxin A or A and B by less sensitive immunoassay. Testing two stools on different days will increase sensitivity; toxin testing for test-of-cure is not recommended. Fecal WBCs are present in 30–50% of cases. The toxin is very labile and can be present in infants with no disease. Stool culture is not recommended because non-toxigenic strains occur. Colonoscopy and visualization of characteristic 1–5 mm raised yellow plaques provides the most rapid diagnosis. However, an ultrasound appearance of grossly thickened bowel wall with luminal narrowing or CT findings of thickened bowel wall, presence of an "accordion" sign, heterogeneous contrast enhancement pattern ("target sign"), pericolonic stranding, ascites, pleural effusion, and subcutaneous edema can suggest the diagnosis of pseudomembranous colitis.	Antibiotics cause changes in normal intestinal flora, allowing overgrowth of *C difficile* and elaboration of toxin. Other risk factors for *C difficile*-induced colitis are GI manipulations, advanced age, female sex, inflammatory bowel disease, HIV, chemotherapy, and renal disease. *C difficile* nosocomial infection can be controlled by handwashing. Antibiotic-associated diarrhea may include uncomplicated diarrhea, colitis, or pseudomembranous colitis. Only 10–20% of cases are caused by infection with *C difficile*. Most clinically mild cases are due to functional disturbances of intestinal carbohydrate or bile acid metabolism, to allergic and toxic effects of antibiotics on intestinal mucosa, or to their pharmacologic effects on motility. Radiolog 1996;198:1. Clin Infect Dis 1998;27:702. Dig Dis 1998;16:292. Dis Colon Rectum 1998;41:1435. J Antimicrob Chemother 1998;41 (Suppl C):29, 59. Digestion 1999;60:91. Hepatogastroenterology 1999;46:343.

ABDOMEN	
Diarrhea in HIV	
Diarrhea in the HIV-Infected Host Same as Child-Adult Infectious Colitis with addition of cytomegalovirus, cryptosporidium, *Isospora belli*, microsporidia (*Enterocytozoon bieneusi*), *C difficile*, *Giardia intestinalis*, *Mycobacterium avium-intracellulare* complex (AFB), herpes simplex (HSV), *Entamoeba histolytica*, ?HIV.	Stool for stain for fecal leukocytes, culture (especially for salmonella, shigella, yersinia, and campylobacter), *C difficile* toxin, ova and parasite examination, and AFB smear. Multiple samples are often needed. Proctosigmoidoscopy with fluid aspiration and biopsy is indicated in patients with chronic or recurrent diarrhea or in diarrhea of unknown cause for smears of aspirates (may show organisms) and histologic examination and culture of tissue. Rectal and jejunal biopsies may be necessary, especially in patients with tenesmus or bloody stools. Need modified acid-fast stain for cryptosporidium. Intranuclear inclusion bodies on histologic exam suggest CMV. Immunodiagnosis of giardia, cryptosporidium, and *E histolytical* cysts in stool is highly sensitive and specific.	Most patients with HIV infection will develop diarrhea at some point in their illness. Cryptosporidium causes a chronic debilitating diarrheal infection that rarely remits spontaneously and is still without effective treatment. Diarrhea seems to be the result of malabsorption and produces a cholera-like syndrome. Between 15% and 50% of HIV-infected patients with diarrhea have no identifiable pathogen. J Clin Microbiol 1995;33:745. Gastroenterology 1996;111:1724. Gastrointest Endosc Clin North Am 1998;8:857. J Infect Dis 1999;179(Suppl 3):S454. Am J Gastroenterol 1999;94:596. Arch Intern Med 1999;159:1473.

	ABDOMEN
	Peritonitis

Organism	Specimen / Diagnostic Tests	Comments
Peritonitis	Peritoneal fluid sent for WBC (> 1000/μL in SPB, > 100/μL in CAPD) with PMN (≥ 250/μL SBP and secondary peritonitis, 50% PMN in CAPD): total protein (> 1 gd/L); glucose (< 50 mg/dL) and lactate dehydrogenase (> 225 units/mL) in secondary: pH (< 7.35 in 57% for SBP). Gram stain (22–77% for SBP), and culture of large volumes often in blood culture bottles. (See Ascitic fluid profiles, p 365.)	In nephrotic patients, Enterobacteriaceae and *S aureus* are most frequent. In cirrhotics, 69% of cases are due to Enterobacteriaceae. Cirrhotic patients with low ascitic fluid protein levels (≤ 1 g/dL) and high bilirubin level or low platelet count are at high risk of developing spontaneous bacterial peritonitis.
Spontaneous or primary (associated with nephrosis or cirrhosis) peritonitis (SBP): Enterobacteriaceae (GNR) (69%), *S pneumoniae* (GPC), group A streptococcus (GPC), *S aureus* (GPC), anaerobes (5%).		"Bacterascites," a positive ascitic fluid culture without an elevated PMN count, is seen in 8% of cases of SBP and probably represents early infection.
Secondary (bowel perforation, hospital-acquired, or antecedent antibiotic therapy): Enterobacteriaceae, enterococcus (GPC), bacteroides sp (GNR), *Pseudomonas aeruginosa* (GNR) (3–15%).	Blood cultures for bacteria positive in 75% of SBP cases. Catheter-related infection is associated with a WBC > 500/μL.	In secondary peritonitis, factors influencing the incidence of postoperative complications and death include age, presence of certain concomitant diseases, site of origin of peritonitis, type of admission, and the ability of the surgeon to eliminate the source of infection.
Chronic ambulatory peritoneal dialysis (CAPD): Coagulase-negative staphylococci (GPC) (43%), *S aureus* (14%), streptococcus sp (12%), Enterobacteriaceae (14%), *Pseudomonas aeruginosa*, candida (2%), aspergillus (rare), cryptococcus (rare).		Clin Infect Dis 1998;27:669. Eur J Clin Microbiol Infect Dis 1998;17:542. J Am Soc Nephrol 1998;9:1956. Langenbecks Arch Surg 1999;384:24. Gastroenterology 1999;117:414.

ABDOMEN
Tuberculous Peritonitis/Enterocolitis

| Tuberculous Peritonitis/Enterocolitis

Mycobacterium tuberculosis (MTb, AFB, acid-fast beaded rods). | Ascitic fluid for appearance (clear, hemorrhagic or chylous), RBCs (can be high), WBCs (> 1000/μL, > 70% lymphs), protein (> 2.5 g/dL), serum/ascites albumin gradient (<1.1), LDH (> 90 units/L), AFB culture (<50% positive). (See Ascitic fluid profiles, p 365.) With coexistent chronic liver disease, protein level and SAAG are usually not helpful, but LDH > 90 units/L is a useful predictor.
Culture or AFB smear from other sources (especially from respiratory tract) can help confirm diagnosis.
Abdominal ultrasound may demonstrate free or loculated intra-abdominal fluid, intra-abdominal abscess, ileocecal mass, and retroperitoneal lymphadenopathy. Ascites with fine, mobile septations shown by ultrasound and peritoneal and omental thickening detected by CT strongly suggest tuberculous peritonitis.
Marked elevations of serum CA 125 have been noted; levels decline to normal with anti-tuberculous therapy.
Diagnosis of enterocolitis rests on biopsy of colonic lesions via endoscopy if pulmonary or other extra-pulmonary infection cannot be documented.
Diagnosis is best confirmed by laparoscopy with peritoneal biopsy and culture.
Operative procedure may be needed to relieve obstruction or for diagnosis. | Infection of the intestines can occur anywhere along the GI tract but occurs most commonly in the ileo-cecal area or mesenteric lymph nodes. It often complicates pulmonary infection. Peritoneal infection usually is an extension of intestinal disease. Symptoms may be minimal even with extensive disease.
In the US, 29% of patients with abdominal tuberculosis have a normal chest x-ray.
Presence of AFB in the feces does not correlate with intestinal involvement.
Acta Radiologica 1996;37:517.
AJR Am J Roentgenol 1996;167:743.
Am J Med 1996;100:179.
Rays 1998;23:115.
Eur J Surg 1999;165:158.
South Med J 1999;92:406. |

ABDOMEN

	Organism	Specimen/Diagnostic Tests	Comments
Diverticulitis	Enterobacteriaceae (GNR), bacteroides sp (GNR), enterococcus (GPC in chains).	Identification of organism is not usually sought. Ultrasonography (US) or flat and upright x-rays of abdomen are crucial to rule out perforation (free air under diaphragm) and to localize abscess (air-fluid collections). Barium enema can (82%) show presence of diverticula. Avoid enemas in acute disease because increased intraluminal pressure may cause perforation. Ultrasound (85%) and CT (79–98%) have greater accuracy in the evaluation of patients with diverticulitis. Specificities of barium enema, ultrasound, and CT are 81–84%. Thin-section helical CT is also able to reveal inflamed diverticula in acute diverticulitis by demonstrating an enhancing pattern of the colonic wall. Urinalysis will reveal urinary tract involvement, if present.	Pain usually is localized to the left lower quadrant because the sigmoid and descending colon are the most common sites for diverticula. It is important to rule out other abdominal disease (eg, colon carcinoma, Crohn's disease, ischemic colitis). Acta Radiologica 1997;38:313. Radiology 1997;205:503. Dis Colon Rect 1998;41:1023. Radiology 1998;208:611. N Engl J Med 1998;338:1521. AJR Am J Roentgenol 1999;172:601. Surg Endosc 1999;13:430.
Liver Abscess	Usually polymicrobial: Enterobacteriaceae, especially klebsiella (GNR), enterococcus (GPC in chains), bacteroides sp (GNR), actinomyces (GPR), *S aureus* (GPC in clusters), candida sp, *Entamoeba histolytica*.	CT scan with contrast and ultrasonography are the most accurate tests for the diagnosis of liver abscess. Antibodies against *E histolytica* should be obtained on all patients. (See Amebic serology, p 50.) Complete removal of abscess material obtained via surgery or percutaneous aspiration is recommended for culture and direct examination for *E histolytica*. *E histolytica* has been described with modern techniques as a complex of two species, the commensal parasite *E dispar* and the pathogenic parasite. Stool for antigen detection is sensitive and can distinguish the two species. Chest x-ray is often useful with raised hemidiaphragm, right pleural effusion, or right basilar atelectasis in 41% of patients. Elevation of serum alkaline phosphatase level in 78%.	Travel to and origin in an endemic area are important risk factors for amebic liver abscess. 60% of patients have a single lesion; 40% have multiple lesions. Biliary tract disease is the most common underlying disease, including malignancy (biliary tract or pancreatic), colonic disease (diverticulitis), diabetes mellitus, liver disease, and alcoholism. Clin Radiol 1997;52:912. South Med J 1997;90:23. Ann Emerg Med 1999;34:351. World J Surg 1999;23:102. West J Med 1999;170:104.

ABDOMEN
Cholangitis/Cholecystitis

Cholangitis/Cholecystitis		
Enterobacteriaceae (GNR) (68%), enterococcus (GPC in chains) (14%), *Pseudomonas aeruginosa* (GNR), bacteroides (GNR) (10%), clostridium sp (GPR) (7%), microsporidia (*Enterocytozoon bieneusi*), *Ascaris lumbricoides, Opisthorchis viverrini, O felineus, Clonorchis sinensis, Fasciola hepatica, Echinococcus granulosus, E multilocularis,* hepatitis C virus, hepatitis B virus, cytomegalovirus.	Ultrasonography is the best test to quickly demonstrate gallstones or phlegmon around the gallbladder or dilation of the biliary tree. (See Abdominal Ultrasound, p 258.) CT scanning is useful in cholangitis in detecting the site and cause of obstruction but may fail to detect stones in the common bile duct. In acute cholecystitis, ultrasonography is superior to MR cholangiography in evaluating gallbladder wall thickening. However, MR cholangiography is superior to ultrasound in depicting cystic duct and gallbladder neck stones and in evaluating cystic duct obstruction. Radionuclide scans can demonstrate cystic duct obstruction. (See p 266.) Blood cultures for bacteria.	90% of cases of acute cholecystitis are calculous, 10% are acalculous. Risk factors for acalculous disease include prolonged illness, fasting, hyperalimentation, HIV infection, and carcinoma of the gallbladder or bile ducts. Biliary obstruction and cholangitis can develop before biliary dilation is detected. Common bile duct obstruction secondary to tumor or pancreatitis seldom results in infection (0–15%). There is a high incidence of acalculous cholecystitis in AIDS patients with CD4 counts <200/μL, due to cryptosporidium, cytomegalovirus, yeast, tuberculosis, and *Mycobacterium avium-intracellulare.* Observation of gallbladder contraction on hepatobiliary scintigraphy after intravenous cholecystokinin excludes acalculous cholecystitis. Radiology 1998;209:781. Mayo Clin Proc 1998;73:473, 479. Radiology 1999;211:373.

	GENITOURINARY	
	Urinary Tract Infection	
Organism	**Specimen / Diagnostic Tests**	**Comments**
Urinary Tract Infection (UTI)/Cystitis/Pyuria-Dysuria Syndrome Enterobacteriaceae (GNR, especially *E coli*), *Chlamydia trachomatis*, *Staphylococcus saprophyticus* (GPC) (in young women), enterococcus (GPC), candida sp (yeast), *N gonorrhoeae* (GNCB), HSV, adenovirus, *Corynebacterium glucuronolyticum* (GPR), Urea plasma, *urealyticum* (GPR).	Urinalysis and culture reveal the two most important signs: bacteriuria and pyuria (> 10 WBCs/μL). 30% of patients have hematuria. Cystitis (95%) is diagnosed by ≥ 10^2 CFU/mL of bacteria; other urinary infections (90%) by ≥ 10^5 CFU/mL. Culture is generally not necessary for uncomplicated cystitis in women. However, pregnant women should be screened for asymptomatic bacteriuria and promptly treated. Both Gram stain for bacteria and dipstick analysis for nitrite and leukocyte esterase perform similarly in detecting UTI in children and are superior to microscopic analysis for pyuria. Intravenous pyelogram and cystoscopy should be performed in women with recurrent or childhood infections, all young boys with UTI, men with recurrent or complicated infection, and patients with symptoms suggestive of obstruction or renal stones. (See Intravenous pyelogram, p 273.)	Most men with urinary tract infections have a functional or anatomic genitourinary abnormality. In catheter-related UTI, cure is unlikely unless the catheter is removed. In asymptomatic catheter-related UTI, antibiotics should be given only if patients are at risk for sepsis (old age, underlying disease, diabetes mellitus, pregnancy). Up to one-third of cases of acute cystitis have "silent" upper tract involvement. Infect Dis Clin North Am 1997;11:13 Infect Dis Clin North Am 1997;11:609. Pediatrics 1999;103(4 Part 1):843. Urol Clin North Am 1999;26:821. Nephrol Dial Transplant 1999;14:2746. Am J Med 1999;106:636. Postgrad Med 1999;105:181. BMJ 1999;318:770.

GENITOURINARY		
Prostatitis		
Prostatitis		
Acute and Chronic: Enterobacteriaceae (GNR), pseudomonas sp (GNR), enterococcus (GPC in chains), cytomegalovirus (CMV).	Urinalysis shows pyuria. Urine culture usually identifies causative organism. Prostatic massage is useful in chronic prostatitis to retrieve organisms but is contraindicated in acute prostatitis (it may cause bacteremia). Bacteriuria is first cleared by antibiotic treatment. Then urine cultures are obtained from first-void, bladder, and post-prostatic massage urine specimens. A higher organism count in the post-prostatic massage specimen localizes infection to the prostate (91%).	Acute prostatitis is a severe illness characterized by fever, dysuria, and a boggy or tender prostate. Chronic prostatitis often has no symptoms of dysuria or perineal discomfort and a normal prostate examination. Nonbacterial prostatitis (prostatodynia) represents 90% of prostatitis cases. Its etiology is unknown, although chlamydia antigen can be found in up to 25% of patients. Int J STD AIDS 1997;8:475. Clin Microbiol Rev 1998;11:604. Int J Clin Pract 1998;52:540. Am J Med 1999;106:327. Sex Transm Infect 1999;75(Suppl 1):S46. Urol Clin North Am 1999;26:737.

	GENITOURINARY	
	Pyelonephritis	**Perinephric Abscess**

Organism	Specimen/Diagnostic Tests	Comments
Pyelonephritis Acute, uncomplicated (usually young women): Enterobacteriaceae (especially *E coli*) (GNR). Complicated (older women, men; post-catheterization, obstruction, post-renal transplant): Enterobacteriaceae (especially *E coli*), *Pseudomonas aeruginosa* (GNR), enterococcus (GPC), *Staphylococcus saprophyticus* (GPC).	Urine culture is indicated when pyelonephritis is suspected. Urinalysis will usually show pyuria (≥ 5 WBC/hpf) and may show WBC casts. Blood cultures for bacteria if sepsis is suspected. In uncomplicated pyelonephritis, ultrasonography is not necessary. In severe cases, however, ultrasound is the optimal procedure for ruling out urinary tract obstruction, pyonephrosis, and calculi. Doppler ultrasonography (88%) has a specificity of 100% for acute pyelonephritis. Intravenous pyelogram in patients with recurrent infection will show irregularly outlined renal pelvis with caliectasis and cortical scars. (See Intravenous pyelogram, p 273.)	Patients usually present with fever, chills, nausea, vomiting, and costovertebral angle tenderness. 20–30% of pregnant women with untreated bacteriuria develop pyelonephritis. Brit J Urol 1998;81:360. Int J Antimicrob Ag 1999;11:257. Clin Obstet Gynecol 1998;41:515. Urol Clin North Am 1999;26:753.
Perinephric Abscess Associated with staphylococcal bacteremia: *Staphylococcus aureus* (GPC). Associated with pyelonephritis: Enterobacteriaceae (GNR), candida sp (yeast), coagulase-negative staphylococci (GPC).	CT scan with contrast is more sensitive than ultrasound in imaging abscess and confirming diagnosis. (See Abdominal CT, p 259.) Urinalysis may be normal or may show pyuria. Urine culture (positive in 60%). Blood cultures for bacteria (positive in 20–40%). Bacterial culture of abscess fluid via needle aspiration or drainage (percutaneous or surgical).	Most perinephric abscesses are the result of extension of an ascending urinary tract infection. Often they are very difficult to diagnose. They should be considered in patients who fail to respond to antibiotic therapy, in patients with anatomic abnormalities of the urinary tract, and in patients with diabetes mellitus. Hosp Pract (Off Ed) 1997;32(6):40. Infect Dis Clin North Am 1997;11:663.

GENITOURINARY

	Urethritis	Epididymitis/Orchitis

Urethritis (Gonococcal and Nongonococcal)

Organisms:
Gonococcal (GC): Neisseria gonorrhoeae (GNDC).
Nongonococcal (NGU): Chlamydia trachomatis (50%), Ureaplasma urealyticum, Trichomonas vaginalis, herpes simplex (HSV), Mycoplasma genitalium, unknown (35%).

Specimen/Diagnostic Tests:
Urethral discharge collected with urethral swab usually shows ≥4 WBCs per oil immersion field, Gram stain (identify gonococcal organisms as gram-negative intracellular diplococci), PMNs (in GC, >95% of WBCs are PMNs, in NGU usually <80% are PMNs).
Urethral discharge for culture (80%) or nucleic acid assay (97%) for GC (usually not needed for diagnosis); urine (80–92%) or urethral discharge (97%) for detection of C trachomatis by nucleic acid amplification or wet mount for T vaginalis. Culture or nonamplified assays are considerably less sensitive for diagnosis of C trachomatis.
VDRL should be checked in all patients because of high incidence of associated syphilis.

Comments:
About 50% of patients with GC will have concomitant NGU infection.
Always treat sexual partners. Recurrence may be secondary to failure to treat partners. Half of the cases of nongonococcal urethritis (NGU) are not due to Chlamydia trachomatis; frequently, no pathogen can be isolated.
Persistent or recurrent episodes with adequate treatment of patient and partners may warrant further evaluation for other causes (eg, prostatitis).
MMWR Morb Mortal Wkly Rep 1998;47(RR-1):1.
Dermatol Clinic 1998;16:723.
Sex Transm Infect 1999;75(Suppl 1):S9
Aust Fam Physician 1999;28:333.
Clin Infect Dis 1999;28(Suppl 1):S66.
FEMS Immunol Med Microbiol 1999;24:437.

Epididymitis/Orchitis

Organisms:
Age <35 years, homosexual men: Chlamydia trachomatis, N gonorrhoeae (GNDC).
Age >35 years, or children: Enterobacteriaceae (especially E coli) (GNR), pseudomonas sp (GNR), salmonella (GNR), Haemophilus influenzae (GNCB), varicella (VZV), mumps.
Immunosuppression: H influenzae, Mycobacterium tuberculosis (AFB), candida sp (yeast), cytomegalovirus (CMV).

Specimen/Diagnostic Tests:
Urinalysis may reveal pyuria. Patients aged >35 years will often have midstream pyuria and scrotal edema.
Culture urine and expressible urethral discharge when present.
Prostatic secretions for Gram stain and bacterial culture are helpful in older patients.
When testicular torsion is considered, Doppler ultrasound or radionuclide scan can be useful in diagnosis.
Ultrasonography in tuberculous epididymitis shows enlargement of the epididymis (predominantly the tail) and marked heterogeneity in texture. Other sonographic findings include a hypoechoic lesion of the testis with associated sinus tract or extratesticular calcifications.

Comments:
Testicular torsion is a surgical emergency that is often confused with orchitis or epididymitis.
Sexual partners should be examined for signs of sexually transmitted diseases.
In non-sexually transmitted disease, evaluation for underlying urinary tract infection or structural defect is recommended.
Clin Nucl Med 1996;21:479.
J Urol 1997;158:2158.
J Clin Ultrasound 1997;25:390.
Clin Infect Dis 1998;26:942.
Sex Transm Infect 1999;75(Suppl 1):S51.
BJU Int 1999;84:827.

	GENITOURINARY	
	Vaginitis/Vaginosis	
Organism	**Specimen/Diagnostic Tests**	**Comments**
Vaginitis/Vaginosis Candida sp. *Trichomonas vaginalis*, *Gardnerella vaginalis* (GPR), bacteroides (non-*fragilis* GNR), mobiluncus (GPR), peptostreptococcus (GPC), *Mycoplasma hominis*, groups A and B streptococci (GPC), herpes simplex (HSV).	Vaginal discharge for appearance (in candidiasis, area is pruritic with thick "cheesy" discharge; in trichomoniasis, copious foamy discharge), pH (about 4.5 for candida; 5.0–6.0 in trichomonas; 5.0–6.0 with bacterial), saline ("wet") preparation (motile organisms seen in trichomonas; cells covered with organisms—"clue" cells—in gardnerella; yeast and hyphae in candida, "fishy" odor on addition of KOH with gardnerella infection). Vaginal fluid pH as a screening test for bacterial vaginosis showed a sensitivity of 74.3%, but combined with clinical symptoms and signs its sensitivity increased to 81.3%. (See Vaginitis table, p 397.) Atrophic vaginitis is seen in postmenopausal patients, often with bleeding, scant discharge, and pH 6.0–7.0 Cultures for gardnerella are not useful and are not recommended. Culture for *T vaginalis* has greater sensitivity than wet mount. Culture for groups A and B streptococci and rare causes of bacterial vaginosis may be indicated.	Bacterial vaginosis results from massive overgrowth of anaerobic vaginal bacterial flora (especially gardnerella). Serious infectious sequelae associated with bacterial vaginosis include abscesses, endometritis and pelvic inflammatory disease. There is also a danger of miscarriage, premature rupture of the membranes, and premature labor. Am J Obstet Gynecol 1991;165(4 Part 2):1161. N Engl J Med 1997;337:1896. J Gen Intern Med 1998;13:335. Pediatr Clin North Am 1999;46:733. Int J Gynaecol Obstet 1999;66:143. Sex Transm Infect 1999;75(Suppl 1):S16, S21.

GENITOURINARY		
Cervicitis		
Cervicitis, Mucopurulent *Chlamydia trachomatis* (50%), *N gonorrhoeae* (GNDC) (8%).	Cervical swab specimen for appearance (yellow or green purulent material), cell count (>10 WBCs per high-power oil immersion field and culture (58–80%) or nucleic acid assay (93%) for GC; urine for nucleic acid assay (93%) for GC; urine (80–92%) or cervical swab (97%) for detection of *C trachomatis* by nucleic acid amplification. Culture (52%) or nonamplified assays (50–80%) are considerably less sensitive for diagnosis of *C trachomatis*.	Because of the danger of false-positive amplified nucleic acid assays, culture is the preferred method in cases of suspected child abuse. In one study of pregnant women, a wet mount preparation of endocervical secretions with <10 PMNs per high-power field had a negative predictive value of 99% for gonococcus-induced cervicitis and of 96% for *C trachomatis*-induced cervicitis. In family planning clinics, however, a mucopurulent discharge with > 10 PMNs/hpf had a low positive predictive value of 29.2% for *C trachomatis*-related cervicitis. Mucopurulent discharge may persist for 3 months or more even after appropriate therapy. Curr Probl Dermatol 1996;24:110. CMAJ 1998;158:41. J Clin Microbiol 1998;36:1630. Am J Obstet Gynecol 1999;181:283. Eur J Clin Microbiol Infect Dis 1999;18:142.

	GENITOURINARY	
	Salpingitis	**Chorioamnionitis/Endometritis**

Organism

Salpingitis/Pelvic Inflammatory Disease (PID)

Usually polymicrobial: *N gonorrhoeae* (GNDC), *Chlamydia trachomatis*, bacteroides, peptostreptococcus, *G vaginalis*, and other anaerobes, Enterobacteriaceae (GNR), streptococci (GPC in chains), *Mycoplasma hominis* (debatable).

Specimen/Diagnostic Tests

Gram stain and culture or amplified nucleic acid assays of urethral or endocervical exudate. Ultrasonographic findings include thickened fluid-filled tubes, polycystic-like ovaries, and free pelvic fluid. MRI imaging findings for PID (95%) include fluid-filled tube, pyosalpinx, tubo-ovarian abscess, or polycystic-like ovaries and free fluid. Laparoscopy supplemented by microbiologic tests and fimbrial biopsy is the diagnostic standard for PID. Transvaginal ultrasonography (81%) has a lower specificity than MRI. Laparoscopy should be checked in all patients because of the high incidence of PID. VDRL should be checked in all patients because of the high incidence of associated syphilis.

Comments

PID typically progresses from cervicitis to endometritis to salpingitis. PID is a sexually transmitted disease in some cases, not in others. All sexual partners should be examined. All IUDs should be removed. Some recommend that all patients with PID be hospitalized. A strategy of identifying, testing, and treating women at increased risk for cervical chlamydial infection can lead to a reduced incidence of PID. N Engl J Med 1996;334:1362. Hum Reprod 1997;12(11 Suppl):121. Dermatol Clin 1998;16:747. Lippincott Primary Care 1998;2:307. Radiology 1999;210:209. Clin Infect Dis 1999;28 (Suppl 1):S29.

Chorioamnionitis/Endometritis

Group B streptococcus (GPC), *Escherichia coli* (GNR), *Listeria monocytogenes* (GPR), *Mycoplasma hominis, Ureaplasma urealyticum, Gardnerella vaginalis,* enterococci (GPC), viridans streptococci (GPC), bacteroides (GNR), prevotella (GNR), and other anaerobic flora, *Chlamydia trachomatis,* group A streptococcus (GPC)

Amniotic fluid for Gram stain, leukocyte esterase, glucose levels <10–20 mg/dL, and aerobic and anaerobic culture; blood for culture. Sonographic evaluation of fetus can be helpful, but findings are nonspecific.

Risk factors include bacterial vaginosis, preterm labor, duration of labor, parity, internal fetal monitoring. Infect Dis Clin North Am 1997;11:177;203. Semin Perinatol 1998;22:242. Pediatrics 1999;103:78.

BONE		
Osteomyelitis		
Osteomyelitis	Blood cultures for bacteria are positive in about 60%. Cultures of percutaneous needle biopsy or open bone biopsy are needed if blood cultures are negative and osteomyelitis is suspected.	Hematogenous or contiguous infection (eg, infected prosthetic joint, chronic cutaneous ulcer) may lead to osteomyelitis in children (metaphyses of long bones) or adults (vertebrae, metaphyses of long bones).
Staphylococcus aureus (GPC) (about 60% of all cases).	Imaging with bone scan or gallium/indium scan (sensitivity 95%, specificity 60–70%) can localize areas of suspicion. Technetium (^{99m}Tc)-Methylene diphosphonate (MDP) bone scan can suggest osteomyelitis days or weeks before plain bone films. Plain bone films are abnormal in acute cases after about 2 weeks of illness (33%). Indium-labeled WBC scan is useful in detecting abscesses. Ultrasound to detect subperiosteal abscesses and ultrasound-guided aspiration can assist in diagnosis and management of osteomyelitis. Ultrasound can differentiate acute osteomyelitis from vaso-occlusive crisis in patients with sickle cell disease. CT scan aids in detecting sequestra. When bone x-rays and scintigraphy are negative, MRI (98%) is useful for detecting early osteomyelitis (specificity 89%), in defining extent, and in distinguishing osteomyelitis from cellulitis. Myelography, CT, or MRI is indicated to rule out epidural abscess in vertebral osteomyelitis.	Hematogenous osteomyelitis in drug addicts occurs in unusual locations (vertebrae, clavicle, ribs). In infants, osteomyelitis is often associated with contiguous joint involvement. Acta Radiologica 1998;39:523. J Pediatr Orthop 1998;18:552. J Comput Assist Tomogr 1998;22:437. Clin Radiol 1999;54:636. Pediatr Surg Int 1999;15:363.
Infant: *S aureus*, Enterobacteriaceae (GNR), groups A and B streptococci (GPC).		
Child (<3 years): *H influenzae* (GNCB), *S aureus*, streptococci.		
Child (>3 years) to Adult: *S aureus*, *Pseudomonas aeruginosa*.		
Postoperative: *S aureus*, Enterobacteriaceae, pseudomonas sp (GNR), *Bartonella henselae* (GNR).		
Joint prosthesis: Coagulase-negative staphylococci, peptostreptococcus (GPC), *Propionibacterium acnes* (GPR), viridans streptococci (GPC in chains).		

	JOINT	
	Bacterial/Septic Arthritis	

Organism	Specimen/Diagnostic Tests	Comments
Bacterial/Septic Arthritis Infant (<3 months): *S aureus* (GPC), Enterobacteriaceae (GNR), *Kingella kingae* (GNCB), *Haemophilus influenzae* (GNCB). Child (3 months to 6 years): *S aureus* (35%), *H influenzae*, group A streptococcus (GPC), Enterobacteriaceae (6%), *Borrelia burgdorferi* (Lyme). Adult, STD not likely: *S aureus* (40%), group A streptococcus (27%), Enterobacteriaceae (23%), *Streptobacillus moniliformis* (GNR), brucella (GNR), *Mycobacterium marinum* (AFB). Adult, STD likely: *N gonorrhoeae* (GNDC) (disseminated gonococcal infection, DGI). Prosthetic joint, postoperative or following intraarticular injection: Coagulase-negative staphylococci (40%), *S aureus* (20%), viridans streptococci (GPC in chains), enterococci (GPC), peptostreptococcus (GPC), *Propionibacterium acnes* (GPR), Enterobacteriaceae, pseudomonas sp.	Joint aspiration (synovial) fluid for WBCs (in non-gonococcal infection, mean WBC is 100,000/μL). Gram stain (best on centrifuged concentrated specimen; positive in one-third of cases), culture (non gonococcal infection in adults [85–95%], DGI [25%]). (See Synovial fluid profiles, p 389.) Yield of culture is greatest if 10 mL of synovial fluid is inoculated into a large volume of culture media, such as a blood culture bottle, within 1 hour after collection. Blood cultures for bacteria may be useful, especially in infants; nongonococcal infection in adults (50%); DGI (13%). *B burgdorferi* serology for Lyme disease. Genitourinary, throat, or rectal culture: DGI may be diagnosed by positive culture from a nonarticular source and by a compatible clinical picture. In difficult cases, MRI can help differentiate septic arthritis from transient synovitis.	It is important to obtain synovial fluid and blood for culture before starting antimicrobial treatment. Septic arthritis is usually hematogenously acquired. Prosthetic joint and diminished host defenses secondary to cancer, HIV, liver disease, or hypogammaglobulinemia are common predisposing factors. Nongonococcal bacterial arthritis is usually monarticular (and typically affects one knee joint). DGI is the most common cause of septic arthritis in urban centers and is usually polyarticular with associated tenosynovitis. Radiol Clin North Am 1996;34:293. Rheumat Dis Clin North Am 1997;23:239. Lancet 1998;351:197. Am J Orthop 1999;28:168. Radiology 1999;211:459. Pediatr Emerg Care 1999;15:40.

	MUSCLE	SKIN
	Gas Gangrene	**Impetigo**
Gas Gangrene *Clostridium perfringens* (GPR), (80–95%), other clostridium sp.	Diagnosis should be suspected in areas of devitalized tissue when gas is discovered by palpation (subcutaneous crepitation) or x-ray. Gram stain of foul-smelling, brown or blood-tinged watery exudate can be diagnostic with gram-positive rods and a remarkable absence of neutrophils. Anaerobic culture of discharge is confirmatory.	Gas gangrene occurs in the setting of a contaminated wound. *Clostridium perfringens* produces potent exotoxins, including alpha toxin and theta toxin, which depresses myocardial contractility, induces shock, and causes direct vascular injury at the site of infection. Infections with enterobacter or *E coli* and anaerobic infections can also cause gas formation. These agents cause cellulitis rather than myonecrosis. Postgrad Med 1996;99:217. Clin Infect Dis 1999;28:159.
Impetigo Infant (impetigo neonatorum): Staphylococcus (GPC). Nonbullous or "vesicular": *S pyogenes* (GPC), *S aureus* (GPC), anaerobes. Bullous: *S aureus*.	Gram stain, culture, and smear for HSV and VZV antigen detection by direct fluorescent antibody (DFA) of scrapings from lesions may be useful in differentiating impetigo from other vesicular or pustular lesions (HSV, VZV, contact dermatitis). DFA smear can be performed by scraping the contents, base, and roof of vesicle and applying to glass slide. After fixing, the slide is stained with direct fluorescent antibody (DFA) for identification of HSV or VZV.	Impetigo neonatorum requires prompt treatment and protection of other infants (isolation). Polymicrobial aerobic-anaerobic infections are present in some patients. Patients with recurrent impetigo should have cultures of the anterior nares to exclude carriage of *S aureus*. Pediatr Dermatol 1997;14:192. Practitioner 1998;242:405. Aust Fam Physician 1998;27:735.

SKIN

Cellulitis

Organism	Specimen/Diagnostic Tests	Comments
Cellulitis Spontaneous, traumatic wound: Polymicrobial: *S aureus* (GPC), groups A, C, and G streptococci (GPC), enterococci (GPC), Enterobacteriaceae (GNR), *Clostridium perfringens* (GPR), *Clostridium tetani*, pseudomonas sp (GNR) (if water exposure). Postoperative wound (not GI or GU): *S aureus*, group A streptococcus, Enterobacteriaceae, pseudomonas sp. Postoperative wound (GI or GU): Must add bacteroides sp, anaerobes, enterococcus (GPC), groups B or C streptococci. Diabetes mellitus: Polymicrobial: *S pyogenes*, enterococcus, *S aureus*, Enterobacteriaceae, anaerobes. Bullous lesions, sea water contaminated abrasion, after raw seafood consumption: *Vibrio vulnificus* (GNR). Vein graft donor site: Streptococcus. Decubitus ulcers: Polymicrobial: *S aureus*, anaerobic streptococci, Enterobacteriaceae, pseudomonas sp, bacteroides sp. Necrotizing fasciitis, type 1: Streptococcus, anaerobes, Enterobacteriaceae; type 2: Group A streptococcus (hemolytic streptococcal gangrene).	Skin culture: In spontaneous cellulitis, isolation of the causative organism is difficult. In traumatic and postoperative wounds, Gram stain may allow rapid diagnosis of staphylococcal or clostridial infection. Culture of wound or abscess material after disinfection of the skin site will almost always yield the diagnosis. MRI can aid in diagnosis of secondary abscess formation, necrotizing fasciitis, or pyomyositis. Frozen section of biopsy specimen may be useful.	Cellulitis has long been considered to be the result of an antecedent bacterial invasion with subsequent bacterial proliferation. However, the difficulty in isolating putative pathogens from cellulitic skin has cast doubt on this theory. Predisposing factors for cellulitis include diabetes mellitus, edema, peripheral vascular disease, venous insufficiency, leg ulcer or wound, tinea pedis, dry skin, obesity, and prior history of cellulitis. Consider updating antitetanus prophylaxis for all wounds. In the diabetic, and in postoperative and traumatic wounds, consider prompt surgical debridement for necrotizing fasciitis. With abscess formation, surgical drainage is the mainstay of therapy and may be sufficient. Hemolytic streptococcal gangrene may follow minor trauma and involves specific strains of streptococcus. AJR Am J Roentgenol 1998;170:615. Diagn Microbiol Infect Dis 1999;34:325. Lippincott Primary Care Pract 1999;3:59. BMJ 1999;318:1591.

BLOOD

Bacteremia of Unknown Source

Bacteremia of Unknown Source		
Bacteremia of Unknown Source Neonate <4 days): Group B strepto-cocci (GPC), *E coli* (GNR), kleb-siella (GNR), enterobacter (GNR), *S aureus* (GPC), coagulase-negative staphylococci (GPC). Neonate (> 5 days): Add *H influenzae* (GNCB). Child (nonimmunocompromised): *H influenzae, S pneumoniae* (GPDC), *N meningitidis* (GNDC), *S aureus.* Adult (IV drug use): *S aureus* or viri-dans streptococci (GPC). Adult (catheter-related, "line" sepsis): *S aureus,* coagulase-negative staphy-lococci, *Corynebacterium jeikeium* (GPR), pseudomonas sp, candida sp, *Malassezia furfur* (yeast). Adult (splenectomized): *S pneumo-niae, H influenzae, N meningitidis.* Neutropenia (<500 PMN): Enterobac-teriaceae, pseudomonas sp, *S aureus,* coagulase-negative staphylococci, viridans group streptococcus. Parasites: Babesia, ehrlichia, plasmo-dium sp, filarial worms. Immunocompromised: Bartonella sp (GNR), herpesvirus 8 (HHV8), *Mycobacterium avium-intracellulare* (AFB).	Blood cultures are mandatory for all patients with fever and no obvious source of infection. Often they are negative, especially in neonates. Cultures should be drawn at onset of febrile episode. Culture should never be drawn from an IV line or from a femoral site. Culture and Gram stain of urine, wounds, and other potentially infected sites provide a more rapid diagnosis than blood cultures.	Occult bacteremia affects approximately 5% of febrile children ages 2–36 months. In infants, the findings of an elevated total WBC count (>15,000) and absolute neutrophil count (ANC >10,000) were equally sensitive in predicting bacteremia, but the ANC was more specific. Predisposing factors in adults include IV drug use, neutropenia, cancer, diabetes mellitus, venous catheterization, hemodialysis, and plasmapheresis. Catheter-related infection in patients with long-term venous access (Broviac, Hickman, etc) may be treated successfully without removal of the line, but recurrence of bacteremia is frequent. Switching needles during blood cultures does not decrease contamination rates and increases the risk of needle-stick injuries. Am J Clin Pathol 1998;109:221. Pediatrics 1998;102(1 Part 1):67. Ann Emerg Med 1998;31:679. Infect Dis Clin North Am 1999;13:397. Infect Dis Clin North Am 1999;13:483.

6

Diagnostic Imaging:
Test Selection and Interpretation

Sean Perini, MD, and Susan D. Wall, MD

HOW TO USE THIS SECTION

Information in this chapter is arranged anatomically from superior to inferior. It would not be feasible to include all available imaging tests in one chapter in a book this size, but we have attempted to summarize the essential features of those examinations that are most frequently ordered in modern clinical practice or those that may be associated with difficulty or risk. Indications, advantages and disadvantages, contra-indications, and patient preparation are presented. Costs of the studies are approximate and represent averages reported from several large medical centers.

$$\$ = < \$250$$
$$\$\$ = \$250–\$750$$
$$\$\$\$ = \$750–\$1000$$
$$\$\$\$\$ = > \$1000$$

RISKS OF INTRAVENOUS CONTRAST STUDIES

While intravenous contrast is an important tool in radiology, it is not without substantial risks. Minor reactions (nausea, vomiting, hives) occur with an overall incidence between 1% and 12%. Major reactions (laryngeal edema, bronchospasm, cardiac arrest) occur in 0.16 to 2 cases per 1000 patients. Deaths have been reported in 1 : 170,000 to 1 : 40,000 cases. Patients with an allergic history (asthma, hay fever, allergy to foods or drugs) are at increased risk. A history of reaction to contrast material is associated with an increased risk of a subsequent severe reaction. Prophylactic measures that may be required in such cases include H_1 and H_2 blockers and corticosteroids.

In addition, there is a risk of contrast-induced renal failure, which is usually mild and reversible. Persons at increased risk for potentially *irreversible* renal damage include patients with preexisting renal disease (particularly diabetics with high serum creatinine concentrations), multiple myeloma, and severe hyperuricemia.

In summary, intravenous contrast should be viewed in the same manner as other medications—ie, risks and benefits must be balanced before an examination using this pharmaceutical is ordered.

	HEAD			
Test	**Indications**	**Advantages**	**Disadvantages/Contraindications**	**Preparation**
	CT			
HEAD **Computed tomography (CT)** $$$	Evaluation of acute craniofacial trauma, acute neurologic dysfunction (<72 hours) from suspected intracranial or subarachnoid hemorrhage. Further characterization of intracranial masses identified by MRI (presence or absence of calcium or involvement of the bony calvarium). Evaluation of sinus disease and temporal bone disease.	Rapid acquisition makes it the modality of choice for trauma. Superb spatial resolution. Superior to MRI in detection of hemorrhage within the first 24–48 hours.	Artifacts from bone may interfere with detection of disease at the skull base and in the posterior fossa. Generally limited to transaxial views. Direct coronal images of paranasal sinuses and temporal bones are routinely obtained if patient can lie prone. **Contraindications and risks:** Contraindicated in pregnancy because of the potential harm of ionizing radiation to the fetus. See Risks of Intravenous Contrast Studies, page 244.	Normal hydration. Sedation of agitated patients. Recent serum creatinine determination if intravenous contrast is to be used.
	MRI			
HEAD **Magnetic resonance imaging (MRI)** $$$$	Evaluation of essentially all intracranial disease except those listed above for CT.	Provides excellent tissue contrast resolution, multiplanar capability. Can detect flowing blood and cryptic vascular malformations. Can detect demyelinating and dysmyelinating disease. No beam-hardening artifacts such as can be seen with CT. No ionizing radiation.	Subject to motion artifacts. Inferior to CT in the setting of acute trauma because it is insensitive to acute hemorrhage, incompatible with traction devices, inferior in detection of bony injury and foreign bodies, and requires longer imaging acquisition time. Special instrumentation required for patients on life support. **Contraindications and risks:** Contraindicated in patients with cardiac pacemakers, intraocular metallic foreign bodies, intracranial aneurysm clips, cochlear implants, and some artificial heart valves.	Sedation of agitated patients. Screening CT or plain radiograph images of orbits if history suggests possible metallic foreign body in the eye.

	BRAIN	
	MRA/MRV	**Brain Scan**

Test	Indications	Advantages	Disadvantages/Contraindications	Preparation
BRAIN **Magnetic resonance angiography/venography (MRA/MRV)** $$$$	Evaluation of cerebral arteriovenous malformations, intracranial aneurysm, and blood supply of vascular tumors as an aid to operative planning (MRA). Evaluation of dural sinus thrombosis (MRV).	No ionizing radiation. No iodinated contrast needed.	Subject to motion artifacts. Special instrumentation required for patients on life support. **Contraindications and risks:** Contraindicated in patients with cardiac pacemakers, intraocular metallic foreign bodies, intracranial aneurysm clips, cochlear implants, and some artificial heart valves.	Sedation of agitated patients. Screening CT or plain radiograph images of orbits if history suggests possible metallic foreign body in the eye.
BRAIN **Brain scan (radionuclide)** $$	Confirmation of brain death.	Confirmation of brain death not impeded by hypothermia or barbiturate coma. Can be portable.	Limited resolution. Delayed imaging required with some agents. Cannot be used alone to establish diagnosis of brain death. Must be used in combination with clinical examination or cerebral angiography to establish diagnosis. **Contraindications and risks:** Caution in pregnancy because of the potential harm of ionizing radiation to the fetus.	Sedation of agitated patients. Premedicate with potassium perchlorate when using TcO_4 in order to block choroid plexus uptake.

BRAIN			
	Brain PET/SPECT		**Cisternography**
BRAIN **Positron emission tomography** (PET)/single photon emission (SPECT) brain scan $$$	Evaluation of suspected dementia. Evaluation of medically refractory seizures.	Provide functional information. Can localize seizure focus prior to surgical excision. Up to 82% positive predictive value for Alzheimer's dementia in appropriate clinical settings. Provide cross-sectional images and therefore improved lesion localization compared with planar imaging techniques.	Limited resolution compared with MRI and CT. Limited application in workup of dementia due to low specificity of images and fact that test results do not alter clinical management. **Contraindications and risks:** Caution in pregnancy because of potential harm of ionizing radiation to the fetus.	Requires lumbar puncture to deliver radiopharmaceutical.
BRAIN **Cisternography** (radionuclide) $$	Evaluation of hydrocephalus (particularly normal pressure), CSF rhinorrhea or otorrhea, and ventricular shunt patency.	Provides functional information. Can help distinguish normal pressure hydrocephalus from senile atrophy. Can detect CSF leaks.	Requires multiple delayed imaging sessions up to 48–72 hours after injection. **Contraindications and risks:** Caution in pregnancy because of the potential harm of ionizing radiation to the fetus.	Sedation of agitated patients. For suspected CSF leak, pack the patient's nose or ears with cotton pledgets prior to administration of dose. Must follow strict sterile precautions for intrathecal injection.

		NECK	
		MRI	**MRA**
Test	**Indications**	**Advantages**	**Disadvantages/Contraindications**	**Preparation**

Test	Indications	Advantages	Disadvantages/Contraindications	Preparation
NECK **Magnetic resonance imaging** (MRI) $$$$	Evaluation of the upper aero-digestive tract. Staging of neck masses. Differentiation of lymphadenopathy from blood vessels. Evaluation of head and neck malignancy, thyroid nodules, parathyroid adenoma, lymphadenopathy, retropharyngeal abscess, brachial plexopathy.	Provides excellent tissue contrast resolution. Tissue differentiation of malignancy or abscess from benign tumor often possible. Sagittal and coronal planar imaging possible. Multiplanar capability especially advantageous regarding brachial plexus. No iodinated contrast needed to distinguish lymphadenopathy from blood vessels.	Subject to motion artifacts, particularly those of carotid pulsation and swallowing. Special instrumentation required for patients on life support. **Contraindications and risks:** Contraindicated in patients with cardiac pacemakers, intraocular metallic foreign bodies, intracranial aneurysm clips, cochlear implants, and some artificial heart valves.	Sedation of agitated patients. Screening CT or plain radiograph images of orbits if history suggests possible metallic foreign body in the eye.
NECK **Magnetic resonance angiography** (MRA) $$$$	Evaluation of carotid bifurcation atherosclerosis, cervicocranial arterial dissection.	No ionizing radiation. No iodinated contrast needed. MRA of the carotid arteries can be a sufficient preoperative evaluation regarding critical stenosis when local expertise exists.	Subject to motion artifacts, particularly from carotid pulsation and swallowing. Special instrumentation required for patients on life support. **Contraindications and risks:** Contraindicated in patients with cardiac pacemakers, intraocular metallic foreign bodies, intracranial aneurysm clips, cochlear implants, and some artificial heart valves.	Sedation of agitated patients. Screening CT or plain radiograph images of orbits if history suggests possible metallic foreign body in the eye.

	NECK		THYROID
	CT	**Ultrasound**	**Ultrasound**
NECK **Computed tomography (CT)** $$$$	Evaluation of the upper aero-digestive tract. Staging of neck masses for patients who are not candidates for MRI. Evaluation of suspected abscess.	Rapid. Superb spatial resolution. Can guide percutaneous fine-needle aspiration of possible tumor or abscess.	Adequate intravenous contrast enhancement of vascular structures is mandatory for accurate interpretation. **Contraindications and risks:** Contraindicated in pregnancy because of the potential harm of ionizing radiation to the fetus. See Risks of Intravenous Contrast Studies, page 244.	Normal hydration. Sedation of agitated patients. Recent serum creatinine determination.
NECK **Ultrasound (US)** $$	Patency and morphology of arteries and veins. Evaluation of thyroid and parathyroid. Guidance for percutaneous fine-needle aspiration biopsy of neck lesions.	Can detect and monitor atherosclerotic stenosis of carotid arteries noninvasively and without iodinated contrast.	Technically demanding, operator-dependent. Patient must lie supine and still for 1 hour.	None.
THYROID **Ultrasound (US)** $$	Determination as to whether a palpable nodule is a cyst or solid mass and whether single or multiple nodules are present. Assessment of response to suppressive therapy. Screening patients with a history of prior radiation to the head and neck. Guidance for biopsy.	Noninvasive. No ionizing radiation. Can be portable. Can image in all planes.	Cannot distinguish between benign and malignant lesions unless local invasion is demonstrated. Technique very operator-dependent. **Contraindications and risks:** None.	None.

	THYROID
	Thyroid uptake and scan

Test	Indications	Advantages	Disadvantages/Contraindications	Preparation
THYROID	Uptake indicated for evaluation of clinical hypothyroidism, hyperthyroidism, thyroiditis, effects of thyroid-stimulating and suppressing medications, and for calculation of therapeutic radiation dosage.	Demonstrates both morphology and function. Can identify ectopic thyroid tissue and "cold" nodules that have a greater risk of malignancy.	Substances interfering with test include iodides in vitamins and medicines, antithyroid drugs, steroids, and intravascular contrast agents. Delayed imaging is required with iodides (^{123}I, 6 hours and 24 hours; ^{131}I total body, 72 hours).	Administration of dose after a 4- to 6-hour fast aids absorption. Discontinue all interfering substances prior to test, especially thyroid-suppressing medications: T_3 (1 week), T_4 (4–6 weeks), propylthiouracil (2 weeks).
Thyroid uptake and scan (radionuclide)				
$$	Scanning indicated for above as well as evaluation of palpable nodules, mediastinal mass, and screening of patients with history of head and neck irradiation. Total body scanning used for postoperative evaluation of thyroid metastases.	Imaging of total body with one dose (^{131}I).	Test may not visualize thyroid gland in subacute thyroiditis. **Contraindications and risks:** Not advised in pregnancy because of the risk of ionizing radiation to the fetus (iodides cross placenta and concentrate in fetal thyroid). Significant radiation exposure occurs in total body scanning with ^{131}I; patients should be instructed about precautionary measures by nuclear medicine personnel.	

	THYROID			PARATHYROID
	Radionuclide therapy			Radionuclide scan
THYROID **Thyroid therapy** (radionuclide) $$$	Hyperthyroidism and some thyroid carcinomas (papillary and follicular types are amenable to treatment, whereas medullary and anaplastic types are not).	Noninvasive alternative to surgery.	Rarely, radiation thyroiditis may occur 1–3 days after therapy. Hypothyroidism occurs commonly as a long-term complication. Higher doses that are required to treat thyroid carcinoma may result in pulmonary fibrosis. **Contraindications and risks:** Contraindicated in pregnancy and lactation. Contraindicated in patients with metastatic disease to the brain, because treatment may result in brain edema and subsequent herniation, and in those <20 years of age because of possible increased risk of thyroid cancer later in life. After treatment, a patient's activities are restricted to limit total exposure of any member of the general public until radiation level is ≤0.5 rem. High doses for treatment of thyroid carcinoma may necessitate hospitalization.	After treatment, patients must isolate all bodily secretions from household members.
PARA-THYROID **Parathyroid scan** (radionuclide) $$	Evaluation of suspected parathyroid adenoma.	Identifies hyperfunctioning tissue, which is useful when planning surgery.	Small adenomas (<500 mg) may not be detected. **Contraindications and risks:** Caution in pregnancy is advised because of the risk of ionizing radiation to the fetus.	Requires strict patient immobility during scanning.

		CHEST	
		Chest radiograph	CT

Test	Indications	Advantages	Disadvantages/Contraindications	Preparation
CHEST **Chest radiograph** $	Evaluation of pleural and parenchymal pulmonary disease, mediastinal disease, cardiogenic and noncardiogenic pulmonary edema, congenital and acquired cardiac disease. Screening for traumatic aortic rupture (though angiogram is the standard and spiral computed tomography is playing an increasing role). Evaluation of possible pneumothorax (expiratory upright film) or free flowing fluid (decubitus views).	Inexpensive. Widely available.	Difficult to distinguish between causes of hilar enlargement (ie, vasculature versus adenopathy). **Contraindications and risks:** Caution in pregnancy because of the potential harm of ionizing radiation to the fetus.	None.
CHEST **Computed tomography (CT)** $$$	Differentiation of mediastinal and hilar lymphadenopathy from vascular structures. Evaluation and staging of primary and metastatic lung neoplasm. Characterization of pulmonary nodules. Differentiation of parenchymal versus pleural process (ie, lung abscess versus empyema). Evaluation of interstitial lung disease (1 mm thin sections), aortic dissection, and aneurysm.	Rapid. Superb spatial resolution. Can guide percutaneous fine-needle aspiration of possible tumor or abscess.	Patient cooperation required for appropriate breath-holding. Generally limited to transaxial views. **Contraindications and risks:** Contraindicated in pregnancy because of the potential harm of ionizing radiation to the fetus. See Risks of Intravenous Contrast Studies, page 244.	Preferably NPO for 2 hours prior to study. Normal hydration. Sedation of agitated patients. Recent serum creatinine determination.

	CHEST			LUNG
	MRI			**Ventilation-perfusion scan**
CHEST **Magnetic resonance imaging** (MRI) $$$$	Evaluation of mediastinal masses. Discrimination between hilar vessels and enlarged lymph nodes. Tumor staging (especially when invasion of vessels or pericardium is suspected). Evaluation of aortic dissection, aortic aneurysm, congenital and acquired cardiac disease.	Provides excellent tissue contrast resolution and multiplanar capability. No beam-hardening artifacts such as can be seen with CT. No ionizing radiation.	Subject to motion artifacts. **Contraindications and risks:** Contraindicated in patients with cardiac pacemakers, intraocular metallic foreign bodies, intracranial aneurysm clips, cochlear implants, and some artificial heart valves.	Sedation of agitated patients. Screening CT of the orbits if history suggests possible metallic foreign body in the eye.
LUNG **Ventilation-perfusion scan** (radionuclide) $\dot{V}$ = $$ $\dot{Q}$ = $$ $\dot{V} + \dot{Q}$ = $$$–$$$$	Evaluation of pulmonary embolism or burn inhalation injury. Preoperative evaluation of patients with chronic obstructive pulmonary disease and of those who are candidates for pneumonectomy.	Noninvasive. Provides functional information in preoperative assessment. Permits determination of differential and regional lung function in preoperative assessment. Documented pulmonary embolism is extremely rare with normal perfusion scan.	Patients must be able to cooperate for ventilation portion of the examination. There is a high proportion of intermediate probability studies in patients with underlying lung disease. The likelihood of pulmonary embolism ranges from 20% to 80% in these cases. A patient who has a low probability scan still has a chance ranging from nil to 19% of having a pulmonary embolus. **Contraindications and risks:** Patients with severe pulmonary artery hypertension or significant right-to-left shunts should have fewer particles injected. Caution advised in pregnancy because of risk of ionizing radiation to the fetus.	Current chest radiograph is mandatory for interpretation.

	LUNG
	CT

Test	Indications	Advantages	Disadvantages/Contraindications	Preparation
LUNG **Spiral computed tomography** (CT) $$$	Evaluation of clinically suspected pulmonary embolism.	Rapid. Sensitivity and specificity values likely about 90% for the CT diagnosis of pulmonary emboli involving main to segmental artery branches in unselected patients. Overall, spiral CT sensitivity may be higher than ventilation/perfusion scintigraphy.	Accuracy of spiral CT in diagnosing pulmonary embolism depends on the size of the pulmonary artery involved and the size of the thrombus. Sensitivity and accuracy of CT decreases for small, subsegmental emboli (sensitivity rates of 53–63% have been reported). Respiratory motion artifacts can be a problem in dyspneic patients. High-quality study requires breath-holding of approximately 20 seconds. Specific imaging protocol utilized which limits diagnostic information for other abnormalities. **Contraindications and risks:** Contraindicated in pregnancy because of potential harm of ionizing radiation to fetus. See Risks of Intravenous Contrast Studies, page 244.	Large gauge intravenous access (minimum 20-gauge) required. Prebreathing oxygen may help dyspneic patients perform adequate breath hold. Normal hydration. Preferably NPO for 2 hours prior to study. Recent serum creatinine determination.

LUNG			
Pulmonary angiography			
LUNG **Pulmonary angiography** $$$$	Suspected pulmonary embolism with equivocal results on ventilation/perfusion scan or when definitive diagnosis especially important because of contraindication to anticoagulation. Arteriovenous malformation, pulmonary sequestration, vasculitides, vascular occlusion by tumor or inflammatory disease.	Remains the standard for diagnosis of acute and chronic pulmonary embolism.	Invasive. Requires catheterization of the right heart and pulmonary artery. **Contraindications:** Elevated pulmonary artery pressure (> 70 mm Hg) or elevated right ventricular end-diastolic pressure (> 20 mm Hg). Pulmonary artery hypertension.	Ventilation/perfusion scan for localization of right versus left lung. Electrocardiogram, especially to exclude left bundle branch block (in such cases, temporary cardiac pacemaker should be placed before the catheter is introduced into the pulmonary artery).

		BREAST		
		Mammogram		
Test	Indications	Advantages	Disadvantages/Contraindications	Preparation
BREAST Mammo-gram $	Screening for breast cancer in asymptomatic women: (1) every 1–2 years between ages 40 and 49; (2) every year after age 50. If prior history of breast cancer, mammogram should be performed yearly at any age. Indicated at any age for symptoms (palpable mass, bloody discharge) or before breast surgery.	Newer film screen techniques generate lower radiation doses (0.1–0.2 rad per film, mean glandular dose). A 23% lower mortality has been demonstrated in patients screened with combined mammogram and physical exam compared to physical exam alone. In a screening population, more than 40% of cancers are detected by mammography alone and cannot be palpated on physical exam.	Detection of breast masses is more difficult in patients with radiographically dense breasts. Breast compression may cause patient discomfort. In a screening population, 9% of cancers are detected by physical examination alone and are not detectable by mammography. **Contraindications and risks:** Radiation from repeated mammograms can theoretically cause breast cancer; however, the benefits of screening mammograms greatly outweigh the risks.	None.

HEART			Thallium scan	Ventriculography
HEART **Myocardial perfusion scan** (thallium scan, technetium-99m methoxyisobutyl isonitrile (sestamibi) scan, others) $–$$–$$$ (broad range)	Evaluation of atypical chest pain. Detection of presence, location, and extent of myocardial ischemia.	Highly sensitive for detecting physiologically significant coronary stenosis. Noninvasive. Able to stratify patients according to risk for myocardial infarction. Normal examination associated with average risk of cardiac death or nonfatal myocardial infarction of <1% per year.	The patient must be carefully monitored during treadmill or pharmacologic stress—optimally, under the supervision of a cardiologist. False-positive results may be caused by exercise-induced spasm, aortic stenosis, or left bundle branch block; false-negative results may be caused by inadequate exercise, mild or distal disease, or balanced diffuse ischemia. **Contraindications and risk:** Aminophylline (inhibitor of dipyridamole) is a contraindication to the use of dipyridamole. Treadmill or pharmacologic stress carries a risk of arrhythmia, ischemia, infarct, and, rarely, death. Caution in pregnancy because of the risk of ionizing radiation to the fetus.	Patient should be able to exercise on a treadmill. In case of severe peripheral vascular disease, severe pulmonary disease, or musculoskeletal disorder, pharmacologic stress with dipyridamole or other agents may be used. Tests should be performed in the fasting state. Patient should not exercise between stress and redistribution scans.
HEART **Radionuclide ventriculography** (multigated acquisition [MUGA]) $$–$$$–$$$$	Evaluation of patients with ischemic heart disease and other cardiomyopathies. Evaluation of response to pharmacologic therapy and effects of cardiotoxic drugs.	Noninvasive. Ejection fraction is a reproducible index that can be used to follow course of disease and response to therapy.	Gated data acquisition may be difficult in patients with severe arrhythmias. **Contraindications and risks:** Recent infarct is a contraindication to exercise ventriculography (arrhythmia, ischemia, infarct, and rarely death may occur with exercise). Caution is advised in pregnancy because of the risk of ionizing radiation to the fetus.	Requires harvesting, labeling, and re-injecting the patient's red blood cells. Sterile technique required in handling of red cells.

		ABDOMEN	
		KUB	**Ultrasound**
Preparation		None.	NPO for 6 hours.
Disadvantages/Contraindications		Supine film alone is inadequate to rule out pneumoperitoneum (see indications). Obstipation may obscure lesions. **Contraindications and risks:** Contraindicated in pregnancy because of the risk of ionizing radiation to the fetus.	Technique very operator-dependent. Organs (particularly pancreas and distal aorta) may be obscured by bowel gas. Presence of barium obscures sound waves. **Contraindications and risks:** None.
Advantages		Inexpensive. Widely available.	Noninvasive. No ionizing radiation. Can be portable. Imaging in all planes. Can guide percutaneous fine-needle aspiration of tumor or abscess.
Indications		Assessment of bowel gas patterns (eg, to distinguish ileus from obstruction). To rule out pneumoperitoneum, order an upright abdomen and chest radiograph (acute abdominal series).	Differentiation of cystic versus solid lesions of the liver and kidneys, intra- and extrahepatic biliary ductal dilation, cholelithiasis, gallbladder wall thickness, pericholecystic fluid, peripancreatic fluid and pseudocyst, primary and metastatic liver carcinoma, hydronephrosis, abdominal aortic aneurysm, appendicitis, ascites.
Test		**ABDOMEN** **Abdominal plain radiograph** (KUB [kidneys, ureters, bladder] x-ray) $	**ABDOMEN** **Ultrasound** (US) $$

ABDOMEN			
		CT	
ABDOMEN **Computed tomography** (CT) $$$–$$$$	Morphologic evaluation of all abdominal and pelvic organs. Differentiation of intraperitoneal versus retroperitoneal disorders. Evaluation of abscess, trauma, mesenteric and retroperitoneal lymphadenopathy, bowel wall thickening, obstructive biliary disease, pancreatitis, site of gastrointestinal obstruction, appendicitis, peritonitis, and carcinomatosis, splenic infarction, retroperitoneal hemorrhage, aortoenteric fistula. Staging of renal cell carcinoma, carcinomas of the gastrointestinal tract, and metastatic liver disease. Sensitive in predicting that pancreatic carcinoma is unresectable. Excellent screening tool for evaluation of suspected renal and ureteral calculi. Spiral CT angiography valuable in the evaluation of the aorta and its branches. Can provide preoperative assessment of abdominal aortic aneurysm to determine aneurysm size, proximal and distal extent, relationship to renal arteries, and presence of anatomic anomalies.	Rapid. Superb spatial resolution. Not limited by overlying bowel gas, as with ultrasound. Can guide fine-needle aspiration and percutaneous drainage procedures. Noncontrast spiral CT is superior to plain abdominal radiography, ultrasound, and intravenous urography in determination of size and location of renal and ureteral calculi.	Barium or Hypaque, surgical clips, and metallic prostheses can cause artifacts and degrade image quality. **Contraindications and risks:** Contraindicated in pregnancy because of the potential harm of ionizing radiation to the fetus. See Risks of Intravenous Contrast Studies, page 244.	Preferably NPO for 4–6 hours. Normal hydration. Opacification of gastrointestinal tract with water-soluble oral contrast (Gastrografin). Sedation of agitated patients. Recent serum creatinine determination.

	ABDOMEN
	MRI

Test	Indications	Advantages	Disadvantages/Contraindications	Preparation
ABDOMEN **Magnetic resonance imaging (MRI)** $$$$	Clarification of CT findings when surgical clip artifacts are present. Differentiation of retroperitoneal lymphadenopathy from blood vessels or the diaphragmatic crus. Preoperative staging of renal cell carcinoma. Differentiation of benign nonhyperfunctioning adrenal adenoma from malignant adrenal mass. Complementary to CT in evaluation of liver lesions (especially metastatic disease and possible tumor invasion of hepatic or portal veins). Differentiation of benign cavernous hemangioma (> 2 cm in diameter) from malignancy.	Provides excellent tissue contrast resolution, multiplanar capability. No beam-hardening artifacts such as can be seen with CT. No ionizing radiation.	Subject to motion artifacts. Gastrointestinal opacification not yet readily available. Special instrumentation required for patients on life support. **Contraindications and risks:** Contraindicated in patients with cardiac pacemakers, intraocular metallic foreign bodies, intracranial aneurysm clips, cochlear implants, and some artificial heart valves.	NPO for 4–6 hours. Intramuscular glucagon to inhibit peristalsis. Sedation of agitated patients. Screening CT or plain radiograph images of orbits if history suggests possible metallic foreign body in the eye.

ABDOMEN			
Mesenteric angiography			
ABDOMEN **Mesenteric angiography** $$$$	Gastrointestinal hemorrhage that does not resolve with conservative therapy and cannot be treated endoscopically. Localization of gastrointestinal bleeding site. Acute mesenteric ischemia, intestinal angina, splenic or other splanchnic artery aneurysm. Evaluation of possible vasculitis, such as polyarteritis nodosa. Detection of islet cell tumors not identified by other studies. Abdominal trauma.	Therapeutic embolization of gastrointestinal hemorrhage is often possible.	Invasive. Patient must remain supine with leg extended for 6 hours following the procedure in order to protect the common femoral artery at the catheter entry site. **Contraindications and risks:** Allergy to iodinated contrast material may require corticosteroid and H_1 blocker or H_2 blocker premedication. Contraindicated in pregnancy because of the potential harm of ionizing radiation to the fetus. Contrast nephrotoxicity, especially with preexisting impaired renal function due to diabetes mellitus or multiple myeloma; however, any creatinine elevation following the procedure is usually reversible (see page 244).	NPO for 4–6 hours. Good hydration to limit possible renal insult due to iodinated contrast material. Recent serum creatinine determination, assessment of clotting parameters, reversal of anticoagulation. Performed with conscious sedation. Requires cardiac, respiratory, blood pressure, and pulse oximetry monitoring.

		GASTROINTESTINAL	
		UGI	Enteroclysis

Test	Indications	Advantages	Disadvantages/Contraindications	Preparation
GI **Upper GI study** (UGI) $$	Double-contrast barium technique demonstrates esophageal, gastric, and duodenal mucosa for evaluation of inflammatory disease and other subtle mucosal abnormalities. Single-contrast technique is suitable for evaluation of possible outlet obstruction, peristalsis, gastroesophageal reflux and hiatal hernia, esophageal cancer and varices. Water-soluble contrast (Gastrografin) is suitable for evaluation of anastomotic leak or gastrointestinal perforation.	Good evaluation of mucosa with double-contrast examination. No sedation required. Less expensive than endoscopy.	Aspiration of water-soluble contrast material may occur, resulting in severe pulmonary edema. Leakage of barium from a perforation may cause granulomatous inflammatory reaction. Identification of a lesion does not prove it to be the site of blood loss in patients with gastrointestinal bleeding. Barium precludes endoscopy and body CT examination. Retained gastric secretions prevent mucosal coating with barium. **Contraindications and risks:** Contraindicated in pregnancy because of the potential harm of ionizing radiation to the fetus.	NPO for 8 hours.
GI **Enteroclysis** $$	Barium fluoroscopic study for location of site of intermittent partial small bowel obstruction. Evaluation of extent of Crohn's disease or small bowel disease in patient with persistent gastrointestinal bleeding and normal upper gastrointestinal and colonic evaluations. Evaluation of metastatic disease to the small bowel.	Clarifies lesions noted on more traditional barium examination of the small bowel. Best means of establishing small bowel as normal. Controlled high rate of flow of barium can dilate a partial obstruction.	Requires nasogastric or orogastric tube placement and manipulation to beyond the ligament of Treitz. **Contraindications and risks:** Radiation exposure is substantial, since lengthy fluoroscopic examination is required. Therefore, the test is contraindicated in pregnant women and should be used sparingly in children and women of childbearing age.	Clear liquid diet for 24 hours. Colonic cleansing.

GASTROINTESTINAL			
Peroral pneumocolon		**Barium enema**	
GI **Peroral pneumocolon** $	Fluoroscopic evaluation of the terminal ileum by insufflating air per rectum after orally ingested barium has reached the cecum.	Best evaluation of the terminal ileum. Can be performed concurrently with upper GI series.	Undigested food in the small bowel interferes with the evaluation. **Contraindications and risk:** Contraindicated in pregnancy because of the potential harm of ionizing radiation to the fetus.
			Clear liquid diet for 24 hours.
GI **Barium enema** (BE) $$	Double-contrast technique for evaluation of colonic mucosa in patients with suspected inflammatory bowel disease or neoplasm. Single-contrast technique for investigation of possible fistulous tracts, bowel obstruction, large palpable masses in the abdomen, and diverticulitis and for examination of debilitated patients. Least invasive colon cancer screening technique.	Good mucosal evaluation. No sedation required.	Retained fecal material limits study. Requires patient cooperation. Marked diverticulosis precludes evaluation of possible neoplasm in that area. Evaluation of right colon occasionally incomplete or limited by reflux of barium across ileocecal valve and overlapping opacified small bowel. Use of barium delays subsequent colonoscopy and body CT. **Contraindications and risks:** Contraindicated in patients with toxic megacolon and immediately after full-thickness colonoscopic biopsy.
			Colon cleansing with enemas, cathartic, and clear liquid diet (1 day in young patients, 2 days in older patients). Intravenous glucagon (which inhibits peristalsis) sometimes given to distinguish colonic spasm from a mass lesion.

		GASTROINTESTINAL	
		Hypaque enema	**Esophageal reflux study**
Test		GI **Hypaque enema** $$	GI **Esophageal reflux study** (radio-nuclide) $$
Indications		Water-soluble contrast for fluoroscopic evaluation of sigmoid or cecal volvulus, anastomotic leak or other perforation. Differentiation of colonic versus small bowel obstruction. Therapy for obstipation.	Evaluation of heartburn, regurgitation, recurrent aspiration pneumonia.
Advantages		Water-soluble contrast medium is evacuated much faster than barium because it does not adhere to the mucosa. Therefore, Hypaque enema can be followed immediately by oral ingestion of barium for evaluation of possible distal small bowel obstruction.	Noninvasive and well tolerated. More sensitive for reflux than fluoroscopy, endoscopy, and manometry; sensitivity similar to that of acid reflux test. Permits quantitation of reflux. Can also identify aspiration into the lung fields.
Disadvantages/Contraindications		Demonstrates only colonic morphologic features and not mucosal changes. **Contraindications and risks:** Contraindicated in patients with toxic megacolon. Hypertonic solution may lead to fluid imbalance in debilitated patients and children.	Incomplete emptying of esophagus may mimic reflux. Abdominal binder—used to increase pressure in the lower esophagus—may not be tolerated in patients who have undergone recent abdominal surgery. **Contraindications and risks:** Contraindicated in pregnancy because of the potential harm of ionizing radiation to the fetus.
Preparation		Colonic cleansing is desirable but not always necessary.	NPO for 4–6 hours. During test, patient must be able to consume 300 mL of liquid.

GASTROINTESTINAL	
Gastric emptying study	**GI bleeding scan**
Evaluation of dumping syndrome, vagotomy, gastric outlet obstruction due to inflammatory or neoplastic disease, effects of drugs, and other causes of gastroparesis (eg, diabetes mellitus).	Evaluation of upper or lower gastrointestinal blood loss.
Gives functional information not available by other means.	Noninvasive compared with angiography. Longer period of imaging possible, which aids in detection of intermittent bleeding. Labeled red cells and sulfur colloid can detect bleeding rates as low as 0.05–0.10 mL/min (angiography requires rate of about 0.5 mL/min). Ninety percent sensitivity for blood loss >500 mL/24 h.
Reporting of meaningful data requires adherence to standard protocol and establishment of normal values. **Contraindications and risks:** Contraindicated in pregnancy because of the potential harm of ionizing radiation to the fetus.	Bleeding must be active during time of imaging. Presence of free TcO_4 (poor labeling efficiency) can lead to gastric, kidney, and bladder activity that can be misinterpreted as sites of bleeding. Uptake in hepatic hemangioma, varices, arteriovenous malformation, abdominal aortic aneurysm, and bowel wall inflammation can also lead to false-positive examination. **Contraindications and risks:** Contraindicated in pregnancy because of the potential harm of ionizing radiation to the fetus.
NPO for 4–6 hours. During test, patient must be able to eat a 300 g meal consisting of both liquids and solids.	Sterile technique required during in vitro labeling of red cells.

Row labels (left margin):

GI
Gastric emptying study (radionuclide)
$$

GI
GI bleeding scan (labeled red cell scan, radionuclide)
$$–$$$

	GALLBLADDER	
	Ultrasound	**HIDA scan**

Test	Indications	Advantages	Disadvantages/Contraindications	Preparation
GALL-BLADDER **Ultrasound** (US) $	Demonstrates cholelithiasis (95% sensitive), gallbladder wall thickening, pericholecystic fluid, intra- and extrahepatic biliary dilation.	Noninvasive. No ionizing radiation. Can be portable. Imaging in all planes. Can guide fine-needle aspiration, percutaneous transhepatic cholangiography, and biliary drainage procedures.	Technique very operator-dependent. Presence of barium obscures sound waves. Difficult in obese patients. **Contraindications and risks:** None.	Preferably NPO for 6 hours to enhance visualization of gallbladder.
GALL-BLADDER **Hepatic iminodiacetic acid scan** (HIDA) $$	Evaluation of suspected acute cholecystitis or common bile duct obstruction. Evaluation of bile leaks, biliary atresia, and biliary enteric bypass patency.	Ninety-five percent sensitivity and 99% specificity for diagnosis of acute cholecystitis. Hepatobiliary function assessed. Defines pathophysiology underlying acute cholecystitis. Rapid. Can be performed in patients with elevated serum bilirubin. No intravenous contrast used.	Does not demonstrate the cause of obstruction (eg, tumor or gallstone). Not able to evaluate biliary excretion if hepatocellular function is severely impaired. Sensitivity may be lower in acalculous cholecystitis. False-positive results can occur with hyperalimentation, prolonged fasting, and acute pancreatitis. **Contraindications and risks:** Contraindicated in pregnancy because of the potential harm of ionizing radiation to the fetus.	NPO for at least 4 hours but preferably less than 24 hours. Premedication with cholecystokinin (CCK) can prevent false-positive examination in patients who are receiving hyperalimentation or who have been fasting longer than 24 hours. Avoid administration of morphine prior to examination if possible.

	PANCREAS/BILIARY TREE			LIVER
	ERCP			**Ultrasound**
PANCREAS/ BILIARY TREE **Endoscopic retrograde cholangiopancreatography** (ERCP) $$	Primary sclerosing cholangitis, AIDS-associated cholangitis, and cholangiocarcinomas. Demonstrates cause, location, and extent of extrahepatic biliary obstruction (eg, choledocholithiasis). Can diagnose chronic pancreatitis.	Avoids surgery. Less invasive than percutaneous transhepatic cholangiography. If stone is suspected, ERCP offers therapeutic potential (sphincterotomy and extraction of common bile duct stone). Finds gallstones in up to 14% of patients with symptoms but negative ultrasound. Plastic or metallic stent placement may be possible in patients with obstruction.	Requires endoscopy. May cause pancreatitis (1%), cholangitis (<1%), peritonitis, hemorrhage (if sphincterotomy performed), and death (rare). **Contraindications and risks:** Relatively contraindicated in patients with concurrent or recent (<6 weeks) acute pancreatitis or suspected pancreatic pseudocyst. Contraindicated in pregnancy because of the potential harm of ionizing radiation to the fetus.	NPO for 6 hours. Sedation required. Vital signs should be monitored by the nursing staff. Not possible in patient who has undergone Roux-en-Y hepaticojejunostomy.
LIVER **Ultrasound** (US) $	Differentiation of cystic versus solid intrahepatic lesions. Evaluation of intra- and extrahepatic biliary dilation, primary and metastatic liver tumors, and ascites. Evaluation of patency of portal vein, hepatic arteries, and hepatic veins.	Noninvasive. No radiation. Can be portable. Imaging in all planes. Can guide fine-needle aspiration, percutaneous transhepatic cholangiography, and biliary drainage procedures.	Technique very operator-dependent. Presence of barium obscures sound waves. More difficult in obese patients. The presence of fatty liver or cirrhosis can limit the sensitivity of ultrasound for focal mass lesions. **Contraindications and risks:** None.	Preferably NPO for 6 hours.

	LIVER	
	CT	CTAP

Test	Indications	Advantages	Disadvantages/Contraindications	Preparation
LIVER **Computed tomography (CT)** $$$–$$$$	Suspected metastatic or primary tumor, gallbladder carcinoma, biliary obstruction, abscess.	Excellent spatial resolution. Can direct percutaneous fine-needle aspiration biopsy.	Requires iodinated contrast material administered intravenously. **Contraindications and risks:** Contraindicated in pregnancy because of the potential harm of ionizing radiation to the fetus. See Risks of Intravenous Contrast Studies, page 244.	NPO for 4–6 hours. Recent creatinine determination. Administration of oral contrast material for opacification of stomach and small bowel. Specific hepatic protocol with arterial, portal venous, and delayed images used for evaluation of neoplasm.
LIVER **Computed tomographic arterial portography (CTAP)** $$$$	Assessment of number, location, and resectability of metastatic liver tumors.	Sensitive to number of liver lesions (good for lesion detection). Provides cross-sectional imaging for segmental localization of liver tumors.	Invasive, requiring percutaneous catheter placement in the superior mesenteric artery. Patient must remain supine with leg extended for 6 hours following the procedure to protect the common femoral artery at the catheter entry site. Useful for lesion detection but does not permit characterization of lesions. May not be possible in patients with cirrhosis where portal hypertension limits delivery of contrast material to liver.	NPO for 4–6 hours. Recent creatinine determination. Requires some conscious sedation.

| | LIVER | | |
	MRI		
LIVER **Magnetic resonance imaging (MRI)** $$$$	Characterization of focal hepatic lesion, including suspected cyst, hepatocellular carcinoma, focal nodular hyperplasia, and metastasis. Suspected metastatic or primary tumor. Differentiation of benign cavernous hemangioma from malignant tumor. Evaluation of hemochromatosis, hemosiderosis, fatty liver, and suspected focal fatty infiltration.	Requires no iodinated contrast material. Provides excellent tissue contrast resolution, multiplanar capability.	Subject to motion artifacts, particularly those of respiration. Special instrumentation required for patients on life support. **Contraindications and risks:** Contraindicated in patients with cardiac pacemakers, intraocular metallic foreign bodies, intracranial aneurysm clips, cochlear implants, some artificial heart valves.	Screening CT or plain radiograph images of orbits if history suggests possible metallic foreign body in the eye. Intramuscular glucagon is used to inhibit intestinal peristalsis.

| | LIVER | | | |
| | PTC | | | |
Test	Indications	Advantages	Disadvantages/Contraindications	Preparation
LIVER/ BILIARY TREE **Percutaneous transhepatic cholangiogram (PTC)** $$$	Evaluation of biliary obstruction in patients in whom ERCP has failed or patients with Roux-en-Y hepaticojejunostomy.	Best examination to assess site and morphology of obstruction close to the hilum (as opposed to endoscopic retrograde cholangiopancreatography [ERCP], which is better for distal obstruction). Can characterize the nature of diffuse intrahepatic biliary disease such as primary sclerosing cholangitis. Provides guidance and access for percutaneous transhepatic biliary drainage (PTBD) and possible stent placement to treat obstruction.	Invasive; requires special training. Performed with conscious sedation. Ascites may present a contraindication.	NPO for 4–6 hours. Sterile technique, assessment of clotting parameters, correction of coagulopathy. Performed with conscious sedation.

	LIVER	LIVER/SPLEEN
	Hepatic angiography	**Liver, spleen scan**
LIVER **Hepatic angiography** $$$$	Preoperative evaluation for liver transplantation, vascular malformations, trauma, Budd-Chiari syndrome, portal vein patency (when ultrasound equivocal) prior to transjugular intrahepatic portosystemic shunt (TIPS) procedure. In some cases, evaluation of hepatic neoplasm or transcatheter embolotherapy of hepatic malignancy.	Best assessment of hepatic arterial anatomy, which is highly variable. More accurate than ultrasound with respect to portal vein patency when the latter suggests occlusion.	Invasive. Patient must remain supine with leg extended for 6 hours following the procedure in order to protect the common femoral artery at the catheter entry site. **Contraindications and risks:** Allergy to iodinated contrast material may require corticosteroid and H_1 blocker or H_2 blocker premedication. Contraindicated in pregnancy because of the potential harm of ionizing radiation to the fetus. Contrast nephrotoxicity may occur, especially with preexisting impaired renal function due to diabetes mellitus or multiple myeloma; however, any creatinine elevation following the procedure is usually reversible.	NPO for 4–6 hours. Good hydration to limit possible renal insult due to iodinated contrast material. Recent serum creatinine determination, assessment of clotting parameters, reversal of anticoagulation. Performed with conscious sedation. Requires cardiac, respiratory, blood pressure, and pulse oximetry monitoring.
LIVER, SPLEEN **Liver, spleen scan** (radionuclide) $$	Identification of functioning splenic tissue to localize an accessory spleen or evaluate suspected functional asplenia. Assessment of size, shape, and position of liver and spleen. Characterization of a focal liver mass with regard to inherent functioning reticuloendothelial cell activity (with the exception of focal nodular hyperplasia mass lesions, which are more often "cold" than "hot"). Confirmation of patency and distribution of hepatic arterial perfusion catheters.	May detect isodense lesions missed by CT.	Diminished sensitivity for small lesions (less than 1.5–2 cm) and deep lesions. Single photon emission computed tomography (SPECT) increases sensitivity (can detect lesions of 1–1.5 cm). Nonspecific; unable to distinguish solid versus cystic or inflammatory versus neoplastic tissue. Lower sensitivity for diffuse hepatic tumors. **Contraindications and risks:** Caution in pregnancy advised because of the risk of ionizing radiation to the fetus.	None.

	PANCREAS		ADRENAL
	CT	**Ultrasound**	**MIBG scan**
Test			
PANCREAS **Computed tomography (CT)** $$$–$$$$			
PANCREAS **Ultrasound (US)** $			
ADRENAL **MIBG (meta-iodobenzyl-guanidine) (radionuclide)** $$$$			

Test	Indications	Advantages	Disadvantages/Contraindications	Preparation
PANCREAS **Computed tomography (CT)** $$$–$$$$	Evaluation of biliary obstruction and possible adenocarcinoma. Staging of pancreatic carcinoma. Diagnosis and staging of acute pancreatitis.	Can guide fine-needle biopsy or placement of a drainage catheter. Can identify early necrosis in pancreatitis.	Optimal imaging requires special protocol, including precontrast plus arterial and venous phase contrast-enhanced images. **Contraindications and risks:** Contraindicated in pregnancy because of the potential harm of ionizing radiation to the fetus. See Risks of Intravenous Contrast Studies, page 244.	Preferably NPO for 4–6 hours. Normal hydration. Opacification of gastrointestinal tract with Gastrografin. Sedation of agitated patients. Recent serum creatinine determination.
PANCREAS **Ultrasound (US)** $	Identification of peripancreatic fluid collections, pseudocysts, and pancreatic ductal dilation.	Noninvasive. No radiation. Can be portable. Imaging in all planes. Can guide fine-needle aspiration or placement of drainage catheter.	Pancreas may be obscured by overlying bowel gas. Technique very operator-dependent. Presence of barium obscures sound waves. Less sensitive than CT. **Contraindications and risks:** None.	Preferably NPO for 6 hours.
ADRENAL **MIBG (meta-iodobenzyl-guanidine) (radionuclide)** $$$$	Suspected pheochromocytoma when CT is negative or equivocal. Also useful in evaluation of neuroblastoma, carcinoid, and medullary carcinoma of thyroid.	Test is useful for localization of pheochromocytomas (particularly extra-adrenal). Eighty to 90 percent sensitive for detection of pheochromocytoma.	High radiation dose to adrenal gland. High cost and limited availability of MIBG. Delayed imaging (at 1, 2, and 3 days) necessitates return of patient. **Contraindications and risks:** Contraindicated in pregnancy because of the risk of ionizing radiation to the fetus. Because of the relatively high dose of ^{131}I, patients should be instructed about precautionary measures by nuclear medicine personnel.	Administration of Lugol's iodine solution (to block thyroid uptake) prior to and following administration of MIBG.

GENITOURINARY		
IVP	**Ultrasound**	**MRI**
GENITO-URINARY **Intravenous pyelogram (IVP)** $$$	GENITO-URINARY **Ultrasound (US)** $$	GENITO-URINARY **Magnetic resonance imaging (MRI)** $$$$
Fluoroscopic evaluation of uro-epithelial neoplasm, calculus, papillary necrosis, and medullary sponge kidney. Screening for urinary system injury after trauma.	Evaluation of renal morphology, hydronephrosis, size of prostate, and residual urine volume. Differentiation of cystic versus solid renal lesions.	Staging of cancers of the uterus, cervix, and prostate. Can provide information additional to what is obtained by CT in some cases of cancer of the kidney and urinary bladder.
Permits evaluation of collecting system in less invasive manner than retrograde pyelogram. Can assess both renal morphology and function.	Noninvasive. No radiation. Can be portable. Imaging in all planes. Can guide fine-needle aspiration or placement of drainage catheter.	Provides excellent tissue contrast resolution, multiplanar capability. No beam-hardening artifacts such as can be seen with CT. No ionizing radiation.
Suboptimal evaluation of the renal parenchyma. Does not adequately evaluate cause of ureteral deviation. **Contraindications and risks:** Caution in pregnancy is advised because of the risk of ionizing radiation to the fetus. See Risks of Intravenous Contrast Studies, page 244.	Technique very operator-dependent. More difficult in obese patients. **Contraindications and risks:** None.	Subject to motion artifacts. Gastrointestinal opacification not yet readily available. Special instrumentation required for patients on life support. **Contraindications and risks:** Contraindicated in patients with cardiac pacemakers, intracranial metallic foreign bodies, intracranial aneurysm clips, cochlear implants, and some artificial heart valves.
Adequate hydration. Colonic cleansing is preferred but not essential. Recent serum creatinine determination.	Preferably NPO for 6 hours. Full urinary bladder required for pelvic studies.	Sedation of agitated patients. Screening CT or plain radiograph images of orbits if history suggests possible metallic foreign body in the eye.

	GENITOURINARY
	Radionuclide scan

Test	Indications	Advantages	Disadvantages/Contraindications	Preparation
GENITO-URINARY	Evaluation of suspected renal vascular hypertension. Differentiation of a dilated but non-obstructed system from one that has a urodynamically significant obstruction. Evaluation of renal blood flow and function in acute or chronic renal failure. Evaluation of both medical and surgical complications of renal transplant. Estimation of glomerular filtration rate (GFR) and effective renal plasma flow (ERPF). Determination of relative renal function prior to nephrectomy.	Provides functional information without risk of iodinated contrast used in IVP. Provides quantitative information not available by other means.	Finding of poor renal blood flow does not pinpoint an etiologic diagnosis. Limited utility when renal function is extremely poor. Estimation of glomerular filtration rate and renal plasma flow often is inaccurate. **Contraindications and risks:** Caution in pregnancy because of the risk of ionizing radiation to the fetus.	Normal hydration needed for evaluation of suspected obstructive uropathy since dehydration may result in false-positive examination. Blood pressure should be monitored and an intravenous line started when an angiotensin-converting enzyme (ACE) inhibitor is used to enhance test sensitivity in the evaluation of renal vascular hypertension. Patient should discontinue ACE inhibitor medication for at least 48 hours prior to examination if possible.
Renal scan (radionuclide) $$				

PELVIS		
	Ultrasound	**MRI**

PELVIS **Ultrasound (US)** $$	Evaluation of palpable ovarian mass, enlarged uterus, vaginal bleeding, pelvic pain, possible ectopic pregnancy, and infertility. Monitoring of follicular development. Localization of intrauterine device.	Use of a vaginal probe enables very early detection of intrauterine pregnancy and ectopic pregnancy and does not require a full bladder.	Transabdominal scan has limited sensitivity for uterine or ovarian pathology. Vaginal probe has limited field of view and therefore may miss large masses outside the pelvis. **Contraindications and risks:** None.	Distended bladder required (only in transabdominal examination).
PELVIS **Magnetic resonance imaging (MRI)** $$$$	Evaluation of gynecologic malignancies, particularly endometrial, cervical, and vaginal carcinoma. Evaluation of prostate, bladder, and rectal carcinoma. Evaluation of congenital anomalies of the genitourinary tract. Useful in distinguishing lymphadenopathy from vasculature.	Provides excellent tissue contrast resolution, multiplanar capability. No beam-hardening artifacts such as can be seen with CT. No ionizing radiation.	Subject to motion artifacts. Special instrumentation required for patients on life support. **Contraindications and risks:** Contraindicated in patients with cardiac pacemakers, intraocular metallic foreign bodies, intracranial aneurysm clips, cochlear implants, and some artificial heart valves.	Intramuscular glucagon is used to inhibit intestinal peristalsis. Sedation of agitated patients. Screening CT or plain radiograph images of orbits if history suggests possible metallic foreign body in the eye. An endorectal device (radiofrequency coil) is used for prostate MRI.

| | BONE | | | |
| | Bone scan | | | |
Test	Indications	Advantages	Disadvantages/Contraindications	Preparation
BONE **Bone scan, whole body** (radionuclide) $$–$$$	Evaluation of primary or metastatic neoplasm, osteomyelitis, arthritis, metabolic disorders, trauma, avascular necrosis, joint prosthesis, and reflex sympathetic dystrophy. Evaluation of clinically suspected but radiographically occult fractures. Identification of stress fractures.	Can examine entire osseous skeleton or specific area of interest. Highly sensitive compared with plain film radiography for detection of bone neoplasm. In osteomyelitis, bone scan may be positive much earlier (24 hours) than plain film (10–14 days).	Nonspecific. Correlation with plain film radiographs often necessary. Limited utility in patients with poor renal function. Poor resolution in distal extremities, head, and spine; in these instances, single photon emission computed tomography (SPECT) is often useful. Sometimes difficult to distinguish osteomyelitis from cellulitis or septic joint; dual imaging with gallium or with indium-labeled leukocytes can be helpful. False-negative results for osteomyelitis can occur following antibiotic therapy and within the first 24 hours after trauma. In avascular necrosis, bone scan may be "hot," "cold," or normal, depending on the stage. **Contraindications and risks:** Caution in pregnancy because of the risk of ionizing radiation to the fetus.	Patient should be well hydrated and void frequently after the procedure.

SPINE				
SPINE **Computed tomography** (CT) $$$	Evaluation of structures that are not well visualized on MRI, including ossification of the posterior longitudinal ligament, tumoral calcification, osteophytic spurring, retropulsed bone fragments after trauma. Also used for patients in whom MRI is contraindicated.	Rapid. Superb spatial resolution. Can guide percutaneous fine-needle aspiration of possible tumor or abscess.	Generally limited to transaxial views. Coronal and sagittal reformation images can be generated. MRI unequivocally superior in evaluation of the spine and cord except for conditions mentioned in Indications. Artifacts from metal prostheses degrade images. **Contraindications and risks:** Contraindicated in pregnancy because of the potential harm of ionizing radiation to the fetus. See Risks of Intravenous Contrast Studies, page 244.	Normal hydration. Sedation of agitated patients.
SPINE **Magnetic resonance imaging** (MRI) $$$$	Diseases involving the spine and cord except where CT is superior (ossification of the posterior longitudinal ligament, tumoral calcification, osteophytic spurring, retropulsed bone fragments after trauma).	Provides excellent tissue contrast resolution, multiplanar capability. No beam-hardening artifacts such as can be seen with CT. No ionizing radiation.	Less useful in detection of calcification, small spinal vascular malformations, acute spinal trauma (because of longer acquisition time, incompatibility with life support devices, and inferior detection of bony injury). Subject to motion artifacts. Special instrumentation required for patients on life support. **Contraindications and risks:** Contraindicated in patients with cardiac pacemakers, intraocular metallic foreign bodies, intracranial aneurysm clips, cochlear implants, and some artificial heart valves.	Sedation of agitated patients. Screening CT or plain radiograph images of orbits if history suggests possible metallic foreign body in the eye.

Test	Indications	Advantages	Disadvantages/Contraindications	Preparation
	MUSCULOSKELETAL			**VASCULATURE**
	MRI			**Ultrasound**
MUSCULO-SKELETAL SYSTEM **Magnetic resonance imaging (MRI)** $$$$	Evaluation of joints except where a prosthesis is in place. Extent of primary or malignant tumor (bone and soft tissue). Evaluation of aseptic necrosis, bone and soft tissue infections, marrow space disease, and traumatic derangements.	Provides excellent tissue contrast resolution, multiplanar capability. No beam-hardening artifacts such as can be seen with CT. No ionizing radiation.	Subject to motion artifacts. Less able than CT to detect calcification, ossification, and periosteal reaction. Special instrumentation required for patients on life support. **Contraindications and risks:** Contraindicated in patients with cardiac pacemakers, intraocular metallic foreign bodies, intracranial aneurysm clips, cochlear implants, and some artificial heart valves.	Sedation of agitated patients. Screening CT or plain radiograph images of orbits if history suggests possible metallic foreign body in the eye.
VASCU-LATURE **Ultrasound (US)** $$	Evaluation of deep venous thrombosis, extremity grafts, patency of inferior vena cava, portal vein, and hepatic veins. Carotid doppler indicated for symptomatic carotid bruit, atypical transient ischemic attack, monitoring after endarterectomy, and baseline prior to major vascular surgery. Surveillance of transjugular intrahepatic portosystemic shunt (TIPS) patency and flow.	Noninvasive. No radiation. Can be portable. Imaging in all planes.	Technique operator-dependent. Ultrasound not sensitive to detection of ulcerated plaque. May be difficult to diagnose tight stenosis versus occlusion (catheter angiography may be necessary). May be difficult to distinguish acute from chronic deep venous thrombosis. **Contraindications and risks:** None.	None.

AORTA			
Angiography			
AORTA AND ITS BRANCHES **Angiography** $$$	Peripheral vascular disease, abdominal aortic aneurysm, renal artery stenosis (atherosclerotic and fibromuscular disease), polyarteritis nodosa, visceral ischemia, thoracic aortic dissection, gastrointestinal hemorrhage, thromboangiitis obliterans (Buerger's disease), popliteal entrapment syndrome, cystic adventitial disease, abdominal tumors, arteriovenous malformations, abdominal trauma. Preoperative evaluation for aorto-femoral bypass reconstructive surgery. Postoperative assessment of possible graft stenosis, especially femoral to popliteal or femoral to distal (foot or ankle).	Can localize atherosclerotic stenosis and assess the severity by morphology, flow, and pressure gradient. Provides assessment of stenotic lesions and access for percutaneous transluminal balloon dilation as well as stent treatment of iliac stenoses. Provides access for thrombolytic therapy of acute or subacute occlusion of native artery or bypass graft.	Invasive. Patient must remain supine with leg extended for 6 hours following the procedure in order to protect the common femoral artery at the catheter entry site. **Contraindications and risks:** Allergy to iodinated contrast material may require corticosteroid and H_1 blocker or H_2 blocker premedication. Contraindicated in pregnancy because of the potential harm of ionizing radiation to the fetus. Contrast nephrotoxicity may occur, especially with preexisting impaired renal function due to diabetes mellitus or multiple myeloma; however, any creatinine elevation that occurs after the procedure is usually reversible.	NPO for 4–6 hours. Good hydration to limit possible renal insult due to iodinated contrast material. Recent serum creatinine determination, assessment of clotting parameters, reversal of anticoagulation. Performed with conscious sedation. Requires cardiac, respiratory, blood pressure, and pulse oximetry monitoring as well as noninvasive studies of peripheral vascular disease to verify indication for angiography and to guide the examination.

	AORTA			
	MRA			
Test	Indications	Advantages	Disadvantages/Contraindications	Preparation
AORTA AND ITS BRANCHES **Magnetic resonance angiography (MRA)** $$$$	Can provide preoperative assessment of abdominal aortic aneurysm size, proximal and distal extent, relationship to renal arteries, and presence of anatomic anomalies. Permits evaluation of the hemodynamic and functional significance of renal artery stenosis.	No ionizing radiation. No iodinated contrast needed.	Subject to motion artifacts. Special instrumentation required for patients on life support. **Contraindications and risks:** Contraindicated in patients with cardiac pacemakers, intraocular metallic foreign bodies, intracranial aneurysm clips, cochlear implants, and some artificial heart valves.	Sedation of agitated patients. Screening CT or plain radiograph images of orbits if history suggests possible metallic foreign body in the eye.

BLOOD			
Indium scan			
BLOOD **Leukocyte scan** (indium scan, labeled white blood cell [WBC] scan, technetium-99m hexamethylpropyleneamine oxime [Tc99m-HMPAO]-labeled WBC scan, radionuclide) $$-$$$	Evaluation of fever of unknown origin, suspected abscess, pyelonephritis, osteomyelitis, and inflammatory bowel disease. Examination of choice for evaluation of suspected vascular graft infection.	Highly specific (98%) for infection (in contrast to gallium). Highly sensitive in detecting abdominal source of infection. In patients with fever of unknown origin, total body imaging is advantageous compared with CT scan or ultrasound. Preliminary imaging as early as 4 hours is possible with indium but less sensitive (30–50% of abscesses are detected at 24 hours).	24-hour delayed imaging may limit the utility of indium scan in critically ill patients. False-negative scans occur with antibiotic administration or in chronic infection. Perihepatic or splenic infection can be missed because of normal leukocyte accumulation in these organs; liver and spleen scan is necessary adjunct in this situation. False-positive scans occur with swallowed leukocytes, bleeding, indwelling tubes and catheters, surgical skin wound uptake, and bowel activity due to inflammatory processes. Pulmonary uptake is nonspecific and has low predictive value for infection. Patients must be able to hold still during relatively long acquisition times (5–10 minutes). Tc99m-HMPAO WBC may be suboptimal for detecting infection involving the genitourinary and gastrointestinal tracts because of normal distribution of the agent to these organs. **Contraindications and risks:** Contraindicated in pregnancy because of the hazard of ionizing radiation to the fetus. High radiation dose to spleen.	Leukocytes from the patient are harvested, labeled in vitro, and then reinjected; process requires 12 hours. Scanning takes place 24 hours after injection of indium-labeled WBC and 1–2 hours after injection of Tc99m-HMPAO WBC. Homologous donor leukocytes should be used in neutropenic patients.

7

Basic Electrocardiography*

G. Thomas Evans, Jr., MD

HOW TO USE THIS SECTION

This chapter includes criteria for the diagnosis of basic electrocardiographic waveforms and cardiac arrhythmias. It is intended for use as a reference and assumes a basic understanding of the electrocardiogram (ECG).

Electrocardiographic interpretation is a "stepwise" procedure, and the first steps are to study and characterize the cardiac rhythm.

Step One

Categorize what you see in the 12-lead ECG or rhythm strip, using the three major parameters that allow for systematic analysis and subsequent diagnosis of the rhythm:

1. Mean rate of the QRS complexes (slow, normal, or fast).
2. Width of the QRS complexes (wide or narrow).
3. Rhythmicity of the QRS complexes (characterization of spaces between QRS complexes) (regular or irregular).

---

*Adapted, with permission, from Evans GT Jr.: *ECG Interpretation Cribsheets,* 4th ed. Ring Mountain Press, 1999.

Based upon this categorization, refer to pages 286–299 for specific categories of rhythms. If the rhythm is irregularly irregular, go directly to page 288 (atrial fibrillation). For specific criteria for atrial flutter, go to page 288.

Step Two

Step 2 consists of examining and characterizing the morphology of the cardiac waveforms.

1. Examine for atrial abnormalities and bundle branch blocks (BBBs) (pages 301–302).

2. Assess the QRS axis and the causes of axis deviations (pages 304–306).

3. Examine for signs of left ventricular hypertrophy (pages 306–307).

4. Examine for signs of right ventricular hypertrophy (pages 307–308).

5. Examine for signs of myocardial infarction, if present (pages 310–320).

6. Bear in mind conditions that may alter the ability of the ECG to diagnose a myocardial infarction (page 320).

7. Examine for abnormalities of the ST segment or T wave (pages 320–323).

8. Assess the QT interval (pages 324–327).

9. Examine for miscellaneous conditions (pages 327–330).

STEP 1: DIAGNOSIS OF THE CARDIAC RHYTHM

A. APPROACH TO DIAGNOSIS OF THE CARDIAC RHYTHM

Most electrocardiograph machines display 10 seconds of data in a standard tracing. A rhythm is defined as three or more successive P waves or QRS complexes.

Categorize the patterns seen in the tracing according to a systematic method. This method proceeds in three steps that lead to a diagnosis based upon the most likely rhythm producing a particular pattern:

1. What is the mean rate of the QRS complexes?
   Slow (<60 bpm): The easiest way to determine this is to count the total number of QRS complexes in a 10-second period. If there are no more than 9, the rate is slow.

TABLE 7–1. SUSTAINED REGULAR RHYTHMS.

Rate	Fast	Normal	Slow

Narrow QRS duration	Sinus tachycardia
	Atrial tachycardia
	Atrial flutter
	    (2 : 1 AV conduction)
		Sinus rhythm
		Ectopic atrial rhythm
		Atrial flutter
		    (4 : 1 conduction)
			Sinus bradycardia
			Ectopic atrial bradycardia

Wide QRS duration	All rhythms listed above under narrow QRS duration, but with BBB or intraventricular conduction delay (IVCD) patterns		
	Ventricular tachycardia	Accelerated ventricular rhythm	Ventricular escape rhythm

> **Normal** (60–100 bpm): If there are 10–16 complexes in a 10-second period, the rate is normal.
>
> **Fast** (>100 bpm): If there are ≥17 complexes in a 10-second period, the rate is fast.

2. Is the duration of the dominant QRS morphology narrow (≤0.119 s) or wide (≥0.12 s)? (Refer to the section below on the QRS duration.)

3. What is the "rhythmicity" of the QRS complexes (defined as the spacing between QRS complexes)? Regular or irregular? (Any change in the spacing of the R-R intervals defines an irregular rhythm.)

Using the categorization above, refer to Tables 7–1 and 7–2 to select a specific diagnosis for the cardiac rhythm.

TABLE 7–2. SUSTAINED IRREGULAR RHYTHMS.

Rate	Fast	Normal	Slow

Narrow QRS duration	Atrial fibrillation
	Atrial flutter (variable
	    AV conduction)
	Multifocal atrial tachycardia
	Atrial tachycardia with
	    AV block (rare)
		Atrial fibrillation
		Atrial flutter (variable
		    AV conduction)
		Multiform atrial rhythm
		Atrial tachycardia with
		    AV block (rare)
			Atrial fibrillation
			Atrial flutter (variable
			    AV conduction)
			Multiform atrial rhythm

Wide QRS duration	All rhythms listed above under narrow QRS duration, but with BBB or IVCD patterns		

	Rarely, anterograde conduc-
	    tion of atrial fibrillation
	    over an accessory
	    pathway in patients with
	    WPW syndrome		

B. CATEGORIES OF QRS RHYTHM IRREGULARITY

A Dominant Regular Rhythm With Interruptions

This is the most common category of irregularity. Diagnoses include the following:

A. An **atrial pause,** defined as occasional abrupt pauses not initiated by premature QRS activity (and accompanied by a change in the P-P interval). Causes include: a nonconducted premature atrial complex (PAC) (most common); sinus pause (less common); atypical sinus arrhythmia (less common); and sinoatrial exit block (rare).

B. During **tachycardia,** occasional lengthening of the R–R cycle, unmasking the presence of either regular atrial activity or flutter waves.

C. **Premature QRS activity** that initiates a pause, called a **postextrasystolic pause,** with either (1) a narrow QRS complex (most common) due to either a normally conducted premature atrial complex (PAC) or, rarely, a premature junctional complex (PJC); or (2) a wide or abnormal QRS complex, due to a premature ventricular complex (PVC), the most common cause of a de novo wide QRS complex; aberrant ventricular conduction of a premature supraventricular impulse (either a PAC or PJC); or, rarely, a PAC that conducts over an accessory pathway.

Aberrant Ventricular Conduction

Aberrant ventricular conduction is defined as an abnormal QRS complex formed by premature activation of the His-Purkinje system that results in block of the impulse in one of the bundle branches. Aberrant conduction is usually a normal phenomenon and does not imply disease of the conduction system. The PR interval of a PAC that causes aberrant ventricular conduction is commonly prolonged.

An Irregularly Irregular Rhythm

Irregularly irregular rhythms have successive RR intervals that occur in random patterns. One method of ascertaining this pattern is to place calipers on the first RR interval at the start of the tracing and to precisely adjust the calipers to each successive RR interval throughout the 10-second period. If there are random changes in the intervals, the rhythm is irregularly irregular.

An irregularly irregular rhythm is usually the QRS "footprint" of (1) atrial fibrillation (most common sustained abnormal cardiac rhythm), (2) atrial flutter (with variable AV conduction), (3) multifocal atrial tachycardia (MAT), (4) atrial tachycardia with AV block, or (5) other less common rhythms.

Regularly Irregular Rhythm ("Group Beating")

Group beating is defined as clusters of regularly spaced QRS complexes, separated by pauses of identical duration. Whenever there is group beating, consider some form of Wenckebach periodicity, either during AV block or during junctional tachycardia with exit block in digitalis toxicity. Causes of group beating include the following:

A. Second-degree AV block, type I (Wenckebach) or type II (Mobitz II): There are usually single—but rarely multiple—nonconducted P waves in the setting of a constant PP interval.
B. PVCs in a repetitive pattern (ventricular trigeminy, quadrigeminy).
C. PACs or PJCs in a repetitive pattern (atrial trigeminy, etc).

Accelerating-Decelerating Rhythm

Causes include **sinus arrhythmia** (most common), defined as PP intervals that vary by > 10%; and **sinoatrial exit block** in a Wenckebach pattern (rare).

C. SINUS RHYTHMS

Sinus rhythms are defined by upright P waves in leads I, II, and aVF (present in 94% of normals) and are classified in Table 7–3.

D. ATRIAL RHYTHMS

Atrial rhythms, by definition, have nonsinus P waves. **Focal atrial arrhythmias** are defined as arrhythmias with a single focus (Table 7–4).

Multifocal Atrial Tachycardia (MAT)

Defined as having P waves with three or more morphologies per lead, with variable P-R intervals, and a mean atrial rate > 100/min. There is

TABLE 7–3. SINUS RHYTHMS.

Sinus rhythm	Rate 60–100 bpm
Sinus bradycardia	Rate <60 bpm (or <55 in persons age >65)
Sinus tachycardia	Rate >100 bpm
Sinus arrhythmia	Sinus P waves with >10% variation in PP intervals (due to respiration)

TABLE 7–4. ATRIAL RHYTHMS.

Ectopic atrial bradycardia	Rate <60 bpm
Ectopic atrial rhythm	Rate 60–100 bpm
Atrial tachycardia	Rate >100 bpm, but usually <240–250 bpm

commonly nonconducted atrial activity. The baseline between T waves and P waves is isoelectric. The cause is COPD (60% of cases).

Atrial Fibrillation

Atrial fibrillation is the most common sustained abnormal cardiac rhythm. It is defined by the presence of fibrillatory waves that have a small amplitude and very rapid rate and are characterized by an inconstancy of morphology. They are best seen in leads V_1, V_2, II, aVF, and III.

Atrial Flutter

Classic atrial flutter, seen in two-thirds of patients, produces the waveforms shown below, usually at an atrial rate of 250–350/min.

| II, aVF, III | | "Sawtooth" morphology |
| V_1 | | Discrete upright "P" waves |

E. JUNCTIONAL RHYTHMS

"Junctional rhythm" is not recommended terminology for a final rhythm diagnosis because the specific subtypes have clinical implications.

Definition of Junctional Complexes

There are three possible relationships between the P waves and QRS complexes during junctional complexes or rhythms:

A. A constant PR interval ≥0.08 s with a 1:1 AV ratio.
B. No discernible P wave activity (P waves buried in the QRS complexes).
C. A retrograde P wave following the QRS complex.

Definition of an Escape Complex or Rhythm

An escape complex or rhythm occurs when a lower down, subsidiary (secondary) pacemaking site assumes the role of cardiac pacemaker

TABLE 7–5. THREE TYPES OF JUNCTIONAL RHYTHM.

Rhythm	Rate	Clinical Correlates
Junctional escape rhythm	Rate <60 bpm	Sinus node dysfunction or drug side effects
Accelerated junctional rhythm	Rate 61–100 bpm	Digitalis toxicity, post cardiac surgery, rheumatic fever, infections of the AV node area, idiopathic
Junctional tachycardia	Rate >100 bpm	Same as accelerated junctional rhythm

because of failure of a primary pacer site anatomically superior to the escape focus. *Note:* "Escape" always implies normal function of the structure that is escaping and that an anatomically superior pacemaker has failed. Escape rhythms are usually very regular.

Definition of an Accelerated Complex or Rhythm

In contrast, an accelerated rhythm always implies abnormal function of the structure that is accelerated. The lower rate limit of accelerated rhythms equals the upper rate limit of the escape rate of the structure but is <101 bpm. Accelerated rhythms are usually very regular.

Classification of Junctional Rhythms

Table 7–5 summarizes a useful classification of junctional rhythms.

F. VENTRICULAR RHYTHMS

Definition of Ventricular Complexes

Ventricular complexes are not initiated by atrial activity and have a morphology that is inconsistent with that of typical RBBB or LBBB. The QRS duration is ≥0.12 s, usually between 0.14 s and 0.16 s. There are three major types of ventricular rhythms (Table 7–6).

TABLE 7–6. MAJOR TYPES OF VENTRICULAR RHYTHMS.[1]

Ventricular escape rhythm	Rate 25–40 bpm
Accelerated ventricular rhythm	Rate 41–100
Ventricular tachycardia	Rate >100 bpm

[1] *Refer to definitions of escape and accelerated rhythms, above.*

G. WIDE QRS COMPLEX TACHYCARDIA WITH A REGULAR RHYTHM (WCT-RR)

The most common cause of a wide QRS complex tachycardia with a regular rhythm (WCT-RR) is sinus tachycardia with either RBBB or LBBB. However, if a patient with structural heart disease presents with WCT-RR, one assumes a worst-case scenario and the presumptive diagnosis becomes ventricular tachycardia (VT). If the QRS complex in WCT-RR does not fit the typical pattern of either LBBB or RBBB, the diagnosis defaults to VT.

VT usually originates in an area at the border of infarcted and normal myocardium. Therefore, it does not require normal activation via the bundle branches or Purkinje system and produces an abnormal QRS complex.

Diagnosis of VT

Many criteria will diagnose VT with good performance, but no method will diagnose VT with 100% accuracy. Three methods—the "Quick" method, the Brugada algorithm, and the Griffith method (see below)—are commonly used but may yield different answers (VT or SVT). In some methods, 83% of VTs can be diagnosed using only the morphology of the QRS complex.

AV Dissociation in WCT-RR

The presence of AV dissociation or VA block in WCT-RR supersedes all other QRS morphologic criteria and is diagnostic of VT. However, during wide QRS complex tachycardia, it may be very difficult to identify atrial activity.

Regularity of RR Intervals in Ventricular Tachycardia

In ventricular tachycardia induced in the electrophysiology laboratory, the RR intervals were noted to be regular after 30 QRS complexes in 50% of patients and regular after 50 QRS complexes in 93% of patients. The mean rate of VT in these patients was 170 bpm. Therefore, a fast, wide, irregularly irregular rhythm that persists after 50 QRS complexes (about 18 seconds) is not likely to be ventricular tachycardia.

1. METHOD 1: QUICK METHOD FOR DIAGNOSIS OF VT (REQUIRES LEADS I, V_1, AND V_2)

This method derives from an analysis of typical waveforms of RBBB or LBBB as seen in leads I, V_1, and V_2. If the waveforms do not conform to either the common or uncommon typical morphologic patterns, the diagnosis defaults to VT.

Step One

Determine the morphologic classification of the wide QRS complexes (RB type or LB type), using the criteria below.

A. **Determination of the Morphologic Type of Wide QRS Complexes:** Use lead V_1 only to determine the type of bundle branch block morphology of abnormally wide QRS complexes.

1. **RBBB and RBB type QRS complexes as seen in lead V_1:** A wide QRS complex with a net positive area under the QRS curve is called the right bundle branch "type" of QRS. This does not mean that the QRS conforms exactly to the morphologic criteria for RBBB. Typical morphologies seen in RBBB are shown in the box at left below. Atypical morphologies at the right are most commonly seen in PVCs or during VT.

2. **LBBB and LBB-type QRS complexes as seen in lead V_1:** A wide QRS complex with a net negative area under the QRS curve is called a left bundle branch "type" of QRS. This does not mean that the QRS conforms exactly to the morphologic criteria for LBBB. Typical morphologies of LBBB are shown in the box at left below. Atypical morphologies at the right are most commonly seen in PVCs or during VT.

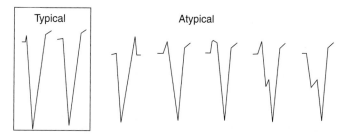

Step Two

Apply criteria for common and uncommon normal forms of either RBBB or LBBB, as described below. The waveforms may not be identical, but the morphologic descriptions must match. If the QRS complexes do not match, the rhythm is probably VT.

   A. RBBB: Lead I must have a terminal broad S wave, but the R/S ratio may be <1.

    In lead V_1, the QRS complex is usually triphasic but sometimes is notched and monophasic. The latter must have notching on the ascending limb of the R wave, usually at the lower left.

   B. LBBB: Lead I must have a monophasic, usually notched R wave and may not have Q waves or S waves.

    Both lead V_1 and lead V_2 must have a dominant S wave, usually with a small, narrow R wave. S descent must be rapid and smooth, without notching.

2. METHOD 2: THE BRUGADA ALGORITHM FOR DIAGNOSIS OF VT

(Requires All Six Precordial Leads)

Brugada and coworkers reported on a total of 554 patients with WCT-RR whose mechanism was diagnosed in the electrophysiology laboratory. Patients included 384 (69%) with VT and 170 (31%) with SVT with aberrant ventricular conduction.

1. **Is there absence of an RS complex in ALL precordial leads?**
    If Yes (n = 83), VT is established diagnosis. (Sensitivity 21%, Specificity 100%.) *Note:* Only QR, Qr, qR, QS, QRS, monophasic R, or rSR′ are present. qRs complexes were not mentioned in the Brugada study.
    If No (n = 471), proceed to next step.
2. **Is the RS interval > 100 ms in ANY ONE precordial lead?**
    If Yes (n = 175), VT is established diagnosis. (Sensitivity 66%, Specificity 98%.) *Note:* The onset of R to the nadir of S is > 100 ms (> 2.5 small boxes) in a lead with an RS complex.

    If No (n = 296), proceed to next step.
3. **Is there AV dissociation?**
    If Yes (n = 59), VT is established diagnosis. (Sensitivity 82%, Specificity 98%.) *Note:* VA block also implies the same diagnosis.
    If No (n = 237), proceed to next step. *Note:* Antiarrhythmic drugs were withheld from patients in this study. Clinically, drugs that prolong the QRS duration may give a false-positive sign of VT using this criterion.
4. **Are morphologic criteria for VT present?**
    If Yes (n = 59), VT is established diagnosis. (Sensitivity 99%, Specificity 97%.) *Note:* RBBB type QRS in V$_1$ versus LBBB type QRS in V$_1$ should be assessed as shown in the boxes below.

If No (n = 169)—and if there are no matches for VT in the boxes below—the diagnosis is SVT with aberration. (Sensitivity 97%, Specificity 99%.)

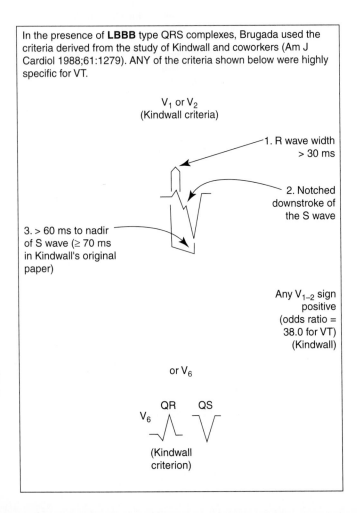

In the presence of **LBBB** type QRS complexes, Brugada used the criteria derived from the study of Kindwall and coworkers (Am J Cardiol 1988;61:1279). ANY of the criteria shown below were highly specific for VT.

V_1 or V_2
(Kindwall criteria)

1. R wave width > 30 ms

2. Notched downstroke of the S wave

3. > 60 ms to nadir of S wave (≥ 70 ms in Kindwall's original paper)

Any V_{1-2} sign positive (odds ratio = 38.0 for VT) (Kindwall)

or V_6

V_6 QR   QS

(Kindwall criterion)

In the presence of **RBBB** type QRS complexes (dominant positive in V_1), a diagnosis of VT can be made by examination of both V_1 and V_6.

V_1 only	V_6
Monophasic R wave	QS or QR
QR or RS	R/S < 1 (seen with LAD)

3. METHOD 3: THE GRIFFITH METHOD FOR DIAGNOSIS OF VT (REQUIRES LEADS V_1 AND V_6)

This method derives from an analysis of typical waveforms of RBBB or LBBB as seen in both leads V_1 and V_6. If the waveforms do not conform to the typical morphologic patterns, the diagnosis defaults to VT.

Step One

Determine the morphologic classification of the wide QRS complexes (RB type or LB type), using the criteria above.

Step Two

Apply criteria for normal forms of either RBBB or LBBB, as described below. A negative answer to any of the three questions is inconsistent with either RBBB or LBBB, and the diagnosis defaults to VT.

   A. For QRS Complexes With RBBB Categorization:
      1. Is there an rSR′ morphology in lead V_1?

2. Is there an RS complex in V₆ (may have a small septal Q wave)?

3. Is the R/S ratio in lead V₆ > 1?

B. For QRS Complexes With LBBB Categorization:
  1. Is there an rS or QS complex in leads V₁ and V₂?

V₁ and V₂
either morphology
is acceptable

2. Is the onset of the QRS to the nadir of the S wave in lead V₁ <70 ms?
3. Is there an R wave in lead V₆, without a Q wave?

Torsade de Pointes

Torsade de pointes ("twisting of the points") is defined as a pause-dependent polymorphic VT with a characteristic shifting morphology of the QRS complex that occurs in the setting of a prolonged QT interval. Clinical correlations include drug-induced states, congenital long QT syndrome, and hypokalemia.

H. AV BLOCK AND AV DISSOCIATION

1. AV BLOCK

Definitions of AV Block

If an atrial impulse has an "opportunity" to conduct normally and does not, then there is AV block. The relationship of P waves to QRS complexes determines the degree of AV block. An "opportunity" to conduct normally occurs when the P wave or atrial impulse enters the conducting system at a time other than during the effective or relative refractory periods of either the AV node or the bundle branches. The end of the T wave usually delineates the end of this period.

A. **First-degree AV block** is defined as prolongation of the PR interval (>0.21 s) with a 1:1 atrioventricular ratio.

B. **Second-degree AV block** is defined as occasional failure of conduction of a P wave, usually during a period of regular PP intervals. There are two major types of second-degree AV block:

1. **Second-degree AV block type I (Wenckebach type I):** The alerting sign is the presence of group beating, defined as clusters of mathematically spaced QRS complexes separated by pauses of identical duration. Criteria include the following:

   There is usually a constant PP interval.

   There is some, but not necessarily progressive, prolongation of successive PR intervals, leading to a nonconducted P wave that initiates a pause.

   Twice the immediate RR interval that precedes the pause is longer than the RR interval that includes the pause.

   The PR interval that precedes the pause is usually the longest in that Wenckebach cycle.

   The PR interval that terminates the pause is usually the shortest P-R interval in that heart.

2. **Second-degree AV block type II (Mobitz type II)** is defined as sudden failure of conduction of a P wave during a period of regular PP intervals. The PR intervals preceding each conducted P wave are constant, and some P waves do not conduct. Rarely, after prior long RR cycles, the PR intervals may shorten by ≤0.02 s.

3. **Third-degree AV block** is defined as complete failure of conduction of all atrial impulses. The escape pacemaker originates from either the AV junction or the ventricle.

2. AV DISSOCIATION

Complete AV Dissociation

The P waves and QRS complexes are without relationship all of the time.

Incomplete AV Dissociation

The P waves and QRS complexes are without relationship *most* of the time. The two electrocardiographic manifestations of incomplete AV dissociation are the presence of either (1) a **fusion complex,** a blending of waveforms in the same chamber, with usually a waveform produced by an atrial impulse at the same time as one produced by a ventricular impulse; or (2) a **capture complex,** ie, a premature QRS complex produced by a P wave when the majority of QRS complexes are not produced by P waves. The P wave producing the ventricular capture is usually superimposed upon the ST segment or T wave caused by the prior QRS complex.

There are four basic disorders of impulse formation or conduction producing incomplete AV dissociation:

A. **Slowing of the Primary Pacemaker:** An example is sinus bradycardia with a junctional escape rhythm.

B. **Acceleration of a Subsidiary Pacemaker:** Examples are ventricular tachycardia (common); accelerated ventricular rhythm (common; requires no AV block); junctional tachycardia (less common); or accelerated junctional rhythm (less common; requires no AV block).

C. **Third-Degree AV Block:** Defined as complete failure of conduction of all atrial impulses. The escape pacemaker originates from one of two sites: the AV junction, producing the normal QRS complex seen in that heart, including RBBB or LBBB; or the ventricle (sub-His), producing a wide QRS complex lacking the classic pattern of either RBBB or LBBB.

D. **Combinations, Usually of A and B:** An example is relative slowing of the sinus in association with an accelerated junctional rhythm. The diagnostic hallmark is a capture complex.

I. PAROXYSMAL SUPRAVENTRICULAR TACHYCARDIA (PSVT)

This category encompasses several types of tachycardias (rate > 100 bpm) that, by definition, are paroxysmal, ie, have sudden onset. The QRS complex is usually narrow in these arrhythmias, but occasionally it can show preexistent BBB or rate-dependent BBB. Approximately 90% of all

PSVTs are due to either AVRT or AVNRT. The four most common mechanisms of PSVT are as follows.

Atrioventricular Reentry Tachycardia (AVRT)

In this common arrhythmia, also called orthodromic reciprocating tachycardia (ORT), there is a reentrant circuit in which an accessory atrioventricular pathway conducts the impulse, usually in a retrograde direction from the ventricle to the atrium. The AV node-His-Purkinje axis conducts the impulse in an anterograde (orthodromic) direction from atrium to ventricle. The onset of atrial activation occurs just after the end of the QRS complex, producing a P wave located a short distance from the J point (a short-RP tachycardia).

AV Nodal Reentry Tachycardia (AVNRT)

This is a common reentrant rhythm involving tissues in close proximity to the AV node or within the node, some of which conduct rapidly and have a relatively long refractory period ("fast" pathway) and some of which conduct slowly and have a relatively short refractory period ("slow" pathway). About half the time, the P wave is buried within the QRS complex and is hidden, while in the remainder the P wave distorts the end of the QRS complex, producing apparent S waves in the inferior leads (pseudo-S waves) and apparent R′ waves in V_1 (pseudo-R′ waves).

Atrial Tachycardia

This arrhythmia is uncommon.

Atrial Flutter (Usually Atypical Flutter)

In this uncommon arrhythmia, there is either 1:1 or 2:1 AV conduction, which may occasionally be very difficult to diagnose from the surface ECG. In these cases, drugs that block AV nodal conduction and prolong the RR intervals may allow for unmasking of the flutter waves.

STEP 2: MORPHOLOGIC DIAGNOSIS OF THE CARDIAC WAVEFORMS

A. THE NORMAL ECG: TWO BASIC QRST PATTERNS

The most common pattern is illustrated below and is usually seen in leads I or II and V_{5-6}. There is a small "septal" Q wave <30 ms in duration. The T wave is upright. The normal ST segment, which is never normally isoelectric except sometimes at slow rates (<60 bpm), slopes upward into an upright T wave, whose proximal angle is more obtuse than the distal angle. The normal T wave is never symmetric.

The pattern seen in the right precordial leads, usually V_{1-3}, is shown below. There is a dominant S wave. The J point, the junction between the end of the QRS complex and the ST segment, is usually slightly elevated, and the T wave is upright. The T wave in V_1 may occasionally be inverted as a normal finding in up to 50% of young women and 25% of young men, but this finding is usually abnormal in adult males. V_2 usually has the largest absolute QRS and T wave magnitude of any of the 12 electrocardiographic leads.

B. ATRIAL ABNORMALITIES

Right Atrial Enlargement (RAE)

Diagnostic criteria include a positive component of the P wave in lead V_1 or $V_2 \geq 1.5$ mm. Another criterion is a P wave amplitude in lead II >2.5 mm. *Note:* A tall, peaked P in lead II may represent RAE but is more commonly due to either COPD or increased sympathetic tone.

Clinical correlation: RAE is seen with RVH.

Left Atrial Enlargement (LAE)

The most sensitive lead for the diagnosis of LAE is lead V_1, but the criteria for lead II are more specific. Criteria include a terminal negative wave ≥ 1 mm deep and ≥ 40 ms wide (one small box by one small box in area) and >40 ms between the first (right) and second (left) atrial components of the P wave in lead II, or a P wave duration >110 ms in lead II.

Clinical correlations: LVH, coronary artery disease, mitral valve disease, or cardiomyopathy.

C. BUNDLE BRANCH BLOCK

The normal QRS duration in adults ranges from 67 ms to 114 ms (Glasgow cohort). If the QRS duration is ≥ 120 ms (three small boxes or more on the electrocardiographic paper), there is usually an abnormality of conduction of the ventricular impulse. The most common causes are either RBBB or LBBB, shown above, page 291. However, other conditions may also prolong the QRS duration.

RBBB is defined by delayed terminal QRS forces that are directed to the right and anteriorly, producing broad terminal positive waves in leads V_1 and aVR and a broad terminal negative wave in lead I.

LBBB is defined by delayed terminal QRS forces that are directed to the left and posteriorly, producing wide R waves in leads that face the left ventricular free wall and wide S waves in the right precordial leads.

RIGHT BUNDLE BRANCH BLOCK (RBBB)

Diagnostic Criteria

The diagnosis of uncomplicated complete right bundle branch block is made when the following criteria are met:

1. Prolongation of the QRS duration to 120 ms or more.
2. An rsr′, rsR′, or rSR′ pattern in lead V_1 or V_2. The R′ is usually greater than the initial R wave. In a minority of cases, a wide and notched R pattern may be seen.
3. Leads V_6 and I show a QRS complex with a wide S wave (S duration is longer than the R duration, or >40 ms in adults).

(See common and uncommon waveforms for RBBB under Step Two, page 292, above).

ST–T changes in RBBB

In uncomplicated RBBB, the ST–T segment is depressed and the T wave inverted in the right precordial leads with an R′ (usually only in lead V_1 but occasionally in V_2). The T wave is upright in leads I, V_5, and V_6.

LEFT BUNDLE BRANCH BLOCK (LBBB)

Diagnostic Criteria

The diagnosis of uncomplicated complete left bundle branch block is made when the following criteria are met:

1. Prolongation of the QRS duration to 120 ms or more.
2. There are broad and notched or slurred R waves in left-sided precordial leads V_5 and V_6, as well as in leads I and aVL. Occasionally, an RS pattern may occur in leads V_5 and V_6 in uncomplicated LBBB associated with posterior displacement of the left ventricle.
3. With the possible exception of lead aVL, Q waves are absent in the left-sided leads, specifically in leads V_5, V_6, and I.
4. The R peak time is prolonged to >60 ms in lead V_5 or V_6 but is normal in leads V_1 and V_2 when it can be determined.
5. In the right precordial leads V_1 and V_3, there are small initial r waves in the majority of cases, followed by wide and deep S waves. The transition zone in the precordial leads is displaced to the left. Wide QS complexes may be present in leads V_1 and V_2 and rarely in lead V_3.

(See common and uncommon waveforms for LBBB under Step Two, page 292, above).

ST–T changes in LBBB

In uncomplicated LBBB, the ST segments are usually depressed and the T waves inverted in left precordial leads V_5 and V_6 as well as in leads I and aVL. Conversely, ST segment elevations and positive T waves are recorded in leads V_1 and V_2. Only rarely is the T wave upright in the left precordial leads.

D. INCOMPLETE BUNDLE BRANCH BLOCKS

Incomplete LBBB

The waveforms are similar to those in complete LBBB, but the QRS duration is < 120 ms. Septal Q waves are absent in I and V_6. Incomplete LBBB is synonymous with LVH and commonly mimics a delta wave in leads V_5 and V_6.

Incomplete RBBB

The waveforms are similar to those in complete RBBB, but the QRS duration is < 120 ms. This diagnosis suggests RVH. Occasionally, in a normal variant pattern, there is an rSr′ waveform in lead V_1. In this case, the r′ is usually smaller than the initial r wave; this pattern is not indicative of incomplete RBBB.

Intraventricular Conduction Delay or Defect (IVCD)

If the QRS duration is ≥120 ms but typical waveforms of either RBBB or LBBB are not present, there is an intraventricular conduction delay or defect (IVCD). This pattern is common in dilated cardiomyopathy. An IVCD with a QRS duration of ≥170 ms is highly predictive of dilated cardiomyopathy.

E. FASCICULAR BLOCKS (HEMIBLOCKS)

1. LEFT ANTERIOR FASCICULAR BLOCK (LAFB)

Diagnostic Criteria

1. Mean QRS axis from −45 degrees to −90 degrees (possibly −31 to −44 degrees).
2. A qR pattern in lead aVL, with the R peak time, ie, the onset of the Q wave to the peak of the R wave ≥45 ms (slightly more than one small box wide), as shown below.

Clinical correlations: Hypertensive heart disease, coronary artery disease, or idiopathic conducting system disease.

2. LEFT POSTERIOR FASCICULAR BLOCK (LPFB)

Diagnostic Criteria

1. Mean QRS axis from +90 degrees to +180 degrees.
2. A qR complex in leads III and aVF, an rS complex in leads aVL and I, with a Q wave ≥40 ms in the inferior leads.

Clinical correlations: LPFB is a diagnosis of exclusion. It may be seen in the acute phase of inferior myocardial injury or infarction or may result from idiopathic conducting system disease.

F. DETERMINATION OF THE MEAN QRS AXIS

The mean electrical axis is the average direction of the activation or repolarization process during the cardiac cycle. Instantaneous and mean electrical axes may be determined for any deflection (P, QRS, ST–T) in the three planes (frontal, transverse, and sagittal). The determination of the electrical axis of a QRS complex is useful for the diagnosis of certain pathologic cardiac conditions.

The Mean QRS Axis in the Frontal Plane (Limb Leads)

Arzbaecher developed the **hexaxial reference system** that allowed for the display of the relationships among the six frontal plane (limb) leads. A diagram of this system is shown below.

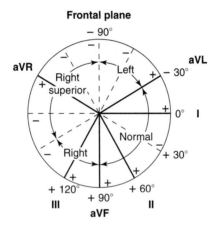

Frontal plane

The normal range of the QRS axis in adults is −30 degrees to +90 degrees.

It is rarely important to precisely determine the degrees of the mean QRS. However, the recognition of abnormal axis deviations is critical since it leads to a presumption of disease. The mean QRS axis is derived from the net area under the QRS curves. The most efficient method of determining the mean QRS axis uses the method of Grant, which requires only leads I and II (see below). If the net area under the QRS curves in these leads is positive, the axis falls between −30 degrees and +90 degrees, which is the normal range of axis in adults. (The only exception to this rule is in RBBB, in which the first 60 ms of the QRS is used. Alternatively, one may use the maximal amplitude of the R and S waves in leads I and II to assess the axis in RBBB.) Abnormal axes are shown below.

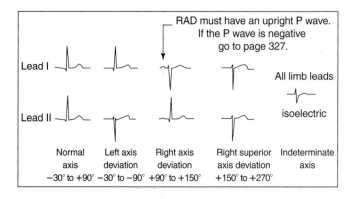

Lead I / Lead II

RAD must have an upright P wave. If the P wave is negative go to page 327.

All limb leads isoelectric

Normal axis	Left axis deviation	Right axis deviation	Right superior axis deviation	Indeterminate axis
−30° to +90°	−30° to −90°	+90° to +150°	+150° to +270°	

Left Axis Deviation (LAD)

The four main causes of left axis deviation (LAD) are as follows:

A. Left Anterior Fascicular Block (LAFB): See criteria above.

B. Inferior MI: There is a pathologic Q wave ≥30 ms either in lead aVF or lead II in the absence of ventricular preexcitation.

C. Ventricular Preexcitation (WPW Pattern): LAD is seen with inferior paraseptal accessory pathway locations. This can mimic inferoposterior MI. The classic definition of the **Wolff-Parkinson-White (WPW) pattern** includes a short PR interval (<120 ms); an initial slurring of the QRS complex, called a **delta wave;** and prolongation of the QRS complex to >120 ms. However, since this pattern may not always be present despite the presence of ventricular preexcitation, a more practical definition is an absent PR segment and an initial slurring of the QRS complex in any lead. The diagnosis of the WPW pattern usually requires sinus rhythm.

D. COPD: LAD is seen in 10% of patients with COPD.

Right Axis Deviation (RAD)

The four main causes of right axis deviation (RAD) are as follows:

A. Right Ventricular Hypertrophy: This is the most common cause (refer to diagnostic criteria, below). However, one must first exclude acute occlusion of the posterior descending coronary artery, causing LPFB, and exclude also items B and C below.

B. Extensive Lateral and Apical MI: Criteria include QS or Qr patterns in leads I and aVL and in leads V_{4-6}.

C. Ventricular Preexcitation (WPW Pattern): RAD seen with left posterosuperior accessory pathway locations. This can mimic lateral MI.

D. Left Posterior Fascicular Block (LPFB): This is a diagnosis of exclusion (see criteria above).

Right Superior Axis Deviation

This category is rare. Causes include RVH, apical MI, ventricular tachycardia, and hyperkalemia. Right superior axis deviation may rarely be seen as an atypical form of LAFB.

G. VENTRICULAR HYPERTROPHY

1. LEFT VENTRICULAR HYPERTROPHY (LVH)

The ECG is very insensitive as a screening tool for LVH, but electrocardiographic criteria are usually specific. Echocardiography is the major resource for this diagnosis.

The best electrocardiographic criterion for the diagnosis of LVH is the Cornell voltage, the sum of the R wave amplitude in lead aVL and the S wave depth in lead V_3, adjusted for sex:

1. RaVL + SV_3 >20 mm (females), >25 mm (males). The R wave height in aVL alone is a good place to start.

2. RaVL >9 mm (females), >11 mm (males).
   Alternatively, application of the following criteria will diagnose most cases of LVH.

3. Sokolow-Lyon criteria: SV_1 + RV_5 or RV_6 (whichever R wave is taller) >35 mm (in patients age >35).

4. Romhilt-Estes criteria: Points are scored for QRS voltage (1 point), the presence of LAE (1 point), typical repolarization abnormalities in the absence of digitalis (1 point), and a few other findings. The combination of LAE (see above) and typical repolarization abnormalities (see below) (score ≥5 points) will suffice for the diagnosis of LVH even when voltage criteria are not met.

5. RV_6 > RV_5 (usually occurs with dilated LV). First exclude anterior MI and establish that the R waves in V_5 are >7 mm tall and that in V_6 they are >6 mm tall before using this criterion.

Repolarization Abnormalities in LVH

Typical repolarization abnormalities in the presence of LVH are an ominous sign of end-organ damage. In repolarization abnormalities in LVH, the ST segment and T wave are directed opposite to the dominant QRS waveform in all leads. However, this directional rule does not apply either in the transitional lead (defined as a lead having an R wave height equal to the S wave depth) or in the transitional zone (defined as leads adjacent to the transitional lead) or one lead to the left in the precordial leads.

Spectrum of Repolarization Abnormalities in LVH

The waveforms below, usually seen in leads I, aVL, V_5, and V_6 but more specifically in leads with dominant R waves, represent hypothetical stages in the progression of LVH.

Normal	LVH voltage	LVH voltage with minor T wave flattening	LVH voltage with minor T wave inversion
CLASSICAL: LVH voltage with typical repol. abnormalities ("strain")	LVH voltage with typical repolarization abnormalities and QRS widening	Incomplete LBBB (absent septal Q in leads I and V_6)	Complete LBBB

2. RIGHT VENTRICULAR HYPERTROPHY (RVH)

The ECG is insensitive for the diagnosis of RVH. In 100 cases of RVH from one echocardiography laboratory, only 33% had RAD because of the confounding effects of LV disease. Published electrocardiographic criteria for RVH are listed below, all of which have ≥97% specificity.

With rare exceptions, right atrial enlargement is synonymous with RVH.

Diagnostic Criteria

Recommended criteria for the electrocardiographic diagnosis of RVH are as follows:

1. Right axis deviation (>90 degrees), or
2. An R/S ratio ≥1 in lead V_1 (absent posterior MI or RBBB), or
3. An R wave >7 mm tall in V_1 (not the R′ of RBBB), or
4. An rsR′ complex in V_1 (R′ ≥10 mm), with a QRS duration of <0.12 s (incomplete RBBB), or
5. An S wave >7 mm deep in leads V_5 or V_6 *(in the absence of a QRS axis more negative than +30 degrees)*, or
6. RBBB with RAD (axis derived from first 60 ms of the QRS). (Consider RVH in RBBB if the R/S ratio in lead I is <0.5.)
   A variant of RVH (type C loop) may produce a false-positive sign of an anterior MI.

Repolarization Abnormalities in RVH

The morphology of repolarization abnormalities in RVH is identical to those in LVH, when a particular lead contains tall R waves reflecting the hypertrophied RV or LV. In RVH, these typically occur in leads V_{1-2} or V_3 and in leads aVF and III. This morphology of repolarization abnormalities due to ventricular hypertrophy is illustrated above. In cases of RVH with massive dilation, all precordial leads may overlie the diseased RV and may exhibit repolarization abnormalities.

H. LOW VOLTAGE OF THE QRS COMPLEX

Low-Voltage Limb Leads Only

Defined as peak-to-peak QRS voltage <5 mm in all limb leads.

Low-Voltage Limb and Precordial Leads

Defined as peak-to-peak QRS voltage <5 mm in all limb leads and <10 mm in all precordial leads. Primary myocardial causes include multiple or massive infarctions; infiltrative diseases such as amyloidosis, sarcoidosis, or hemochromatosis; and myxedema. Extracardiac causes include pericardial effusion, COPD, pleural effusion, obesity, anasarca, and subcutaneous emphysema. When there is COPD, expect to see low voltage in the limb leads as well as in leads V_5 and V_6.

I. PROGRESSION OF THE R WAVE IN THE PRECORDIAL LEADS

The normal R wave height increases from V_1 to V_5. The normal R wave height in V_5 is always taller than that in V_6 because of the attenuating effect of the lungs. The normal R wave height in lead V_3 is usually >2 mm.

"Poor R Wave Progression"

The term "poor wave progression" (PRWP) is a nonpreferred term because most physicians use this term to imply the presence of an anterior MI, though it may not be present. Other causes of small R waves in the right precordial leads include LVH, LAFB, LBBB, cor pulmonale (with the type C loop of RVH), and COPD.

Reversed R Wave Progression (RRWP)

Reversed R wave progression is defined as a loss of R wave height between leads V_1 and V_2 or between leads V_2 and V_3 or between leads V_3 and V_4. In the absence of LVH, this finding suggests anterior MI or precordial lead reversal.

J. TALL R WAVES IN THE RIGHT PRECORDIAL LEADS

Etiology

Causes of tall R waves in the right precordial leads include the following:

A. **Right Ventricular Hypertrophy:** This is the most common cause. There is an R/S ratio ≥ 1 or an R wave height >7 mm in lead V_1.

B. **Posterior MI:** There is an R wave ≥ 6 mm in lead V_1 or ≥ 15 mm in lead V_2. One should distinguish the tall R wave of RVH from the tall R wave of posterior MI in lead V_1. In RVH, there is a downsloping ST segment and an inverted T wave, usually with right axis deviation. In contrast, in posterior MI, there is usually an upright, commonly tall T wave and, because posterior MI is usually associated with concomitant inferior MI, a left axis deviation.

C. **Right Bundle Branch Block:** The QRS duration is prolonged, and typical waveforms are present (see above).

D. The WPW Pattern: Left-sided accessory pathway locations produce prominent R waves with an R/S ratio ≥ 1 in V_1, with an absent PR segment and initial slurring of the QRS complex, usually best seen in lead V_4.

E. Rare or Uncommon Causes: The normal variant pattern of early precordial QRS transition (not uncommon); the reciprocal effect of a deep Q wave in leads V_{5-6} (very rare); Duchenne's muscular dystrophy (very rare); and chronic constrictive pericarditis (very rare); and reversal of the right precordial leads.

K. MYOCARDIAL INJURY, ISCHEMIA, AND INFARCTION

Definitions

A. Myocardial Infarction: Pathologic changes in the QRS complex reflect ventricular activation away from the area of infarction.

B. Myocardial Injury: Injury always points *outward* from the surface that is injured.

  1. Epicardial injury: ST elevation in the distribution of an acutely occluded artery.

  2. Endocardial injury: Diffuse ST segment depression, which is really reciprocal to the primary event, reflected as ST elevation in aVR.

C. Myocardial Ischemia: Diffuse ST segment depression, usually with associated T wave inversion. It usually reflects subendocardial injury, reciprocal to ST elevation in lead aVR. In ischemia, there may only be inverted T waves with a symmetric, sharp nadir.

D. Reciprocal Changes: Passive electrical reflections of a primary event viewed from either the other side of the heart, as in epicardial injury, or the other side of the ventricular wall, as in subendocardial injury.

Steps in the Diagnosis of Myocardial Infarction

The following pages contain a systematic method for the electrocardiographic diagnosis of myocardial injury or infarction, arranged in seven steps. Following the steps will achieve the diagnosis in most cases.

  Step 1: Identify the presence of myocardial injury by ST segment deviations.

  Step 2: Identify areas of myocardial injury by assessing lead groupings.

Step 3: Define the primary area of involvement and identify the culprit artery producing the injury.

Step 4: Identify the location of the lesion in the artery in order to risk-stratify the patient.

Step 5: Identify any electrocardiographic signs of infarction found in the QRS complexes.

Step 6: Determine the age of the infarction by assessing the location of the ST segment in leads with pathologic QRS abnormalities.

Step 7: Combine all observations into a final diagnosis.

STEPS 1 AND 2

Identify presence of and areas of myocardial injury.

The GUSTO study of patients with ST segment elevation in two contiguous leads defined four affected areas as set out in Table 7–7.

Two other major areas of possible injury or infarction were not included in the GUSTO categorization because they do not produce ST elevation in two contiguous standard leads. These are:

1. **Posterior Injury:** The most commonly used sign of posterior injury is ST depression in leads V_{1-3}, but posterior injury may best be diagnosed by obtaining posterior leads V_7, V_8, and V_9.

2. **Right Ventricular Injury:** The most sensitive sign of RV injury, ST segment elevation ≥ 1 mm, is found in lead V_4R. A very specific—but insensitive—sign of RV injury or infarction is ST elevation in V_1, with concomitant ST segment depression in V_2 in the setting of ST elevation in the inferior leads.

STEP 3

Identify the primary area of involvement and the culprit artery.

TABLE 7–7. GUSTO STUDY DEFINITIONS.

Area of ST Segment Elevation	Leads Defining This Area
Anterior (Ant)	V_{1-4}
Apical (Ap)	V_{5-6}
Lateral (Lat)	I, aVL
Inferior (Inf)	II, aVF, III

Primary Anterior Area

ST elevation in two contiguous V_{1-4} leads defines a primary anterior area of involvement. The left anterior descending coronary artery (LAD) is the culprit artery. Lateral (I and aVL) and apical (V_5 and V_6) areas are contiguous to anterior (V_{1-4}), so ST elevation in these leads signifies more myocardium at risk and more adverse outcomes.

Primary Inferior Area

ST segment elevation in two contiguous leads (II, aVF, or III) defines a primary inferior area of involvement. The right coronary artery (RCA) is usually the culprit artery. Apical (V_5 and V_6), posterior (V_{1-3} or V_{7-9}) and right ventricular (V_4R) areas are contiguous to inferior (II, aVF, and III), so ST elevation in these contiguous leads signifies more myocardium at risk and more adverse outcomes (see below).

The Culprit Artery

In the GUSTO trial, 98% of patients with ST segment elevation in any two contiguous V_{1-4} leads, either alone or with associated changes in leads V_{5-6} or I and aVL, had left anterior descending coronary artery obstruction. In patients with ST segment elevation only in leads II, aVF, and III, there was right coronary artery obstruction in 86%.

PRIMARY ANTERIOR PROCESS

Acute occlusion of the LAD coronary artery produces a sequence of changes in the anterior leads (V_{1-4}).

Earliest Findings

  A. **"Hyperacute" Changes:** ST elevation with loss of normal ST segment concavity, commonly with tall, peaked T waves.

  B. **Acute Injury:** ST elevation, with the ST segment commonly appearing as if a thumb has been pushed up into it.

rS
complex
V_2

Evolutionary Changes

A patient who presents to the emergency department with chest pain and T wave inversion in leads with pathologic Q waves is most likely to be in the evolutionary or completed phase of infarction. Successful revascularization usually causes prompt resolution of the acute signs of injury or infarction and results in the electrocardiographic signs of a fully evolved infarction. The tracing below shows QS complexes in lead V_2.

A. Development of Pathologic Q Waves (Infarction): Pathologic Q waves develop within the first hour after onset of symptoms in at least 30% of patients.

QS complexes
V_2 shown

day 1

B. ST Segment Elevation Decreases: T wave inversion usually occurs in the second 24-hour period after infarction.

day 2

C. Fully Evolved Pattern: Pathologic Q waves, ST segment rounded upward, T waves inverted.

chronic

PRIMARY INFERIOR PROCESS

A primary inferior process usually develops after acute occlusion of the right coronary artery, producing changes in the inferior leads (II, III, and aVF).

Earliest Findings

The earliest findings are of acute injury (ST segment elevation). The J point may "climb up the back" of the R wave (a), or the ST segment may rise up into the T wave (b).

Evolutionary Changes

ST segment elevation decreases and pathologic Q waves develop. T wave inversion may occur in the first 12 hours of an inferior MI—in contrast to that in anterior MI.

Right Ventricular Injury or Infarction

With RV injury, there is ST segment elevation, best seen in lead V_4R. With RV infarction, there is a QS complex.

For comparison, the normal morphology of the QRS complex in lead V_4R is shown below. The normal J point averages +0.2 mm.

POSTERIOR INJURY OR INFARCTION

Posterior injury or infarction is commonly due to acute occlusion of the left circumflex coronary artery, producing changes in the posterior leads (V_7, V_8, V_9) or reciprocal ST segment depression in leads V_{1-3}.

Acute Pattern

Acute posterior injury or infarction is shown by ST segment depression in V_{1-3} and perhaps also V_4, usually with upright (often prominent) T waves.

Chronic Pattern

Chronic posterior injury or infarction is shown by pathologic R waves with prominent tall T waves in leads V_{1-3}.

STEP 4

Identify the location of the lesion within the artery in order to risk stratify the patient.

Primary Anterior Process

Aside from an acute occlusion of the left main coronary artery, occlusion of the proximal left anterior descending coronary artery conveys the most adverse outcomes. Four electrocardiographic signs indicate proximal LAD occlusion:

1. ST elevation > 1 mm in lead I, in lead aVL, or in both
2. New RBBB
3. New LAFB
4. New first-degree AV block

Primary Inferior Process

Nearly 50% of patients with IMI have distinguishing features that may produce complications or adverse outcomes unless successfully managed:

1. Precordial ST segment depression in V_{1-3} (suggests concomitant posterior wall involvement);
2. Right ventricular injury or infarction (identifies a proximal RCA lesion);
3. AV block (implies a greater amount of involved myocardium);
4. The sum of ST segment depressions in leads V_{4-6} exceeds the sum of ST segment depressions in leads V_{1-3} (suggests multivessel disease).

Reciprocal Changes in the Setting of Acute MI

ST depressions in leads remote from the primary site of injury are felt to be a purely reciprocal change. With successful reperfusion, the ST depressions usually resolve. If they persist, patients more likely have significant three-vessel disease and so-called ischemia at a distance. Mortality rates are higher in such patients.

STEP 5

Identify Electrocardiographic Signs of Infarction in the QRS Complexes

The 12-lead ECG shown below contains numbers corresponding to pathologic widths for Q waves and R waves for selected leads (see Table 7–8 for more complete criteria).

I ⏐ Q ≥ 30	aVR	V₁ Any Q ⏐ R ≥ 40	V₄ Q ≥ 20
II ⏐ Q ≥ 30	aVL ⏐ Q ≥ 30	V₂ ⏐ R ≥ 50 Any Q	V₅ ⏐ Q ≥ 30
III	aVF ⏐ Q ≥ 30	V₃ Any Q	V₆ ⏐ Q ≥ 30

One can memorize the above criteria by mastering a simple scheme of numbers which represent the durations of pathological Q waves or R waves. Begin with lead V_1 and repeat the numbers in the box below in the following order. The numbers increase from "any" to 50.

Any Q wave in lead V_1, for anterior MI
Any Q wave in lead V_2, for anterior MI
Any Q wave in lead V_3, for anterior MI

20 Q wave ≥ 20 ms in lead V_4, for anterior MI
30 Q wave ≥ 30 ms in lead V_5, for apical MI
30 Q wave ≥ 30 ms in lead V_6, for apical MI

30 Q wave ≥ 30 ms in lead I, for lateral MI
30 Q wave ≥ 30 ms in lead aVL, for lateral MI
30 Q wave ≥ 30 ms in lead II, for inferior MI
30 Q wave ≥ 30 ms in lead aVF, for inferior MI

R40 R wave ≥ 40 ms in lead V_1, for posterior MI
R50 R wave ≥ 50 ms in lead V_2, for posterior MI

Test Performance Characteristics for Electrocardiographic Criteria in the Diagnosis of MI

Haisty and coworkers studied 1344 patients with normal hearts documented by coronary arteriography and 837 patients with documented MI (366 inferior, 277 anterior, 63 posterior, and 131 inferior and anterior) (Table 7–8). (Patients with LVH, LAFB, LPFB, RVH, LBBB, RBBB, COPD, or WPW patterns were excluded from analysis because these conditions can give false-positive results for MI.) Shown below are the

TABLE 7–8. DIAGNOSIS OF MYOCARDIAL INFARCTION.[1]

Infarct Location	ECG Lead	Criterion	Sensitivity	Specificity	Likelihood Ratio (+)	Likelihood Ratio (−)
Inferior	II	Q ≥ 30 ms	45	98	22.5	0.6
	aVF	Q ≥ 30 ms	70	94	11.7	0.3
		Q ≥ 40 ms	40	98	20.0	0.6
		R/Q ≤ 1	50	98	25.0	0.5
Anterior	V_1	Any Q	50	97	16.7	0.5
	V_2	Any Q, or R ≤ 0.1 mV and R ≤ 10 ms, or RV_2 ≤ RV_1	80	94	13.3	0.2
	V_3	Any Q, or R ≤ 0.2 mV, or R ≤ 20 ms	70	93	10.0	0.3
	V_4	Q ≥ 20 ms	40	92	5.0	0.9
		R/Q ≤ 0.5, or R/S ≤ 0.5	40	97	13.3	0.6
Anterolateral (lateral)						
	I	Q ≥ 30 ms R/Q ≤ 1, or R ≤ 2 mm	10 10	98 97	5.0 3.3	0.9 0.9
	aVL	Q ≥ 30 ms	7	97	0.7	1.0
		R/Q ≤ 1	2			
Apical	V_5	Q ≥ 30	5	99	5.0	1.0
		R/Q ≤ 2, or R ≤ 7 mm, or R/S ≤ 2, or notched R	60	91	6.7	0.4
		R/Q ≤ 1, or R/S ≤ 1	25	98	12.5	0.8
	V_6	Q ≤ 30	3	98	1.5	1.0
		R/Q ≤ 3, or R ≤ 6 mm, or R/S ≤ 3, or notched R	40	92	25.0	0.7
		R/Q ≤ 1, or R/S ≤ 1	10	99	10.0	0.9

TABLE 7–8 (CONTINUED).

Infarct Location	ECG Lead	Criterion	Sensitivity	Specificity	Likelihood Ratio (+)	Likelihood Ratio (−)
Posterolateral						
	V_1	R/S ≤ 1	15	97	5.0	0.9
		R ≥ 6 mm, or R ≥ 40 ms	20	93	2.9	0.9
		S ≤ 3 mm	8	97	2.7	0.9
	V_2	R ≥ 15 mm, or R ≥ 50 ms	15	95	3.0	0.9
		R/S ≥ 1.5	10	96	2.5	0.9
		S ≤ 4 mm	2	97	0.7	1.0

[1] *Reproduced, with permission, from Haisty WK Jr et al: Performance of the automated complete Selvester QRS scoring system in normal subjects and patients with single and multiple myocardial infarctions. J Am Coll Cardiol 1992;19:341.*
Key: *Notched R = a notch that begins within the first 40 ms of the R wave; Q = Q wave; R/Q = ratio of R wave height to Q wave depth; R = R wave; R/S ratio = ratio of R wave height to S wave depth; $RV_2 \le RV_1$ = R wave height in V_2 less than or equal to that in V_1; S = S wave.*

sensitivity, specificity, and likelihood ratios for the best-performing infarct criteria. Notice that leads III and aVR are not listed: lead III may normally have a Q wave that is both wide and deep, and lead aVR commonly has a wide Q wave.

Mimics of Myocardial Infarction

Conditions that can produce pathologic Q waves, ST segment elevation, or loss of R wave height in the absence of infarction are set out in Table 7–9.

STEP 6

Determine the Age of the Infarction

An **acute infarction** manifests ST segment elevation in a lead with a pathologic Q wave. The T waves may be either upright or inverted.

An **old** or **age-indeterminate infarction** manifests a pathologic Q wave, with or without slight ST segment elevation or T wave abnormalities.

TABLE 7–9. MIMICS OF MYOCARDIAL INFARCTION.

Condition	Pseudoinfarct Location
WPW pattern	Any, most commonly inferoposterior or lateral
Hypertrophic cardiomyopathy	Lateral-apical (18%), inferior (11%)
LBBB	Anteroseptal, anterolateral, inferior
RBBB	Inferior, posterior (using criteria from leads V_1 and V_2) anterior
LVH	Anterior, inferior
LAFB	Anterior (may cause a tiny Q in V_2)
COPD	Inferior, posterior, anterior
RVH	Inferior, posterior (using criteria from leads V_1 and V_2), anterior, or apical (using criteria for R/S ratios from leads V_{4-6})
Acute cor pulmonale	Inferior, possibly anterior
Cardiomyopathy (nonischemic)	Any, most commonly inferior, (with IVCD pattern) less commonly anterior
Chest deformity	Any
Left pneumothorax	Anterior, anterolateral
Hyperkalemia	Any
Normal hearts	Posterior, anterior

Persistent ST segment elevation ≥ 1 mm after a myocardial infarction is a sign of dyskinetic wall motion in the area of infarct. Half of these patients have ventricular aneurysms.

STEP 7

Combine Observations Into a Final Diagnosis

There are two possibilities for the major electrocardiographic diagnosis: myocardial infarction or acute injury. If there are pathologic changes in the QRS complex, one should make a diagnosis of myocardial infarction—beginning with the primary area, followed by any contiguous areas—and state the age of the infarction. If there are no pathologic changes in the QRS complex, one should make a diagnosis of acute injury of the affected segments—beginning with the primary area and followed by any contiguous areas.

L. ST SEGMENTS

Table 7–10 summarizes major causes of ST segment elevations. Table 7–11 summarizes major causes of ST segment depressions or T wave inversions. The various classes and morphologies of ST–T waves as seen in lead V_2 are shown in Table 7–12.

TABLE 7–10. MAJOR CAUSES OF ST SEGMENT ELEVATION.

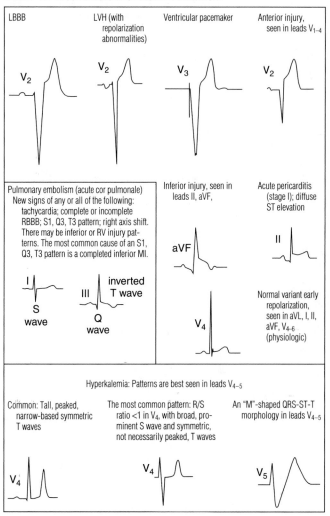

LBBB

V_2

LVH (with repolarization abnormalities)

V_2

Ventricular pacemaker

V_3

Anterior injury, seen in leads V_{1-4}

V_2

Pulmonary embolism (acute cor pulmonale) New signs of any or all of the following: tachycardia; complete or incomplete RBBB; S1, Q3, T3 pattern; right axis shift. There may be inferior or RV injury patterns. The most common cause of an S1, Q3, T3 pattern is a completed inferior MI.

I
S wave

III
inverted T wave
Q wave

Inferior injury, seen in leads II, aVF,

aVF

V_4

Acute pericarditis (stage I); diffuse ST elevation

II

Normal variant early repolarization, seen in aVL, I, II, aVF, V_{4-6} (physiologic)

Hyperkalemia: Patterns are best seen in leads V_{4-5}

Common: Tall, peaked, narrow-based symmetric T waves

V_4

The most common pattern: R/S ratio <1 in V_4, with broad, prominent S wave and symmetric, not necessarily peaked, T waves

V_4

An "M"-shaped QRS-ST-T morphology in leads V_{4-5}

V_5

TABLE 7–11. MAJOR CAUSES OF ST SEGMENT DEPRESSION OR T WAVE INVERSION.

Whenever the ST segment or the T wave is directed counter to an expected repolarization abnormality, consider ischemia, healed MI, or drug or electrolyte effect.

In RBBB, there is an obligatory inverted T wave in right precordial leads with an R′ (usually only in V_1) or its equivalent (a qR complex in septal MI). An upright T in these leads suggests completed posterior MI.

Altered depolarization RBBB — V_1

LBBB — V_5

LVH (with repolarization abnormality) — V_6

Subarachnoid hemorrhage — V_4

RVH — V_{1-3}

Inferior subendocardial injury — II

Posterior subepicardial injury — V_2

Anterior subendocardial injury or non-Q wave MI — V_5

V_4

Hypokalemia — V_4

Digitalis — V_4

Antiarrhythmics — V_4

J point depression secondary to catecholamines — II

When $K^+ \leq 2.8$, 80% have ECG changes

PR interval and ST segment occupy the same curve

TABLE 7–12. VARIOUS CLASSES AND MORPHOLOGIES OF ST-T WAVES AS SEEN IN LEAD V_2.[1]

Normal ST segment (asymmetric upsloping ST segment with concavity, slight ST segment elevation)

Abnormal ST segment elevation or lack of normal upward concavity in the first part of the ST-T segment (as seen in LVH or acute ischemia or injury)

ST-T segment typical of acute or recent myocardial infarction, ie, the ST-T segment appears as though a thumb were pushed up into it

Negative amplitudes in the latter part of the ST-T segment (may be seen in ischemia or old infarction)

Negative T wave (may be a nonspecific sign, but may be seen in ischemia or old MI)

Downward sloping in the first part of the ST-T segment (consider ischemia, digitalis, or hypokalemia)

Flat ST-T segment (a nonspecific sign)

Nonspecific ST segment or T wave abnormalities
By definition, nonspecific abnormalities of either the ST segment (ones that are only slightly depressed or abnormal in contour) or T wave (ones that are either 10% the height of the R wave that produced it, or are either flat or slightly inverted) do not conform to the characteristic waveforms found above or elsewhere.

[1] Adapted from Edenbrandt L, Devine B, Macfarlane PW: Classification of electrocardiographic ST-T segments—human expert vs. artificial neural network. J Electrocardiol 1992;25:167.

M. U WAVES

Normal U Waves

In many normal hearts, low-amplitude positive U waves <1.5 mm tall that range from 160 ms to 200 ms in duration are seen in leads V_2 or V_3. Leads V_2 and V_3 are close to the ventricular mass, and small-amplitude signals may be best seen in these leads.

Cause: Bradycardias.

Abnormal U Waves

Abnormal U waves have increased amplitude or merge with abnormal T waves and produce T–U fusion. Criteria include an amplitude ≥ 1.5 mm or a U wave that is as tall as the T wave that immediately precedes it.

Causes: Hypokalemia, digitalis, antiarrhythmic drugs.

Inverted U Waves

These are best seen in leads V_{4-6}.

Causes: LVH, acute ischemia.

Table 7–13 summarizes various classes and morphologies of ST–T–U abnormalities as seen in lead V_4.

N. QT INTERVAL

A prolonged QT interval conveys adverse outcomes. The QT interval is inversely related to the heart rate. QT interval corrections for heart rate often use Bazett's formula, defined as the observed QT interval divided by the square root of the RR interval in seconds. A corrected QT interval of ≥ 440 ms is abnormal.

Use of the QT Nomogram (Hodges Correction)

Measure the QT interval in either lead V_2 or V_3, where the end of the T wave can usually be clearly distinguished from the beginning of the U wave. If the rate is regular, use the mean rate of the QRS complexes. If the rate is irregular, calculate the rate from the immediately prior R-R cycle, because this cycle determines the subsequent QT interval. Use the numbers you have obtained to classify the QT interval using the

TABLE 7–13. VARIOUS CLASSES AND MORPHOLOGIES OF ST-T-U ABNORMALITIES AS SEEN IN LEAD V$_4$.

Normal		Normal QT interval
Hypokalemia		Depressed, upsloping ST segment, low T wave, prominent U wave
Hypokalemia with T-U fusion (the most common pattern		Depressed, upsloping ST segment, "tent-like" symmetric wide T wave, apparent long QT interval
Class Ia drug: quinidine, procainamide, disopyramide		Wide QRS, horizontally depressed ST segment, low T wave amplitude, prominent U, long QT
Digitalis		Bowl-shaped ST segment, low amplitude T wave, prominent U wave, short QT interval
Digitalis (possible toxicity)		"Checkmark"-shaped ST segment, T low to absent, first-degree AV block, short QT interval
Hypocalcemia		Long, straight ST segment, normal T wave, long QT interval
Hypercalcemia		Abbreviated ST segment, short or normal QT interval

nomogram below. Or remember that at heart rates of ≥40 bpm, an observed QT interval ≥480 ms is abnormal.

Prolonged QT Interval

The four major causes of a prolonged QT interval are as follows:

A. **Electrolyte Abnormalities:** Hypokalemia, hypocalcemia
B. **Drugs:** Also associated with torsade de pointes.
   Class Ia antiarrhythmic agents: Quinidine, procainamide, diso-
      pyramide
   Class Ic agents: Propafenone
   Class III agents: Amiodarone, bretylium, N-acetylprocainamide,
      sotalol
   Antihistamines: Astemizole, terfenadine
   Antibiotics: Erythromycin, trimethoprim-sulfamethoxazole
   Antifungals: Ketoconazole, itraconazole
   Chemotherapeutics: Pentamidine, perhaps anthracyclines
   Psychotropic agents: Tricyclic and heterocyclic antidepressants,
      phenothiazines, haloperidol
   Toxins and poisons: Organophosphate insecticides
   Miscellaneous: Cisapride, prednisone, probucol, chloral hydrate

C. Congenital Long QT Syndromes: Though rare, a congenital long QT syndrome should be considered in any young patient who presents with syncope or presyncope.

D. Miscellaneous Causes:

Third-degree and sometimes second-degree A-V block

At the cessation of ventricular pacing

Left ventricular hypertrophy (usually minor degrees of lengthening)

Myocardial infarction (in the evolutionary stages where there are marked repolarization abnormalities)

Significant active myocardial ischemia

Cerebrovascular accident (subarachnoid hemorrhage)

Hypothermia

Short QT Interval

The four causes of a short QT interval are hypercalcemia, digitalis, thyrotoxicosis, and increased sympathetic tone.

O. MISCELLANEOUS ABNORMALITIES

Right-Left Arm Cable Reversal Versus Mirror Image Dextrocardia

Misplacement of the Right Leg Cable

This error should not occur but it does occur nevertheless. It produces a "far field" signal when one of the bipolar leads (I, II, or III) records the signal between the left and right legs. The lead appears to have no signal except for a tiny deflection representing the QRS complex. There are usually no discernible P waves or T waves. RL–RA cable reversal is shown here.

Early Repolarization Normal Variant ST–T Abnormality

Hypothermia

Hypothermia is usually characterized on the ECG by a slow rate, a long QT, and muscle tremor artifact. An Osborn wave is typically present.

Acute Pericarditis: Stage I
(With PR Segment Abnormalities)

There is usually widespread ST segment elevation with concomitant PR segment depression in the same leads. The PR segment in aVR protrudes above the baseline like a knuckle, reflecting atrial injury.

Differentiating Pericarditis From Early Repolarization

Only lead V_6 is used. If the indicated amplitude ratio A/B is $\geq 25\%$, suspect pericarditis. If A/B $< 25\%$, suspect early repolarization.

Wolff-Parkinson-White Pattern

The WPW pattern is most commonly manifest as an absent PR segment and initial slurring of the QRS complex in any lead. The lead with the best sensitivity is V_4.

A. Left Lateral Accessory Pathway: This typical WPW pattern mimics lateral or posterior MI.

B. Posteroseptal Accessory Pathway: This typical WPW pattern mimics inferoposterior MI.

COPD Pattern, Lead II

The P wave amplitude in the inferior leads is equal to that of the QRS complexes.

Prominent P waves with low QRS voltage

REFERENCES

Braat SH et al: Value of the ST–T segment in lead V_4R in inferior wall acute myocardial infarction to predict the site of coronary arterial occlusion. Am J Cardiol 1985;62:140.

Brugada P et al: A new approach to the differential diagnosis of a regular tachycardia with a wide QRS complex. Circulation 1991; 83:1649.

Edenbrandt L, Devine B, Macfarlane PW: Classification of electro-cardiographic ST–T segments—human expert vs. artificial neural network. J Electrocardiol 1992;25:167.

Haisty WK Jr et al: Performance of the automated complete Selvester QRS scoring system in normal subjects and patients with single and multiple myocardial infarctions. J Am Coll Cardiol 1992;19:341.

Kalbfleisch SJ et al: Differentiation of paroxysmal narrow QRS complex tachycardias using the 12-lead electrocardiogram. J Am Coll Cardiol 1993;21:85.

Kindwall KE, Brown J, Josephson ME: Electrocardiographic criteria for ventricular tachycardia in wide complex left bundle branch morphology tachycardia. Am J Cardiol 1988;61:1279.

Norman JE Jr, Levy D: Improved electrocardiographic detection of echocardiographic left ventricular hypertrophy: Results of a correlated data base approach. J Am Coll Cardiol 1995;26:1022.

Sevilla DC et al: Sensitivity of a set of myocardial infarction screening criteria in patients with anatomically documented single and multiple infarcts. Am J Cardiol 1990;66:792.

Wellens HJJ, Brugada P: Diagnosis of ventricular tachycardia from the 12-lead electrocardiogram. Cardiol Clin 1987;5:511.

Wellens HJJ: The wide QRS tachycardias. Ann Intern Med 1986; 104:879.

Wellens HJJ, Bäar FWHM, Lie KI: The value of the electrocardiogram in the differential diagnosis of a tachycardia with a widened QRS complex. Am J Med 1978;64:27.

Willems JL et al for the WHO/ISFC Ad Hoc Task Force: Criteria for intraventricular conduction disturbances and pre-excitation. J Am Coll Cardiol 1985;5:1261.

8

Diagnostic Testing: Algorithms, Nomograms, and Tables

Stephen J. McPhee, MD, Diana Nicoll, MD, PhD, MPA,
and Michael Pignone, MD, MPH

HOW TO USE THIS SECTION

This section includes algorithms, nomograms, and tables, arranged alphabetically by subject, designed to be used in the selection and interpretation of appropriate laboratory tests.

A conventional algorithm layout is displayed below. Diagnostic tests are enclosed in ovals; diagnoses in italics; and treatment recommendations in rectangles.

SUSPECTED DIAGNOSIS/CLINICAL SITUATION

Abbreviations used throughout this section include the following:

$$
\begin{aligned}
\text{N} &= \text{Normal} \\
\text{Abn} &= \text{Abnormal} \\
\text{Pos} &= \text{Positive} \\
\text{Neg} &= \text{Negative} \\
\text{Occ} &= \text{Occasional} \\
\uparrow &= \text{Increased or high} \\
\downarrow &= \text{Decreased or low}
\end{aligned}
$$

Contents

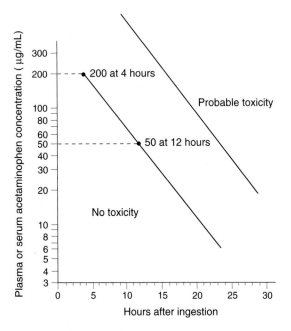

Figure 8–1. ACETAMINOPHEN TOXICITY: Nomogram for prediction of acetaminophen hepatotoxicity following acute overdosage. The upper line defines serum acetaminophen concentrations known to be associated with hepatotoxicity; the lower line defines serum levels 25% below those expected to cause hepatotoxicity. To give a margin for error, the lower line should be used as a guide to treatment. *(Modified and reproduced, with permission, from Rumack BH, Matthew H: Acetaminophen poisoning and toxicity. Pediatrics 1975;55:871. Reproduced by permission of Pediatrics. Copyright © 1975. Permission obtained also from Saunders CE, Ho MT [editors]:* Current Emergency Diagnosis & Treatment, *4th ed. Originally published by Appleton & Lange. Copyright © 1992 by The McGraw-Hill Companies, Inc.)*

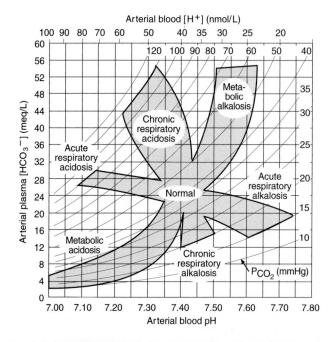

Figure 8–2. ACID-BASE NOMOGRAM: Shown are the 95% confidence limits of the normal respiratory and metabolic compensations for primary acid-base disturbances. *(Reproduced, with permission, from Cogan MG [editor]:* Fluid and Electrolytes: Physiology & Pathophysiology. *Originally published by Appleton & Lange. Copyright © 1991 by The McGraw-Hill Companies, Inc.)*

ADRENOCORTICAL INSUFFICIENCY SUSPECTED

[1] In the rapid ACTH stimulation test, a baseline cortisol sample is obtained; cosyntropin, 10–25 μg, is given IM or IV; and plasma cortisol samples are obtained 30 or 60 minutes later.
[2] The normal response is a cortisol increment >7 μg/dL. If a cortisol level of >18 μg/dL is obtained, the response is normal regardless of the increment.
[3] Administer ACTH, 250 μg every 8 hours, as a continuous infusion for 48 hours, and measure daily urinary 17-hydroxycorticosteroids (17-OHCS) or free cortisol excretion and plasma cortisol. Urinary 17-OHCS excretion of >27 mg during the first 24 hours and >47 mg during the second 24 hours is normal. Plasma cortisol >20 μg/dL at 30 or 60 minutes after infusion is begun and >25 μg/dL 6–8 hours later is normal.
[4] Metyrapone blockade is performed by giving 2–2.5 g metyrapone orally at 12 midnight. Draw cortisol and 11-deoxycortisol levels at 8 AM. 11-Deoxycortisol level <7 μg/dL indicates secondary adrenal insufficiency (as long as there is adequate blockade of cortisol synthesis [cortisol level <10 μg/dL]).

Figure 8–3. ADRENOCORTICAL INSUFFICIENCY: Laboratory evaluation of suspected adrenocortical insufficiency. **ACTH** = adrenocorticotropic hormone. *(Modified, with permission, from Baxter JD, Tyrrell JB: The adrenal cortex. In: Endocrinology and Metabolism, 3rd ed. Felig P, Baxter JD, Frohman LA [editors]. McGraw-Hill, 1995; and from Harvey AM et al: The Principles and Practice of Medicine, 22nd ed. Originally published by Appleton & Lange. Copyright © 1988 by The McGraw-Hill Companies, Inc.)*

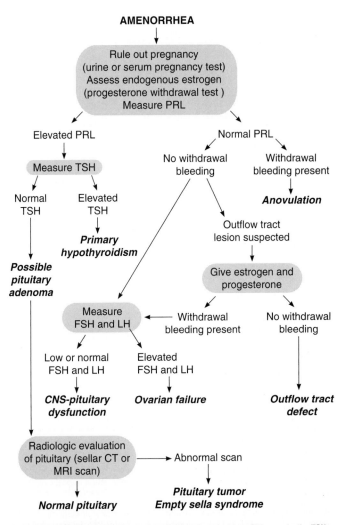

Figure 8–4. AMENORRHEA: Diagnostic evaluation of amenorrhea. **PRL** = prolactin; **TSH** = thyroid-stimulating hormone; **FSH** = follicle-stimulating hormone; **LH** = luteinizing hormone; **CT** = computed tomography; **MRI** = magnetic resonance imaging. *(Modified, with permission, from Greenspan FS, Baxter JD [editors]: Basic & Clinical Endocrinology, 4th ed. Originally published by Appleton & Lange. Copyright © 1994 by The McGraw-Hill Companies, Inc.)*

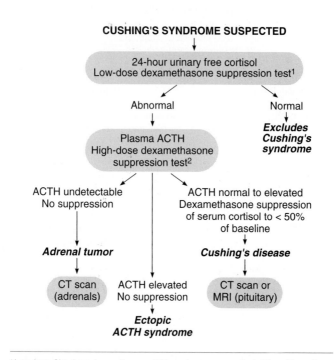

CUSHING'S SYNDROME SUSPECTED

24-hour urinary free cortisol
Low-dose dexamethasone suppression test[1]

Abnormal → Plasma ACTH / High-dose dexamethasone suppression test[2]

Normal → **Excludes Cushing's syndrome**

ACTH undetectable / No suppression → **Adrenal tumor** → CT scan (adrenals)

ACTH elevated / No suppression → **Ectopic ACTH syndrome**

ACTH normal to elevated / Dexamethasone suppression of serum cortisol to < 50% of baseline → **Cushing's disease** → CT scan or MRI (pituitary)

---

[1] Low dose: Give 1 mg dexamethasone at 11 PM; draw serum cortisol at 8 AM. Normally, AM cortisol is <5 µg/dL.

[2] High dose: Give 8 mg dexamethasone at 11 PM; draw serum cortisol at 8 AM or collect 24-hour urinary free cortisol. Normally, AM cortisol is <5 µg/dL or 24-hour urinary free cortisol is <20 µg.

Figure 8–5. CUSHING'S SYNDROME: Diagnostic evaluation of Cushing's syndrome. **ACTH** = adrenocorticotropic hormone; **CT** = computed tomography; **MRI** = magnetic resonance imaging. *(Modified, with permission, from Baxter JD, Tyrrell JB: The adrenal cortex. In: Endocrinology and Metabolism, 3rd ed. Felig P, Baxter JD, Frohman LA [editors]. McGraw-Hill, 1995; from Harvey AM et al [editors]: The Principles and Practice of Medicine, 22nd ed. Appleton & Lange, 1988; and from Greenspan FS, Baxter JD [editors]: Basic & Clinical Endocrinology, 4th ed. Originally published by Appleton & Lange. Copyright © 1994 by The McGraw-Hill Companies, Inc.)*

Nerve root

Peripheral nerve

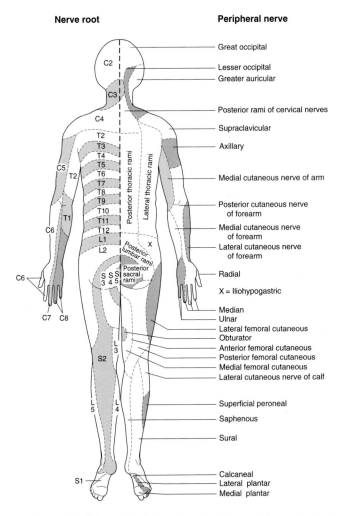

Figure 8–6. DERMATOME CHART: Cutaneous innervation. The segmental or radicular (root) distribution is shown on the left side of the body and the peripheral nerve distribution on the right side. **Above:** posterior view; **next page:** anterior view. *(Reproduced, with permission, from Aminoff MJ, Greenberg DA, Simon RP: Clinical Neurology, 3rd ed. Originally published by Appleton & Lange. Copyright © 1996 by The McGraw-Hill Companies, Inc.)*

Peripheral nerve

Nerve root

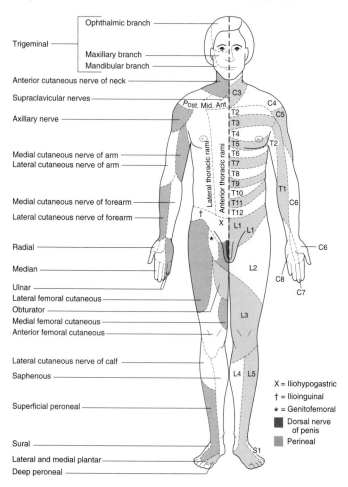

Ophthalmic branch

Trigeminal

Maxillary branch
Mandibular branch

Anterior cutaneous nerve of neck

Supraclavicular nerves

Axillary nerve

Medial cutaneous nerve of arm
Lateral cutaneous nerve of arm

Medial cutaneous nerve of forearm
Lateral cutaneous nerve of forearm

Radial

Median

Ulnar
Lateral femoral cutaneous
Obturator
Medial femoral cutaneous
Anterior femoral cutaneous

Lateral cutaneous nerve of calf
Saphenous

Superficial peroneal

Sural
Lateral and medial plantar
Deep peroneal

Post. Mid. Ant

C3
C4
C5
T2
T3
T4
T5
T6
T7
T8
T9
T10
T11
T12
L1

Lateral thoracic rami
Anterior thoracic rami

†
X
*

L1
L2

L3

L4 L5

S1

C4
C5

T2

T1

C6

C6

C8
C7

X = Iliohypogastric
† = Ilioinguinal
★ = Genitofemoral
█ Dorsal nerve
    of penis
▓ Perineal

Figure 8–6. (*Continued*)

Figure 8–7. **HEPATITIS A:** Usual pattern of serologic changes in hepatitis A. **HA** = hepatitis A; **AST** = aspartate aminotransferase; **ALT** = alanine aminotransferase; **Anti-HAV** = hepatitis A virus antibody; **IgM** = immunoglobulin M; **IgG** = immunoglobulin G. *(Reproduced, with permission, from Harvey AM et al [editors]:* The Principles and Practice of Medicine, *22nd ed. Originally published by Appleton & Lange. Copyright © 1988 by The McGraw-Hill Companies, Inc.)*

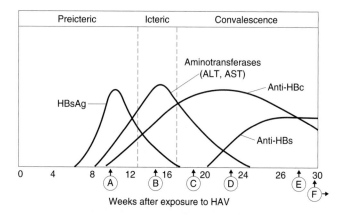

Usual Patterns of Hepatitis B Antigens and Antibodies			
	HBsAg	Anti-HBc	Anti-HBs
A Very early	+	+ or −	−
B Acute	+	+	−
C Active HB with high titer Anti-HBc ("window")	−	+	−
D Convalescence	−	+	+
E Recovery	−	+ or −	+
F Chronic carrier	+	+	−

Figure 8–8. HEPATITIS B: Usual pattern of serologic changes in hepatitis B (HB). **HBV** = hepatitis B virus; **HBsAg** = hepatitis B surface antigen; **Anti-HBc** = hepatitis B core antibody; **Anti-HBs** = hepatitis B surface antibody; **AST** = aspartate aminotransferase; **ALT** = alanine aminotransferase. *(Modified and reproduced, with permission, from Harvey AM et al [editors]: The Principles and Practice of Medicine, 22nd ed. Originally published by Appleton & Lange. Copyright © 1988 by The McGraw-Hill Companies, Inc.)*

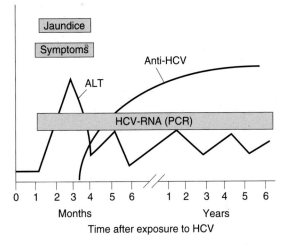

Figure 8–9. HEPATITIS C: The typical course of chronic hepatitis C. **ALT** = alanine amino-transferase; **Anti-HCV** = antibody to hepatitis C virus by enzyme immunoassay; **HCV RNA [PCR]** = hepatitis C viral RNA by polymerase chain reaction.) *(Reproduced, with permission, from Tierney LM Jr, McPhee SJ, Papadakis MA [editors]: Current Medical Diagnosis & Treatment 2000. McGraw-Hill, 2000.)*

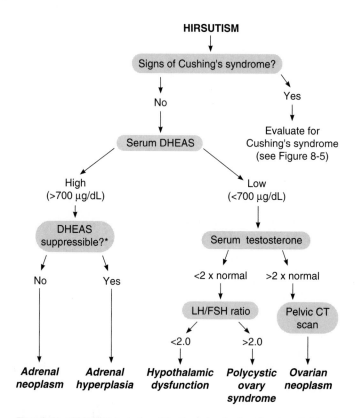

Figure 8–10. HIRSUTISM: Evaluation of hirsutism in females. Exceptions occur that do not fit this algorithm. **CT** = computed tomography; **DHEAS** = dehydroepiandrosterone sulfate; **FSH** = follicle-stimulating hormone; **LH** = luteinizing hormone. (*DHEAS <170 μg/dL after dexamethasone 0.5 mg orally every 6 hours for 5 days, with DHEAS repeated on the fifth day.) *(Reproduced, with permission, from Fitzgerald PA [editor]:* Handbook of Clinical Endocrinology, *2nd ed. Originally published by Appleton & Lange. Copyright © 1992 by The McGraw-Hill Companies, Inc.)*

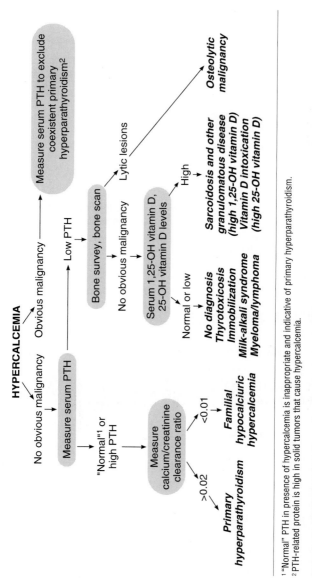

HYPERCALCEMIA

No obvious malignancy → Measure serum PTH

Obvious malignancy → Measure serum PTH to exclude coexistent primary hyperparathyroidism[2]

"Normal"[1] or high PTH → Measure calcium/creatinine clearance ratio

>0.02 → *Primary hyperparathyroidism*

<0.01 → *Familial hypocalciuric hypercalcemia*

Low PTH → Bone survey, bone scan

Lytic lesions → *Osteolytic malignancy*

No obvious malignancy → Serum 1,25-OH vitamin D, 25-OH vitamin D levels

Normal or low → *No diagnosis* *Thyrotoxicosis* *Immobilization* *Milk-alkali syndrome* *Myeloma/lymphoma*

High → *Sarcoidosis and other granulomatous disease (high 1,25-OH vitamin D) Vitamin D intoxication (high 25-OH vitamin D)*

---

[1] "Normal" PTH in presence of hypercalcemia is inappropriate and indicative of primary hyperparathyroidism.
[2] PTH-related protein is high in solid tumors that cause hypercalcemia.

Figure 8–11. HYPERCALCEMIA: Diagnostic approach to hypercalcemia. **PTH** = parathyroid hormone. *(Modified, with permission, from Harvey AM et al [editors]: The Principles and Practice of Medicine, 22nd ed. Originally published by Appleton & Lange. Copyright © 1988 by The McGraw-Hill Companies, Inc.)*

Figure 8–12. HYPERTENSION WITH HYPOKALEMIA: Evaluation of secondary causes of hypertension associated with hypokalemia. (*Studies are performed during a high-sodium intake [120 meq Na+/d.]) (**In addition, plasma aldosterone may be measured at 8 AM supine after overnight recumbency and after 4 hours of upright posture.) *(Reproduced, with permission, from Fitzgerald PA [editor]: Handbook of Clinical Endocrinology, 2nd ed. Originally published by Appleton & Lange. Copyright © 1992 by The McGraw-Hill Companies, Inc.)*

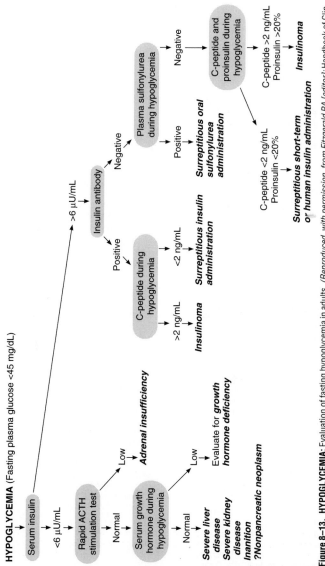

Figure 8–13. HYPOGLYCEMIA: Evaluation of fasting hypoglycemia in adults. *(Reproduced, with permission, from Fitzgerald PA [editor]: Handbook of Clinical Endocrinology, 2nd ed. Appleton & Lange, 1992.)*

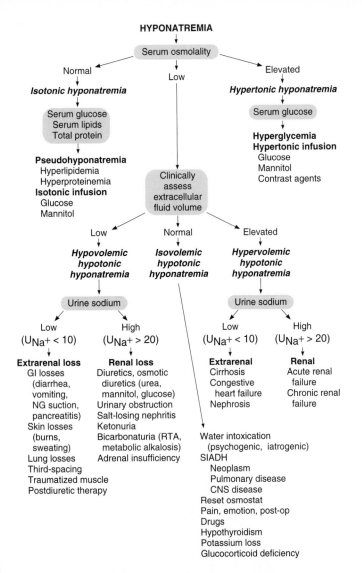

Figure 8–14. HYPONATREMIA: Evaluation of hyponatremia. **SIADH** = syndrome of in-appropriate antidiuretic hormone; U_{Na^+} = urinary sodium (mg/dL). *(Adapted, with permission, from Narins RG et al: Diagnostic strategies in disorders of fluid, electrolyte and acid-base homeostasis. Am J Med 1982;72:496.)*

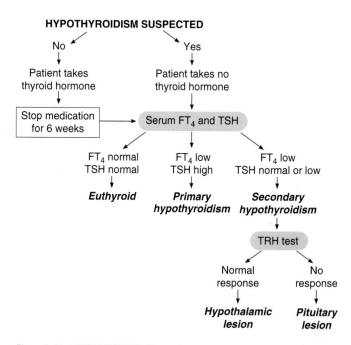

Figure 8–15. HYPOTHYROIDISM: Diagnostic approach to hypothyroidism. **FT$_4$** = free thyroxine index; **TSH** = thyroid-stimulating hormone; **TRH** = thyroid-releasing hormone. *(Modified, with permission, from Greenspan FS, Strewler GJ [editors]: Basic & Clinical Endocrinology, 5th ed. Originally published by Appleton & Lange. Copyright © 1996 by The McGraw-Hill Companies, Inc.)*

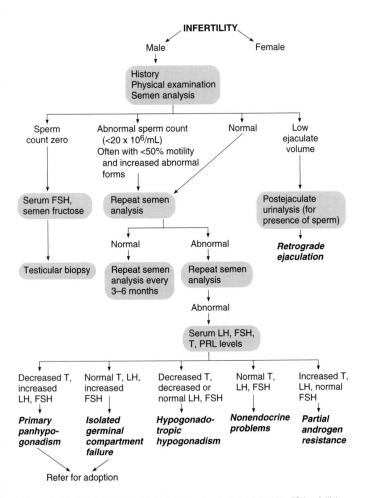

Figure 8–16. MALE INFERTILITY: Evaluation of male factor infertility. **FSH** = follicle-stimulating hormone; **LH** = luteinizing hormone; **PRL** = prolactin; **T** = testosterone. *(Adapted, with permission, from Swerdloff RS, Boyers SM: Evaluation of the male partner of an infertile couple: An algorithmic approach. JAMA 1982;247:2418. Copyright © 1982 by The American Medical Association.)*

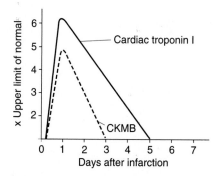

Figure 8–17. MYOCARDIAL ENZYMES: Time course of serum enzyme concentrations after a typical myocardial infarction. **CKMB** = isoenzyme of creatine kinase.

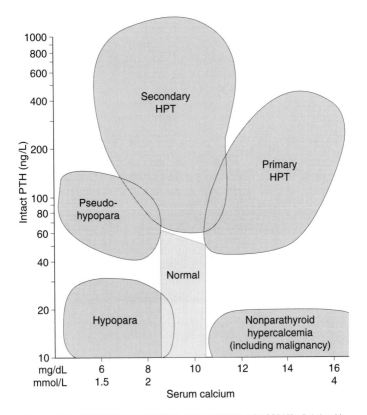

Figure 8–18. PARATHYROID HORMONE AND CALCIUM NOMOGRAM: Relationship between serum intact parathyroid hormone (PTH) and serum calcium levels in patients with hypoparathyroidism, pseudohypoparathyroidism, nonparathyroid hypercalcemia, primary hyperparathyroidism, and secondary hyperparathyroidism. **HPT** = hyperparathyroidism. *(Courtesy of GJ Strewler.)*

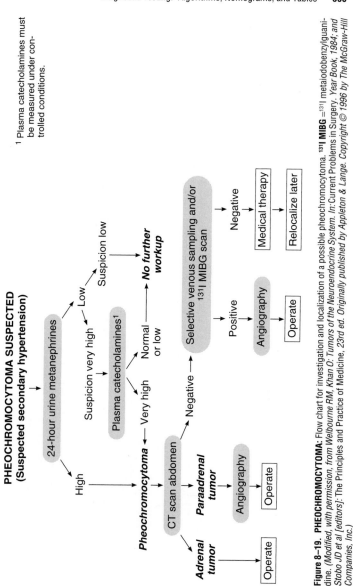

PHEOCHROMOCYTOMA SUSPECTED
(Suspected secondary hypertension)

1 Plasma catecholamines must be measured under controlled conditions.

Figure 8–19. PHEOCHROMOCYTOMA: Flow chart for investigation and localization of a possible pheochromocytoma. **131I MIBG** =131I metaiodobenzylguanidine. *(Modified, with permission, from Welbourne RM, Khan O: Tumors of the Neuroendocrine System. In: Current Problems in Surgery. Year Book, 1984; and Stobo JD et al [editors]: The Principles and Practice of Medicine, 23rd ed. Originally published by Appleton & Lange. Copyright © 1996 by The McGraw-Hill Companies, Inc.)*

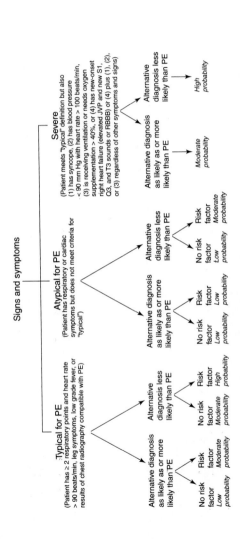

Figure 8–20A. ALGORITHM FOR THE CLINICAL MODEL TO DETERMINE THE PRETEST PROBABILITY OF PULMONARY EMBOLISM (PE): Respiratory points consist of dyspnea or worsening of chronic dyspnea, pleuritic chest pain, chest pain that is nonretrosternal and nonpleuritic, an arterial oxygen saturation <92% while breathing room air that corrects with oxygen supplementation <40%, hemoptysis, and pleural rub. Risk factors are surgery within 12 weeks, immobilization (complete bed rest) for 3 or more days in the 4 weeks before presentation, previous deep venous thrombosis or objectively diagnosed pulmonary embolism, fracture of a lower extremity and immobilization of the fracture within 12 weeks, strong family history of deep venous thrombosis or pulmonary embolism (two or more family members with objectively proved events or a first-degree relative with hereditary thrombophilia), cancer (treatment ongoing, within the past 6 months, or in the palliative stages), the postpartum period, and lower extremity paralysis. **JVP** = jugular venous pressure; **RBBB** = right bundle-branch block. See Figure 8–20B opposite. *(Reproduced, with permission, from Wells PS et al: Use of a clinical model for safe management of patients with suspected pulmonary embolism.* Ann Intern Med 1998;129:997.*)*

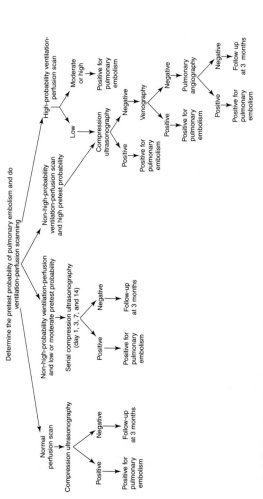

Figure 8–20B. DIAGNOSTIC STRATEGY USED IN PATIENTS WITH SUSPECTED PULMONARY EMBOLISM. See Figure 8–20A opposite. *(Reproduced, with permission, from Wells PS et al: Use of a clinical model for safe management of patients with suspected pulmonary embolism. Ann Intern Med 1998;129:997.)*

Figure 8–21. PULMONARY FUNCTION TESTS: SPIROMETRY. Representative spirograms (upper panel) and expiratory flow-volume curves (lower panel) for normal **(A),** obstructive **(B),** and restrictive **(C)** patterns. *(Reproduced, with permission, from Tierney LM Jr, McPhee SJ, Papadakis MA [editors]:* Current Medical Diagnosis & Treatment 2000. *McGraw-Hill, 2000.)*

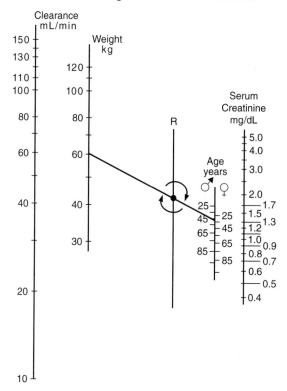

Figure 8–22. RENAL FAILURE: ESTIMATED CREATININE CLEARANCE. Siersback-Nielsen nomogram for estimation of creatinine clearance from serum creatinine.

(1) Identify the axis point along the reference line (R) around which the relation between the patient's serum creatinine and creatinine clearance rotates. To do so, place a straightedge so as to connect the patient's age (in years, for male or female) with the patient's weight (in kilograms).

(2) Put a dot along the reference line where the rule and line intersect.

(3) Rotate the ruler to connect the patient's serum creatinine and this dot, and determine where the ruler falls along the line, estimating the patient's creatinine clearance.

Note: This nomogram is based on the assumption that an increase in weight represents an increase in lean body mass. Substantial error in the estimate occurs when a weight increase reflects obesity rather than increased lean body mass. In addition, the nomogram yields a much more accurate estimate in the presence of moderate to moderately severe renal impairment than in the presence of normal renal function. It should also not be relied upon in severe renal insufficiency (eg, serum creatinine >5 mg/dL or creatinine clearance <15 mL/min). *(Modified, with permission, from Harvey AM et al [editors]: The Principles and Practice of Medicine, 22nd ed. Originally published by Appleton & Lange. Copyright © 1988 by The McGraw-Hill Companies, Inc.)*

Figure 8–23. SALICYLATE TOXICITY: Nomogram for determining severity of salicylate intoxication. Absorption kinetics assume acute ingestion of non-enteric-coated aspirin preparation. *(Modified and reproduced, with permission, from Done AK: Significance of measurements of salicylate in blood in cases of acute ingestion. Pediatrics 1960;26:800. Permission obtained also from Saunders CE, Ho MT [editors]:* Current Emergency Diagnosis & Treatment, *4th ed. Originally published by Appleton & Lange. Copyright © 1992 by The McGraw-Hill Companies, Inc.)*

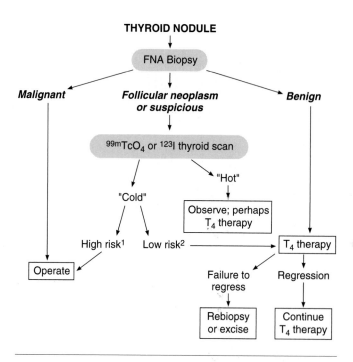

THYROID NODULE

^{1} High risk = child, young adult, male; solitary, firm nodule; family history of thyroid cancer; previous neck irradiation; recent growth of nodule; hoarseness, dysphagia, obstruction; vocal cord paralysis, lymphadenopathy.

^{2} Low risk = older, female; soft nodule; multinodular goiter; family history of benign goiter; residence in endemic goiter area.

Figure 8–24. THYROID NODULE: Laboratory evaluation of a thyroid nodule. **FNA** = fine-needle aspiration; **T_4** = thyroxine. *(Modified, with permission, from Greenspan FS, Strewler GJ [editors]: Basic & Clinical Endocrinology, 5th ed. Originally published by Appleton & Lange. Copyright © 1997 by The McGraw-Hill Companies, Inc.)*

TABLE 8–1. ACID-BASE DISTURBANCES: LABORATORY CHARACTERISTICS OF PRIMARY SINGLE DISTURBANCES OF ACID-BASE BALANCE.[1]

Disturbance	Acute Primary Change	Arterial pH	[K+] (meq/L)	Anion Gap[2] (meq)	Clinical Features
Normal	None	7.35–7.45	3.5–5.0	8–12	None.
Respiratory acidosis	P_{CO_2} retention	↓	↑	N	Dyspnea, polypnea, respiratory outflow obstruction, ↑ anterior-posterior chest diameter, musical rales, wheezes. In severe cases, stupor, disorientation, coma.
Respiratory alkalosis	P_{CO_2} depletion	↑	↓	N or ↓	Anxiety, breathlessness, frequent sighing, lungs usually clear to examination, positive Chvostek and Trousseau signs.
Metabolic acidosis	HCO_3^- depletion	↓	↑ or ↓	N or ↑	Weakness, air hunger, Kussmaul respiration, dry skin and mucous membranes. In severe cases, poor skin turgor, coma, hypotension, death.
Metabolic alkalosis	HCO_3^- retention	↑	↓	N	Weakness, positive Chvostek and Trousseau signs, hyporeflexia.

[1] Reproduced, with permission, from Harvey AM et al (editors): The Principles and Practice of Medicine, 22nd ed. Originally published by Appleton & Lange. Copyright © 1988 by The McGraw-Hill Companies, Inc.

[2] Anion gap = $[Na^+]-([HCO_3^-] + [Cl^-]) = 8–12$ meq normally.

TABLE 8–2. ANEMIA: DIAGNOSIS OF COMMON ANEMIAS BASED ON RED BLOOD CELL (RBC) INDICES. [1]

Type of Anemia	MCV (fL)	MCHC (g/dL)	Common Causes	Common Laboratory Abnormalities	Other Clinical Findings
Microcytic, hypochromic	<80	<32	Iron deficiency	Low reticulocyte count, low serum and bone marrow iron, high TIBC.	Mucositis, blood loss.
			Thalassemias	Reticulocytosis, abnormal red cell morphology, normal serum iron levels.	Asian, African, or Mediterranean descent.
			Chronic lead poisoning	Basophilic stippling of RBCs, elevated lead and free erythrocyte protoporphyrin levels.	Peripheral neuropathy, history of exposure to lead.
			Sideroblastic anemia	High serum iron, ringed sideroblasts in bone marrow.	Population of hypochromic RBCs on smear.
Normocytic, normochromic	81–100	32–36	Acute blood loss	Blood in stool.	Recent blood loss.
			Hemolysis	Haptoglobin low or absent, reticulocytosis, hyperbilirubinemia.	Hemoglobinuria, splenomegaly.
			Chronic disease[2]	Low serum iron, TIBC low or low normal.	Depends on cause.
Macrocytic, normochromic	>101[3]	>36	Vitamin B_{12} deficiency	Hypersegmented PMNs; low serum vitamin B_{12} levels; achlorhydria.	Peripheral neuropathy; glossitis.
			Folate deficiency	Hypersegmented PMNs; low folate levels.	Alcoholism; malnutrition.
			Liver disease	Mean corpuscular volume usually <120 fL; normal serum vitamin B_{12} and folate levels.	Signs of liver disease.
			Reticulocytosis	Marked (>15%) reticulocytosis.	Variable.

[1] Modified, with permission, from Saunders CE, Ho MT (editors): Current Emergency Diagnosis & Treatment, 4th ed. Originally published by Appleton & Lange. Copyright © 1992 by The McGraw-Hill Companies, Inc.

[2] May be microcytic, hypochromic.

[3] If MCV >120–130, vitamin B_{12} or folate deficiency is likely.

MCV = mean corpuscular volume; **MCHC** = mean corpuscular hemoglobin concentration; **TIBC** = total iron-binding capacity, serum; **PMN** = polymorphonuclear cell.

TABLE 8–3. ANEMIA, MICROCYTIC: LABORATORY EVALUATION OF MICROCYTIC, HYPOCHROMIC ANEMIAS.[1]

Diagnosis	MCV (fL)	Serum Iron (μg/dL)	Iron-binding Capacity (μg/dL)	Transferrin Saturation (%)	Serum Ferritin (μg/L)	Free Erythrocyte Protoporphyrin (μg/dL)	Basophilic Stippling	Bone Marrow Iron Stores
Normal	80–100	50–175	250–460	16–60	16–300	<35	Absent	Present
Iron deficiency anemia	↓	<30	↑	<16	<12	↑	Absent	Absent
Anemia of chronic disease	N or ↓	<30	N or ↓	N or ↓	N or ↑	↑	Absent	Present
Thalassemia minor	↓	N	N	N	N	N	Usually present	Present

[1] Modified, with permission, from Harvey AM et al (editors): The Principles and Practice of Medicine, 22nd ed. Originally published by Appleton & Lange. Copyright © 1988 by The McGraw-Hill Companies, Inc.

TABLE 8–4. ASCITES: ASCITIC FLUID PROFILES IN VARIOUS DISEASE STATES. [1]

Diagnosis	Appearance	Fluid Protein (g/dL)	Serum-Ascites Albumin Gradient (SAAG)	Fluid Glucose (mg/dL)	WBC and Differential (per μL)	RBC (per μL)	Bacteriologic Gram Stain and Culture	Cytology	Comments
Normal	Clear	<3.0		Equal to plasma glucose	<250	Few or none	Neg	Neg	
TRANSUDATES[2]									
Cirrhosis	Clear	<3.0	High[3]	N	<250, MN	Few	Neg	Neg	Occasionally turbid, rarely bloody. Fluid LDH/serum LDH ratio <0.6
Congestive heart failure	Clear	<2.5	High[3]	N	<250, MN	Few	Neg	Neg	
Nephrotic syndrome	Clear	<2.5	Low[4]	N	<250, MN	Few	Neg	Neg	
Pseudomyxoma peritonei	Gelatinous	<2.5		N	<250	Few	Neg	Occ Pos	
EXUDATES[5]									
Bacterial peritonitis	Cloudy	>3.0		<50 with perforation	>500, PMN	Few	Pos	Neg	Blood cultures frequently positive
Tuberculous peritonitis	Clear	>3.0	Low[4]	<60	>500, MN	Few, occasionally many	Stain Pos in 25%; culture Pos in 65%	Neg	Occasionally chylous. Peritoneal biopsy positive in 65%.

TABLE 8–4 (CONTINUED).

Diagnosis	Appearance	Fluid Protein (g/dL)	Serum-Ascites Albumin Gradient (SAAG)	Fluid Glucose (mg/dL)	WBC and Differential (per μL)	RBC (per μL)	Bacteriologic Gram Stain and Culture	Cytology	Comments
Malignancy	Clear or bloody	>3.0	Low[4]	<60	>500, MN, PMN	Many	Neg	Pos in 60–90%	Occasionally chylous. Fluid LDH/Serum LDH ratio >0.6. Peritoneal biopsy diagnostic.
Pancreatitis	Clear or bloody	>2.5		N	>500, MN, PMN	Many	Neg	Neg	Occasionally chylous Fluid amylase > 1000 IU/L, sometimes >10,000 IU/L Fluid amylase > serum amylase
Chylous ascites	Turbid	Varies, often >2.5		N	Few	Few	Neg	Neg	Fluid TG > 400 mg/dL (turbid) Fluid TG > serum TG

[1] Modified, with permission, from Harvey AM et al (editors): The Principles and Practice of Medicine, 22nd ed. Originally published by Appleton & Lange. Copyright © 1988 by The McGraw-Hill Companies, Inc.; and from Schiff L, Schiff ER (editors): Diseases of the Liver, 7th ed. Lippincott, 1993.

[2] Transudates have protein concentration <2.5–3 g/dL; fluid LDH/serum LDH ratio <0.6 (may be useful in difficult cases).

[3] High = ≥ 1.1

[4] Low = <1.1

[5] Exudates have fluid protein concentration >2.5–3 g/dL; fluid LDH/serum LDH ratio >0.6 (may be useful in difficult cases).

MN = mononuclear cells; **PMN** = polymorphonuclear cells; **TG** = triglycerides.

TABLE 8–5. AUTOANTIBODIES: ASSOCIATIONS WITH CONNECTIVE TISSUE DISEASES. [1]

Suspected Disease State	Test	Primary Disease Association (Sensitivity, Specificity)	Other Disease Associations (Sensitivity)	Comments
CREST syndrome	Anti-centromere antibody	CREST (70–90%, high)	Scleroderma (10–15%), Raynaud's disease (10–30%).	Predictive value of a positive test is >95% for scleroderma or related disease (CREST, Raynaud's). Diagnosis of CREST is made clinically.
Systemic lupus erythematosus (SLE)	Anti-nuclear antibody (ANA)	SLE (>95%, low)	RA (30–50%), discoid lupus, scleroderma (60%), drug-induced lupus (100%), Sjögren's syndrome (80%), miscellaneous inflammatory disorders.	Often used as a screening test; a negative test virtually excludes SLE; a positive test, while nonspecific, increases posttest probability. Titer does not correlate with disease activity.
	Anti-double-stranded-DNA antibody (anti-ds-DNA)	SLE (60–70%, high)	Lupus nephritis, rarely RA, CTD, usually in low titer.	Predictive value of a positive test is >90% for SLE if present in high titer; a decreasing titer may correlate with worsening renal disease. Titer generally correlates with disease activity.
	Anti-Smith antibody (anti-SM)	SLE (30–40%, high)		SLE-specific. A positive test substantially increases posttest probability of SLE. Test rarely indicated.
Mixed connective tissue disease (MCTD)	Anti-ribonucleoprotein antibody (RNP)	MCTD (95–100%, low) Scleroderma (20–30%, low)	SLE (30%), Sjögren's syndrome, RA (10%), discoid lupus (20–30%).	A negative test essentially excludes MCTD; a positive test in high titer, while nonspecific, increases posttest probability of MCTD.

TABLE 8–5 (CONTINUED).

Suspected Disease State	Test	Primary Disease Association (Sensitivity, Specificity)	Other Disease Associations (Sensitivity)	Comments
Rheumatoid arthritis (RA)	Rheumatoid factor (RF)	Rheumatoid arthritis (50–90%)	Other rheumatic diseases, chronic infections, some malignancies, some healthy individuals, elderly patients.	Titer does not correlate with disease activity.
Scleroderma	Anti-Scl-70 antibody	Scleroderma (15–20%, high)		Predictive value of a positive test is > 95% for scleroderma.
Sjögren's syndrome	Anti-SS-A/Ro antibody	Sjögren's (60–70%, low)	SLE (30–40%), RA (10%), subacute cutaneous lupus, vasculitis.	Useful in counseling women of child-bearing age with known CTD, since a positive test is associated with a small but real risk of neonatal SLE and congenital heart block.
Wegener's granulomatosis	Anti-neutrophil cyto-plasmic antibody (ANCA)	Wegener's granulomatosis (systemic necrotizing vas-culitis) (56–96%, high)	Crescentic glomerulonephritis or other systemic vasculitis (eg, polyarteritis nodosa).	Ability of this assay to reflect disease activity remains unclear.

[1] Modified, with permission, from Harvey AM et al (editors): The Principles and Practice of Medicine, 22nd ed. Appleton & Lange, 1988; from White RH, Robbins DL: Clinical significance and interpretation of antinuclear antibodies. West J Med 1987;147:210; and from Tan EM: Autoantibodies to nuclear antigens (ANA): Their immunobiology and medicine. Adv Immunol 1982;33:173.

RA = rheumatoid arthritis; **SLE** = systemic lupus erythematosus; **CTD** = connective tissue disease; **MCTD** = mixed connective tissue disease; **SSA** = Sjögren's syndrome A antibody; **CREST** = calcinosis, Raynaud's phenomenon, esophageal dysmotility, sclerodactyly and telangiectasia.

TABLE 8–6. CEREBROSPINAL FLUID (CSF): CSF PROFILES IN CENTRAL NERVOUS SYSTEM DISEASE.

Diagnosis	Appearance	Opening Pressure (mm H₂O)	RBC (per µL)	WBC & Diff (per µL)	CSF Glucose (mg/dL)	CSF Protein (mg/dL)	Smears	Culture	Comments
Normal	Clear, colorless	70–200	0	≤5 MN, 0 PMN	45–85	15–45	Neg	Neg	
Bacterial meningitis	Cloudy	↑↑↑	0	200–20,000, mostly PMN	<45	>50	Gram's stain Pos	Pos	PMN predominance may be seen early in course.
Tuberculous meningitis	N or cloudy	↑↑↑	0	100–1000, mostly MN	<45	>50	AFB stain Pos	±	
Fungal meningitis	N or cloudy	N or ↑	0	100–1000, mostly MN	<45	>50		±	Counterimmunoelectrophoresis or latex agglutination may be diagnostic. CSF and serum cryptococcal antigen positive in cryptococcal meningitis.
Viral (aseptic) meningitis	N	N or ↑	0	100–1000, mostly MN	45–85	N or ↑	Neg	Neg	RBC count may be elevated in herpes simplex encephalitis. Glucose may be decreased in herpes simplex or mumps infections. Viral cultures may be helpful.

TABLE 8–6 (CONTINUED).

Diagnosis	Appearance	Opening Pressure (mm H$_2$O)	RBC (per μL)	WBC & Diff (per μL)	CSF Glucose (mg/dL)	CSF Protein (mg/dL)	Smears	Culture	Comments
Parasitic meningitis	N or cloudy	N or ↑	0	100–1000, mostly MN, E	< 45	N or ↑	Amebae may be seen on wet smear	±	
Carcinomatous meningitis	N or cloudy	N or ↑	0	N or 100–1000, mostly MN	< 45	N or ↑	Cytology Pos	Neg	
Cerebral lupus erythematosus	N	N or ↑	0	N or ↑, mostly MN	N	N or ↑	Neg	Neg	
Subarachnoid hemorrhage	Pink-red, supernatant yellow	↑	↑ crenated or fresh	N or 100–1000, mostly PMN	N or ↓		Neg	Neg	Blood in all tubes equally. Pleocytosis and low glucose sometimes seen several days after subarachnoid hemorrhage, reflecting chemical meningitis caused by subarachnoid blood.
"Traumatic" tap	Bloody, supernatant clear	N	↑↑↑ fresh	↑	N	↑	Neg	Neg	Most blood in tube #1, least blood in tube #4.

Spirochetal, early, acute syphilitic meningitis	Clear to turbid	↑	0	25–2000, mostly MN	15–75	>50	Neg	Neg	PMN may predominate early. Positive serum RPR or VDRL. CSF VDRL insensitive. If clinical suspicion is high, institute treatment despite negative CSF VDRL.
Late CNS syphilis	Clear	Usually N	0	N or ↑	N	N or ↑	Neg	Neg	CSF VDRL insensitive.
"Neighborhood" meningeal reaction	Clear or turbid, often xanthochromic	Variable, usually N	Variable	↑	N	N or ↑	Neg	Usually Neg	May occur in mastoiditis, brain abscess, sinusitis, septic thrombophlebitis, brain tumor, intrathecal drug therapy.
Hepatic encephalopathy	N	N	0	≤5	N	N	Neg	Neg	CSF glutamine >15 mg/dL.
Uremia	N	Usually ↑	0	N or ↑	N or ↑	N or ↑	Neg	Neg	
Diabetic coma	N	Low	0	N or ↑	↑	N	Neg	Neg	

MN = mononuclear cells (lymphocytes or monocytes); *PMN* = polymorphonuclear cells; *E* = eosinophils; *CNS* = central nervous system.

TABLE 8–7. RELATIONSHIP OF HEPATIC FUNCTION AND NUTRITION OR PROTHROMBIN TIME TO OPERATIVE DEATH RATE AFTER PORTACAVAL SHUNT.

	Group		
	A	B	C
Child's criteria			
Operative death rate	2%	10%	50%
Serum bilirubin (mg/dL)	<2	2–3	>3
Serum albumin (g/dL)	>3.5	3–3.5	<3
Ascites	None	Easily controlled	Poorly controlled
Encephalopathy	None	Minimal	Advanced
Nutrition[1]	Excellent	Good	Poor
Pugh modification[1] Prothrombin time (seconds prolonged)	1–4	4–6	>6

[1] In the Pugh modification of Child's criteria, prothrombin time is substituted for nutrition.

TABLE 8–8. GENETIC DISEASES DIAGNOSED BY MOLECULAR DIAGNOSTIC TECHNIQUES.

Test/Range/Collection	Physiologic Basis	Interpretation	Comments
Cystic fibrosis mutation PCR + reverse dot blot Blood Lavender $$$$	Cystic fibrosis is caused by a mutation in the cystic fibrosis transmembrane regulator gene (CFTR). Over 600 mutations have been found, with the most common being ΔF508, present in 68% of cases.	Test specificity approaches 100%, so a positive result should be considered diagnostic of a cystic fibrosis mutation. Because of the wide range of mutations, an assay for the ΔF508 mutation alone is 68% sensitive; a combined panel encompassing the 31 most common mutations is about 90% sensitive. The test can distinguish between heterozygous carriers and homozygous patients.	Cystic fibrosis is the most common inherited disease in North American Caucasians, affecting one in 2500 births. Caucasians have a carrier frequency of one in 25. The disease is autosomal recessive. Proc Natl Acad Sci U S A 1989;86;6230. Hum Mutations 1995;5:333. J Lab Clin Med 1995;125:421. J Pediatr 1998;132:589.
Factor V (Leiden) mutation (activated protein C resistance) Blood Lavender or blue $$$$	The Leiden mutation is a single nucleotide base substitution leading to an amino acid substitution (glutamine replaces arginine) at one of the sites where coagulation factor V is cleaved by activated protein C. The mutation causes factor V to be partially resistant to protein C, which is involved in inhibiting coagulation. Factor V mutations may be present in up to half of the cases of unexplained venous thrombosis and are seen in 96% of patients with activated protein C resistance.	**Positive in:** Hypercoagulability secondary to factor V mutation (specificity approaches 100%).	The presence of mutation is only a risk factor for thrombosis, not an absolute marker for disease. Homozygotes have a 50- to 100-fold increase in risk of thrombosis (relative to the general population), and heterozygotes have a 7-fold increase in risk. The current PCR and reverse dot blot assay only detects the Leiden mutation of factor V; other mutations may yet be discovered. There is also increased risk of thrombosis in carriers of the prothrombin $G \rightarrow A^{20210}$ variant and in methylenetetrahydrofolate reductase deficiency. Thromb Hemost 1997;78:523. Ann Intern Med 1998;128:1000. Ann Intern Med 1998;129:89. Ann Intern Med 1999;130:643.

TABLE 8–8 (CONTINUED).

Test/Range/Collection	Physiologic Basis	Interpretation	Comments
Fragile X syndrome Blood, cultured amniocytes Lavender $$$$	Fragile X syndrome results from a mutation in the familial mental retardation–1 gene (*FMR1*), located at Xq27.3. Fully symptomatic patients have abnormal methylation of the gene (which blocks transcription) during oogenesis. The gene contains a variable number of repeating CGG sequences and, as the number of sequences increases, the probability of abnormal methylation increases. The number of copies increases with subsequent generations so that females who are unaffected carriers may have offspring who are affected.	Normal patients have 6–52 CGG repeat sequences. Patients with 52–230 repeat sequences are asymptomatic carriers. Patients with more than 230 repeat sequences are very likely to have abnormal methylation and to be symptomatic.	Fragile X syndrome is the most common cause of inherited mental retardation, occurring in one in 1000–1500 males and one in 2000–2500 females. Full mutations can show variable penetration in females, but most such females will be at least mildly retarded. N Engl J Med 1991;325:1673. Am J Hum Genet 1995;56:1147. Am J Med Genet 1996;64:191. Am J Hum Genet 1997;61:660.
Hemophilia A Southern blot Blood, cultured amniocytes Lavender $$$$	Approximately half of severe hemophilia A cases are caused by an inversion mutation within the factor VIII gene. The resulting rearrangement of *BCL1* sites can be detected by Southern blot hybridization assays.	Test specificity approaches 100%, so a positive result should be considered diagnostic of a hemophilia A inversion mutation. Because of a variety of mutations, however, test sensitivity is only about 50%.	Hemophilia A is one of the most common X-linked diseases in humans, affecting one in 5000 males. Nat Genet 1993;5:236. Hematol Oncol Clin North Am 1998;12:1315.

Huntington's disease PCR + Southern blot Blood, cultured amniocytes, or buccal cells Lavender $$$$	Huntington's disease is an inherited neurodegenerative disorder associated with an autosomal dominant mutation on chromosome 4. The disease is highly penetrant, but symptoms (disordered movements, cognitive decline, and emotional disturbance) are often not expressed until middle age. The mutation results in the expansion of a CAG trinucleotide repeat sequence within the gene.	Normal patients will have fewer than 34 CAG repeats, while patients with disease usually have more than 37 repeats and may have 80 or more. Occasional affected patients can be seen with "high normal" (32–34) numbers of repeats. Tests showing 34–37 repeats are indeterminate.	Huntington's disease testing involves ethical dilemmas. Counseling is recommended prior to testing. Hum Molec Genet 1993;2:633. J Neurol 1998;245:709.
α-Thalassemia PCR + Southern blot Blood, cultured amniocytes, chorionic villi Lavender $$$$	A deletion mutation in the α-globin gene region of chromosome 16 due to unequal crossing-over events can lead to defective synthesis of the α-globin chain of hemoglobin. Normally, there are two copies of the α-globin gene on each chromosome 16, and the severity of disease increases with the number of defective genes.	This assay is highly specific (approaches 100%). Sensitivity, however, can vary since detection of different mutations may require the use of different probes. α-Thalassemia due to point mutations may not be detected.	Patients with one deleted gene are usually normal or very slightly anemic; patients with two deletions usually have a hypochromic microcytic anemia; patients with three deletions have elevated hemoglobin H and a moderately severe hemolytic anemia; patients with four deletions generally die in utero with hydrops fetalis (see Table 8–21). Eur J Clin Invest 1990;20:340. Prenat Diagn 1996;16:1181.

TABLE 8–8 (CONTINUED).

Test/Range/Collection	Physiologic Basis	Interpretation	Comments
β-Thalassemia PCR + reverse dot blot Blood, chorionic villi, cultured amniocytes Lavender $$$$	β-Thalassemia results from a mutation in the gene encoding the β-globin subunit of hemoglobin A (which is composed of a pair of α-chains and a pair of β-chains). A relative excess of α-globin chains precipitates within red blood cells, causing hemolysis and anemia. Over 100 different mutations have been described; testing usually covers a panel of the more common mutations. The test can distinguish between heterozygous and homozygous individuals.	Test specificity approaches 100%, so a positive result should be considered diagnostic of a thalassemia mutation. Because of the large number of mutations, sensitivity can be poor. A panel with the 41 most common mutations has a sensitivity that approaches 95%.	β-Thalassemia is very common; about 3% of the world's population are carriers. The incidence is increased in persons of Mediterranean, African, and Asian descent. The mutations may vary from population to population, and different testing panels may be needed for patients of different ethnicities (see Table 8–22). JAMA 1997;278:1273. J Hum Genet 1998;43:237.

[1] Adapted, with permission, by Lindeman N from Wall J, Chehab F, Kan YW: Clinical Laboratory Manual. *UCSF, 1996.*
PCR (polymerase chain reaction) *is a method for amplifying the amount of a particular DNA sequence in a specimen, facilitating detection by hybridization-based assay (ie, Southern blot, reverse dot blot).*
Southern blot *is a molecular hybridization technique whereby DNA is extracted from the sample and digested by different restriction enzymes. The resulting fragments are separated by electrophoresis and identified by labeled probes.* **Reverse dot blot** *is a molecular hybridization technique in which a specific oligonucleotide probe is bound to a solid membrane prior to reaction with PCR-amplified DNA.*
$$$$ = > $100.00.

TABLE 8–9. HEMOSTATIC FUNCTION: LABORATORY EVALUATION.[1]

Suspected Diagnosis	Platelet Count	PT	PTT	TT	Further Diagnostic Tests
Idiopathic thrombocytopenic purpura, drug sensitivity, bone marrow depression	↓	N	N	N	Platelet antibody, marrow aspirate.
Disseminated intravascular coagulation	↓	↑	↑	↑	Fibrinogen assays, fibrin D-dimers.
Platelet function defect, salicylates, or uremia	N	N	N	N	Bleeding time, platelet aggregation, blood urea nitrogen (BUN), creatinine.
von Willebrand's disease	N	N	↑ or N	N	Bleeding time, factor VIII assay, factor VIII antigen.
Factor VII deficiency or inhibitor	N	↑	N	N	Factor VII assay (normal plasma should correct PT if no inhibitor is present).
Factor V, X, II, I deficiencies as in liver disease or with anticoagulants	N	↑	↑	N or ↑	Liver function tests.
Factor VIII (hemophilia), IX, XI, or XII deficiencies or inhibitor	N	N	↑	N	Inhibitor screen, individual factor assays.
Factor XIII deficiency	N	N	N	N	Urea stabilizing test, factor XIII assay.

[1] Modified with permission, from Tierney LM Jr, McPhee SJ, Papadakis MA (editors): Current Medical Diagnosis & Treatment 1996. Originally published by Appleton & Lange. Copyright © 1996 by the McGraw-Hill Companies, Inc.; and from Harvey AM et al. (editors): The Principles and Practice of Medicine, 22nd ed. Originally published by Appleton & Lange. Copyright © 1988 by The McGraw-Hill Companies, Inc.

Note: In approaching patients with bleeding disorders, try to distinguish clinically between platelet disorders (eg, patient has petechiae, mucosal bleeding) and factor deficiency states (eg, patient has hemarthrosis).

PT = prothrombin time; **PTT** = activated partial thromboplastin time; **TT** = thrombin time.

TABLE 8–10. HEPATIC FUNCTION TESTS.[1]

Clinical Condition	Direct Bilirubin (mg/dL)	Indirect Bilirubin (mg/dL)	Urine Bilirubin	Serum Albumin & Total Protein (g/dL)	Alkaline Phosphatase (IU/L)	Prothrombin time (seconds)	ALT (SGPT); AST (SGOT) (IU/L)
Normal	0.1–0.3	0.2–0.7	None	Albumin, 3.4–4.7 Total protein, 6.0–8.0	30–115 (lab-specific)	11–15 seconds. After vitamin K, 15% increase within 24 hours.	ALT, 5–35; AST, 5–40 (lab specific)
Hepatocellular jaundice (eg, viral, alcoholic hepatitis)	↑↑	↑	↑	↓ Albumin	N to ↑	Prolonged if damage is severe. Does not respond to parenteral vitamin K.	Increased in hepatocellular damage; viral hepatitides; AST/ALT ratio often >2:1 in alcoholic hepatitis
Uncomplicated obstructive jaundice (eg, common bile duct obstruction)	↑↑	↑	↑	N	↑	Prolonged if obstruction marked but responds to parenteral vitamin K.	N to minimally ↑
Hemolysis	N	↑	None	N	N	N	N
Gilbert's syndrome	N	↑	None	N	N	N	N
Intrahepatic cholestasis (drug-induced)	↑↑	↑	↑	N	↑↑	N	AST N or ↑; ALT N or ↑
Primary biliary cirrhosis	↑↑	↑	↑	N ↑ globulin	↑↑	N or ↑	↑

[1] Modified, with permission, from Tierney LM Jr, McPhee SJ, Papadakis MA (editors): Current Medical Diagnosis & Treatment 1996. *Originally published by Appleton & Lange. Copyright © 1996 by The McGraw-Hill Companies, Inc.*; and from Harvey AM et al (editors): The Principles and Practice of Medicine, 22nd ed. *Originally published by Appleton & Lange. Copyright © 1988 by The McGraw-Hill Companies, Inc.*
AST = aspartate aminotransferase; **ALT** = alanine aminotransferase.

TABLE 8–11. HYPERLIPIDEMIA: CHARACTERISTICS AND LABORATORY FINDINGS IN PRIMARY HYPERLIPIDEMIA.[1]

Lipoprotein Disorder	Lipoprotein Abnormalities or Defect	Appearance of Serum[2]	Cholesterol (mg/dL)	Triglyceride (mg/dL)	Clinical Presentation	Comments	Risk of Atherosclerosis
None	None	Clear	<200	<165			Nil
Familial hypercholesterolemia	LDL elevated; decreased or lack of LDL receptors in liver	Clear	Usually 300–600 but may be higher; LDL cholesterol high	Normal	Xanthelasma, tendon and skin xanthomas, accelerated atherosclerosis. Detectable in childhood.	Onset at all ages. Consider hypothyroidism, nephrotic syndrome, hepatic obstruction.	↑↑
Familial combined hyperlipidemia	LDL or VLDL elevated	Turbid or clear	Usually 250–600: LDL cholesterol high	Usually 200–600	Accelerated atherosclerosis. Associated with obesity or diabetes.	Cholesterol or triglyceride or both may be elevated—at different times and in different members of the family.	↑↑
Familial hypertriglyceridemia	VLDL elevated	Turbid	Typically normal	200–5000	Eruptive xanthomas. Triglycerides, if high enough, may cause pancreatitis.	Consider nephrotic syndrome, hypothyroidism, alcoholism, glycogen storage disease, oral contraceptives.	Nil

TABLE 8–11 (CONTINUED).

Lipoprotein Disorder	Lipoprotein Abnormalities or Defect	Appearance of Serum[2]	Cholesterol (mg/dL)	Triglyceride (mg/dL)	Clinical Presentation	Comments	Risk of Athero-sclerosis
Hyper-chylochromemia	Chylomicrons elevated; deficiency of lipoprotein lipase or, less commonly, of C-II apolipoprotein	Creamy, separates into creamy supernate and clear infranate	Increased	Often 1000–10,000; chylomicrons	Eruptive xanthomas, lipemia retinalis, recurrent abdominal pain, hepato-splenomegaly, pancreatitis.	Onset in infancy or childhood. Aggravated by high fat intake, diabetes, alcohol.	Nil
Mixed hyper-triglyceridemia	VLDL and chylomicrons elevated	Creamy, separates into creamy supernate and turbid infranate	300–1000	Usually 500–>10,000; chylomicrons high	Recurrent abdominal pain, hepato-splenomegaly, eruptive xanthomas; glucose intolerance	Symptoms begin in adult life. Sensitive to dietary fat. Alcohol and diabetes aggravated.	Nil to ↑
Dysbetalipo-proteinemia (type III)	VLDL, IDL elevated; apolipoprotein E dysfunction	Turbid	200–500	200–500	Palmar xanthoma typical; other xanthomas common.	Aggravated by alcohol, estrogen.	↑↑

[1] Modified, with permission, from Schroeder SA et al (editors): Current Medical Diagnosis & Treatment 1991. Originally published by Appleton & Lange. Copyright © 1991 by The McGraw-Hill Companies, Inc.; from Harvey AM et al (editors): The Principles and Practice of Medicine, 22nd ed. Originally published by Appleton & Lange. Copyright © 1988 by The McGraw-Hill Companies; and from Siperstein M, 1996. The collaboration of Dr. Marvin D. Siperstein is gratefully acknowledged.

[2] Refrigerated serum overnight at 4°C.

Key: LDL = low-density lipoprotein, calculated as: Total cholesterol—HDL cholesterol—[Triglycerides/5]; **VLDL** = very low density lipoprotein; **IDL** = intermediate density lipoprotein.

TABLE 8–12. THE OSMOLAL GAP IN TOXICOLOGY.[1]

The osmolal gap (Δ osm) is determined by subtracting the calculated serum osmolality from the measured serum osmolality.

$$\text{Calculated osmolality (osm)} = 2\left(Na^+[meq/L]\right) + \frac{\text{Glucose (mg/dL)}}{18} + \frac{\text{BUN (mg/dL)}}{2.8}$$
(mosm/kg H_2O)

Osmolal gap (Δ osm) = Measured osmolality − Calculated osmolality

Serum osmolality may be increased by contributions of circulating alcohols and other low-molecular-weight substances. Since these substances are not included in the calculated osmolality, there will be an osmolal gap directly proportionate to their serum concentration and inversely proportionate to their molecular weight:

$$\text{Serum concentration (mg/dL)} \approx \Delta \text{ osm} \times \frac{\text{Molecular weight of toxin}}{10}$$

For ethanol (the most common cause of Δ osm), a gap of 30 mosm/kg H_2O indicates an ethanol level of:

$$30 \times \frac{46}{10} = 138 \text{ mg/dL}$$

See the following for lethal concentrations of alcohols and their corresponding osmolal gaps.

LETHAL CONCENTRATIONS OF ALCOHOLS AND THEIR CORRESPONDING OSMOLAL GAPS

	Molecular Weight	Lethal Concentration (mg/dL)	Corresponding Osmolal Gap (mosm/kg H_2O)
Ethanol	46	350	75
Methanol	32	80	25
Ethylene glycol	62	200	35
Isopropanol	60	350	60

Note: *Most laboratories use the freezing point method for calculating osmolality. If the vaporization point method is used, alcohols are driven off and their contribution to osmolality is lost.*
[1] *Modified, with permission, from: Tierney LM Jr, McPhee SJ, Papadakis MA (editors):* Current Medical Diagnosis & Treatment 2000. *McGraw-Hill, 2000.*
Na$^+$ = sodium; **BUN** = blood urea nitrogen.

TABLE 8–13. PLEURAL FLUID: PLEURAL FLUID PROFILES IN VARIOUS DISEASE STATES.[1]

Diagnosis	Gross Appearance	Protein (g/dL)	Glucose[2] (mg/dL)	WBC and Differential (per μL)	RBC (per μL)	Microscopic Exam	Culture	Comments
Normal	Clear	1–1.5	Equal to serum	≤1000, mostly MN	0 or Few	Neg	Neg	
TRANSUDATES[3]								
Congestive heart failure	Serous	<3; sometimes ≥3	Equal to serum	<1000	<10,000	Neg	Neg	Most common cause of pleural effusion. Effusion right-sided in 55–70% of patients.
Nephrotic syndrome	Serous	<3	Equal to serum	<1000	<1000	Neg	Neg	Occurs in 20% of patients. Cause is low protein osmotic pressure.
Hepatic cirrhosis	Serous	<3	Equal to serum	<1000	<1000	Neg	Neg	From movement of ascites across diaphragm. Treatment of underlying ascites usually sufficient.
EXUDATES[3]								
Tuberculosis	Usually serous; can be bloody	90% ≥3; may exceed 5 g/dL	Equal to serum; Occ <60	500–10,000, mostly MN	<10,000	Concentrate Pos for AFB in <50%	May yield MTb	PPD usually positive; pleural biopsy positive; eosinophils (>10%) or mesothelial cells (>5%) make diagnosis unlikely.
Malignancy	Usually turbid, bloody; Occ serous	90% ≥3	Equal to serum; <60 in 15% of cases	1000–10,000 mostly MN	>100,000	Pos cytology in 50%	Neg	Eosinophils uncommon; fluid tends to reaccumulate after removal.

Empyema	Turbid to purulent	≥3	Less than serum, often <20	25,000–100,000, mostly PMN	<5,000	Pos	Pos	Drainage necessary; putrid odor suggests anaerobic infection.
Parapneumonic effusion, uncomplicated	Clear to turbid	≥3	Equal to serum	5000–25,000, mostly PMN	<5,000	Neg	Neg	Tube thoracostomy unnecessary; associated infiltrate on chest x-ray; fluid pH ≥7.2.
Pulmonary embolism, infarction	Serous to grossly bloody	≥3	Equal to serum	1000–50,000, MN or PMN	100–>100,000	Neg	Neg	Variable findings; 25% are transudates.
Rheumatoid arthritis or other collagen-vascular disease	Turbid or yellow-green	≥3	Very low (<40 in most); in RA, 5–20 mg/dL	1000–20,000, mostly MN	<1000	Neg	Neg	Rapid clotting time; secondary empyema common.
Pancreatitis	Turbid to serosanguineous	≥3	Equal to serum	1000–50,000, mostly PMN	1000–10,000	Neg	Neg	Effusion usually left-sided; high amylase level.
Esophageal rupture	Turbid to purulent; red-brown	≥3	Usually low	<5000–over 50,000, mostly PMN	<5000	Pos	Pos	Effusion usually left-sided; high fluid amylase level (salivary); pneumothorax in 25% of cases; pH <6.0 strongly suggests diagnosis.

[1] Modified, with permission, from Therapy of pleural effusion. A statement by the Committee on Therapy. Am Rev Respir Dis 1968–97;479; Tierney LM Jr. McPhee SJ, Papadakis MA (editors); Current Medical Diagnosis & Treatment 2000. McGraw-Hill, 2000, and Way LW (editor): Current Surgical Diagnosis & Treatment. 10th ed. Originally published by Appleton & Lange. Copyright © 1974 by The McGraw-Hill Companies, Inc.

[2] Glucose of pleural fluid in comparison to serum glucose.

[3] Exudative pleural effusions meet at least one of the following criteria: (1) pleural fluid protein/serum protein ratio >0.5; (2) pleural fluid LDH/serum LDH ratio >0.6; and (3) pleural fluid LDH >$\frac{2}{3}$ upper normal limit for serum LDH. Transudative pleural effusions meet none of these criteria. Transudative effusions also occur in myxedema and sarcoidosis.

MN = mononuclear cells (lymphocytes or monocytes); **PMN** = polymorphonuclear cells; **AFB** = acid-fast bacilli; **MTb** = Mycobacterium tuberculosis.

TABLE 8–14. PRENATAL DIAGNOSTIC METHODS: AMNIOCENTESIS AND CHORIONIC VILLUS SAMPLING.[1]

Method	Procedure	Laboratory Analysis	Waiting Time for Results	Advantages	Disadvantages
Amniocentesis	Between the 12th and 16th weeks, and by the transabdominal approach, 10–30 mL of amniotic fluid is removed for cytologic and biochemical analysis. Preceding ultrasound locates the placenta and identifies twinning and missed abortion.	**1. Amniotic fluid:** • Alpha-fetoprotein • Limited biochemical analysis • Virus isolation studies **2. Amniotic cell culture:** • Chromosomal analysis	3–4 weeks	Over 35 years of experience.	Therapeutic abortion, if indicated, must be done in the second trimester. (RhoGam should be given to Rh-negative mothers to prevent sensitization.) Risks (approximately 1%): • Fetal: puncture or abortion. • Maternal: infection or bleeding.
Chorionic villus sampling	Between the 8th and 12th week, and with constant ultrasound guidance, the trophoblastic cells of the chorionic villi are obtained by transcervical or transabdominal endoscopic needle biopsy or aspiration.	**1. Direct cell analysis** • Chromosomal studies **2. Cell culture:** • Limited biochemical analysis	1–10 days	Over 15 years of experience. Therapeutic abortion, if indicated, can be done in the first trimester.	Risks (approximately 3%): • Fetal: abortion. • Maternal: bleeding and infection (uncommon).

[1] Modified, with permission, from Schroeder SA et al (editors): Current Medical Diagnosis & Treatment 1990. Originally published by Appleton & Lange. Copyright © 1990 by The McGraw-Hill Companies, Inc.

TABLE 8–15. PULMONARY FUNCTION TESTS: INTERPRETATION IN OBSTRUCTIVE AND RESTRICTIVE PULMONARY DISEASE.[1]

Tests	Units	Definition	Obstructive Disease	Restrictive Disease
SPIROMETRY				
Forced vital capacity (FVC)	L	The volume that can be forcefully expelled from the lungs after maximal inspiration.	N or ↓	↓
Forced expiratory volume in one second (FEV_1)	L	The volume expelled in the first second of the FVC maneuver.	↓	N or ↓
FEV_1/FVC	%		↓	N or ↑
Forced expiratory flow from 25% to 75% of the forced vital capacity (FEF 25–75%)	L/sec	The maximal midexpiratory airflow rate.	↓	N or ↓
Peak expiratory flow rate (PEFR)	L/sec	The maximal airflow rate achieved in the FVC maneuver.	↓	N or ↑
Maximum voluntary ventilation (MVV)	L/min	The maximum volume that can be breathed in 1 minute (usually measured for 15 seconds and multiplied by 4).	↓	N or ↓
LUNG VOLUMES				
Slow vital capacity (SVC)	L	The volume that can be slowly exhaled after maximal inspiration.	N or ↓	↓
Total lung capacity (TLC)	L	The volume in the lungs after a maximal inspiration.	N or ↑	↓
Functional residual capacity (FRC)	L	The volume in the lungs at the end of a normal tidal expiration.	↑	N or ↑
Expiratory reserve volume (ERV)	L	The volume representing the difference between functional residual capacity and residual volume.	N or ↓	N or ↓
Residual volume (RV)	L	The volume remaining in the lungs after maximal expiration.	↑	N or ↑
RV/TLC ratio	...		↑	N or ↑

[1] Modified, with permission, from Tierney LM Jr, McPhee SJ, Papadakis MA (editors): Current Medical Diagnosis & Treatment 2000. McGraw-Hill, 2000.
N = normal; ↓ = less than predicted; ↑ = greater than predicted. Normal values vary according to subject sex, age, body size, and ethnicity.

TABLE 8–16. RANSON'S CRITERIA FOR SEVERITY OF ACUTE PANCREATITIS.[1]

Criteria present at diagnosis or admission
  Age over 55 years
  White blood cell count >16,000/μL
  Blood glucose >200 mg/dL
  Serum LDH >350 IU/L (laboratory-specific)
  AST (SGOT) >250 IU/L (laboratory-specific)

Criteria developing during first 48 hours
  Hematocrit fall >10%
  BUN rise >5 mg/dL
  Serum calcium <8 mg/dL
  Arterial PO_2 <60 mm Hg
  Base deficit >4 meq/L
  Estimated fluid sequestration >6 L

MORTALITY RATES CORRELATE WITH THE NUMBER OF CRITERIA PRESENT:

Number of Criteria	Mortality
0–2	1%
3–4	16%
5–6	40%
7–8	100%

[1] *Modified from Way LW (editor):* Current Surgical Diagnosis & Treatment, *10th ed. Originally published by Appleton & Lange. Copyright © 1994 by the McGraw-Hill Companies, Inc. 1994.*
LDH = *lactic dehydrogenase;* **AST** = *aspartate dehydrogenase;* **BUN** = *blood urea nitrogen.*

TABLE 8–17. CLASSIFICATION AND DIFFERENTIAL DIAGNOSIS OF RENAL FAILURE.[1]

Classification	Prerenal Azotemia	Postrenal Azotemia	Acute Tubular Necrosis (Oliguric or Polyuric)	Intrinsic Renal Disease		
				Acute Glomerulonephritis	Acute Interstitial Nephritis
Etiology	Poor renal perfusion	Obstruction of the urinary tract	Ischemia, nephrotoxins	Poststreptococcal; collagen-vascular disease	Allergic reaction; drug reaction
Urinary indices Serum BUN: Cr ratio	>20:1	>20:1	<20:1	>20:1	<20:1
U_{Na} (meq/L)	<20	Variable	>20	<20	Variable
FE_{Na^+} (%)	<1	Variable	>1	<1	<1; >1
Urine osmolality (mosm/kg)	>500	<400	250–300	Variable	Variable
Urinary sediment	Benign, or hyaline casts	Normal or red cells, white cells, or crystals	Granular casts, renal tubular cells	Dysmorphic red cells and red cell casts	White cells, white cell casts, with or without eosinophils

[1] Reproduced, with permission, from Tierney LM Jr., McPhee SJ, Papadakis MA (editors): Current Medical Diagnosis & Treatment 2000. McGraw-Hill, 2000.

$$FE_{Na^+} = \left(\dfrac{\dfrac{Urine\ Na^+}{Plasma\ Na^+}}{\dfrac{Urine\ creatinine}{Plasma\ creatinine}} \right) \times 100$$

U_{Na} = urine sodium.

TABLE 8–18. RENAL TUBULAR ACIDOSIS (RTA): LABORATORY DIAGNOSIS OF RENAL TUBULAR ACIDOSIS.[1]

Clinical Condition	Renal Defect	GFR	Serum [HCO_3^-] (meq/L)	Serum [K^+] (meq/L)	Minimal Urine pH	Associated Disease States	Treatment
Normal	None	N	24–28	3.5–5	4.8–5.2	None	None
Proximal RTA (type II)	Proximal H^+ secretion	N	15–18	↓	<5.5	Drugs, Fanconi's syndrome, various genetic disorders, dysproteinemic states, secondary hyperparathyroidism, toxins (heavy metals), tubulointerstitial diseases, nephrotic syndrome, paroxysmal nocturnal hemoglobinuria.	$NaHCO_3$, or $KHCO_3$ (10–15 meq/kg/d), thiazides.
Classic distal RTA (type I)	Distal H^+ secretion	N	20–23	↓	>5.5	Various genetic disorders, autoimmune diseases, nephrocalcinosis, drugs, toxins, tubulointerstitial diseases, hepatic cirrhosis, empty sella syndrome.	$NaHCO_3$ (1–3 meq/kg/d).
Buffer deficiency distal RTA (type III)	Distal NH_3 delivery	↓	15–18	N	<5.5	Chronic renal insufficiency, renal osteodystrophy, severe hypophosphatemia.	$NaHCO_3$ (1–3 meq/kg/d).
Generalized distal RTA (type IV)	Distal Na^+ reabsorption, K^+ secretion, and H^+ secretion	↓	24–28	↑	<5.5	Primary mineralocorticoid deficiency (eg, Addison's disease), hyporeninemic hypoaldosteronism (diabetes mellitus, tubulointerstitial diseases, nephrosclerosis, drugs), salt-wasting mineralocorticoid-resistant hyperkalemia.	Fludrocortisone (0.1–0.5 mg/d), dietary K^+ restriction, furosemide (40–160 mg/d), $NaHCO_3$ (1–3 meq/kg/d).

[1] Modified, with permission, from Cogan MG: Fluid & Electrolytes: Physiology & Pathophysiology. Originally published by Appleton & Lange. Copyright © 1991 by the McGraw-Hill Companies, Inc.
GFR = glomerular filtration rate.

TABLE 8–19. SYNOVIAL FLUID: CLASSIFICATION OF SYNOVIAL (JOINT) FLUID.[1]

Type of Joint Fluid	Volume (mL)	Viscosity	Appearance	WBC (per µL)	PMNs	Gram's Stain & Culture	Glucose	Comments
Normal	<3.5	High	Clear, light yellow	<200	<25%	Neg	Equal to serum	Protein 2–3.5 g/dL.
Non-inflammatory (Class I)	Often >3.5	High	Clear, light yellow	200–2000	<25%	Neg	Equal to serum	Protein 2–3.5 g/dL. Degenerative joint disease, trauma, avascular necrosis, osteochondritis dissecans; osteochondromatosis, neuropathic arthropathy, subsiding or early inflammation, hypertrophic osteoarthropathy, pigmented villonodular synovitis.
Inflammatory (Class II)	Often >3.5	Low	Cloudy to opaque, dark yellow	3000–100,000	≥50%	Neg	>25, but lower than serum	Protein >3 g/dL. Rheumatoid arthritis, acute crystal-induced synovitis (gout, pseudogout); Reiter's syndrome, ankylosing spondylitis, psoriatic arthritis, sarcoidosis, arthritis accompanying ulcerative colitis and Crohn's, rheumatic fever, SLE, scleroderma; tuberculous, viral, or mycotic infections. Crystals diagnostic of gout or pseudogout: gout (urate) crystals show negative birefringence, pseudogout (calcium pyrophosphate) show positive birefringence when red compensator filter is used with polarized light microscopy.

TABLE 8–19 (CONTINUED).

Type of Joint Fluid	Volume (mL)	Viscosity	Appearance	WBC (per µL)	PMNs	Gram Stain & Culture	Glucose	Comments
Inflammatory (Class II) (Continued)								Phagocytic inclusions in PMNs suggest rheumatoid arthritis (RA cells). Phagocytosis of leukocytes by macrophages seen in Reiter's syndrome.
Purulent (Class III)	Often >3.5	Low	Cloudy to opaque, dark yellow to green	Usually >40,000, often >100,000	≥75%	Usually positive	<25, much lower than serum	Pyogenic bacterial infection (eg, *N gonorrhoeae*, *S aureus*). Bacteria on culture or Gram-stained smear. Commonest exception: gonococci seen in only about 25% of cases. WBC count and % PMN lower with infections caused by organisms of low virulence or if antibiotic therapy already started.
Hemorrhagic (Class IV)	Often >3.5	Variable	Cloudy, pink to red	Usually >2000	30%	Neg	Equal to serum	Trauma with or without fracture, hemophilia or other hemorrhagic diathesis, neuropathic arthropathy, pigmented villonodular synovitis, synovioma, hemangioma and other benign neoplasms. Many RBCs found also. Fat globules strongly suggest intra-articular fracture.

[1] Modified, with permission, from Rodnan GP: Primer on the rheumatic diseases: Appendix III. JAMA 1973;224(5):802–803. Copyright © 1973 by American Medical Association.

TABLE 8–20. SYPHILIS: LABORATORY DIAGNOSIS IN UNTREATED PATIENTS.[1]

Stage	Onset After Exposure	Persistence	Clinical Findings	Sensitivity of VDRL or RPR[2] (%)	Sensitivity of FTA-ABS[3] (%)	Sensitivity of MHA-TP[4] (%)
Primary	21 days (range 10–90)	2–12 wk	Chancre	72	91	50–60
Secondary	6 wk–6 mo	1–3 mo	Rash, condylomata lata, mucous patches, fever, lymphadenopathy, patchy alopecia	100	100	100
Early latent	<1 yr	Up to 1 yr	Relapses of secondary syphilis	73	97	98
Late latent	>1 yr	Lifelong unless tertiary syphilis appears	Clinically silent	73	97	98
Tertiary	1 yr until death	Until death	Dementia, tabes dorsalis, aortitis, aortic aneurysm, gummas	77	99	98

[1] Modified, with permission, from Harvey AM et al (editors): The Principles and Practice of Medicine, 22nd ed. Originally published by Appleton & Lange. Copyright © 1988 by The McGraw-Hill Companies, Inc.

[2] VDRL is a slide flocculation test for nonspecific (anticardiolipin) antibodies, used for screening, quantitation of titer, and monitoring response to treatment; RPR is an agglutination test for nonspecific antibodies, used primarily for screening.

[3] FTA-ABS is an immunofluorescence test for treponemal antibodies utilizing serum absorbed for nonpathogenic treponemes, used for confirmation of infection, not routine screening.

[4] MHA-TP is a microhemagglutination test similar to the FTA-ABS, but one which can be quantitated and automated.

VDRL = Venereal Disease Research Laboratories test; **RPR** = rapid plasma reagin test; **FTA-ABS** = fluorescent treponemal antibody absorption test; **MHA-TP** = microhemagglutination assay for T pallidum.

TABLE 8–21. ALPHA-THALASSEMIA SYNDROMES.[1,2]

Syndrome	Alpha Globin Genes	Hematocrit	MCV (fL)
Normal	4	N	N
Silent carrier	3	N	N
Thalassemia minor	2	32–40%	60–75
Hemoglobin H disease	1	22–32%	60–75
Hydrops fetalis	0	Fetal death occurs in utero	

[1] Modified, with permission, from Tiemey LM Jr, McPhee SJ, Papadakis MA (editors): Current Medical Diagnosis & Treatment 2000. McGraw-Hill, 2000.
[2] Alpha thalassemias are due primarily to deletion in the alpha globin gene on chromosome 16.

TABLE 8–22. BETA-THALASSEMIA SYNDROMES: FINDINGS ON HEMOGLOBIN ELECTROPHORESIS.[1,2]

Syndrome	Beta Globin Genes	Hb A[3]	Hb A$_2$[4]	Hb F[5]
Normal	Homozygous beta	97–99%	1–3%	<1%
Thalassemia minor	Heterozygous beta^0[6]	80–95%	4–8%	1–5%
	Heterozygous beta$^+$[7]	80–95%	4–8%	1–5%
Thalassemia intermedia	Homozygous beta$^+$ (mild)	0–30%	0–10%	6–100%
Thalassemia major	Homozygous beta^0	0	4–10%	90–96%
	Homozygous beta$^+$		4–10%	

[1] Modified, with permission, from Tierney LM Jr. McPhee SJ, Papadakis MA (editors): Current Medical Diagnosis & Treatment 2000. McGraw-Hill, 2000.
[2] Beta thalassemias are usually caused by point mutations in the beta globin gene on chromosome 11 that result in premature chain terminations or defective RNA transcription, leading to reduced or absent beta globin chain synthesis.
[3] Hb A is composed of two alpha chains and two beta chains: $\alpha_2\beta_2$
[4] Hb A$_2$ is composed of two alpha chains and two delta chains: $\alpha_2\delta_2$.
[5] Hb F is composed of two alpha chains and two gamma chains: $\alpha_2\gamma_2$.
[6] Beta^0 refers to defects that result in absent globin chain synthesis.
[7] Beta$^+$ refers to defects that cause reduced globin chain synthesis.

TABLE 8–23. THYROID FUNCTION TESTS.[1]

	Total T4 (µg/dL)	Free T4 (ng/dL)	Total T3 (ng/dL)	Sensitive Serum TSH (RIA) (µU/mL)	RAI (^{123}) Uptake (at 24 hours)	Comments and Treatment
Normal[2]	5–12	Varies with method	95–190	0.3–5	10–30%	
Hyperthyroidism	↑	↑	↑	↓	↑	In TRH stimulation test, TSH shows no response. Thyroid scan shows increased diffuse activity (Graves' disease) versus "hot" areas (hyperfunctioning nodules). Thyroperoxidase (TPO) and thyroid-stimulating hormone receptor antibodies (TSH-R Ab [stim]) elevated in Graves' disease.
Hypothyroidism	↓	↓	↓	Usually ↑ (primary[3] hypothyroidism, rarely ↓ (secondary[4] hypothyroidism)	N or ↓	TRH stimulation test shows exaggerated response in primary hypothyroidism. In secondary hypothyroidism, TRH test helps to differentiate pituitary from hypothalamic disorders. In pituitary lesions, TSH fails to rise after TRH; in hypothalamic lesion, TSH rises but response is delayed. Antithyroglobulin and thyroperoxidase (TPO) antibodies elevated in Hashimoto's thyroiditis.
HYPOTHYROIDISM ON REPLACEMENT						
T4 replacement	N	N	>	N or ↓	↓	TSH ↓ with 0.1–0.2 mg T4 daily.
T3 replacement	↓	↓	>	N or ↓	↓	TSH ↓ with 50 µg T3 daily.
Euthyroid following injection of radiocontrast dye	N	N or ↑	N	N	↓	Effects may persist for 2 weeks or longer.

TABLE 8–23 (CONTINUED).

	Total T_4 (µg/dL)	Free T_4 (ng/dL)	Total T_3 (ng/dL)	Sensitive Serum TSH (RIA) (µU/mL)	RAI (^{123}I) Uptake (at 24 hours)	Comments and Treatment
PREGNANCY						
Hyperthyroid	↑	↑	↑	↓		Effects may persist for 6–10 weeks post-partum. RAI uptake contraindicated in pregnancy.
Euthyroid	↑	N	↑	N		
Hypothyroid	N or ↓	↓		↑		
Oral contraceptives, estrogens, methadone, heroin	↑	N	↑	N	N	Increased serum thyroid-binding globulin.
Glucocorticoids, androgens, phenytoin, asparaginase, salicylates (high-dose)	↓	N	N or ↓	N	N	Decreased serum thyroid-binding globulin.
Nephrotic syndrome	↓	N	N or ↓	N	N	Loss of thyroid-binding globulin accounts for serum T_4 decrease.
Iodine deficiency	N	N	N	N	↑	Extremely rare in USA.
Iodine ingestion	N	N	N	N	↓	Excess iodine may cause hypothyroidism or hyperthyroidism in susceptible individuals.

Modified, with permission, from Leeper RD: Current Concepts 1972;1:1. Courtesy of Upjohn Co., Kalamazoo, MI.

[1] Normal values vary with laboratory.
[2] Thyroid (end-organ) failure.
[3] Pituitary or hypothalamic lesions.
N = normal; **V** = variable.

TABLE 8–24. URINE COMPOSITION: IN COMMON DISEASE STATES.[1]

Disease	Daily Volume	Specific Gravity	Protein[2] (mg/dL)	Esterase	Nitrite	RBC	WBC	Casts	Other Microscopic Findings
Normal	600–2500 mL	1.003–1.030	0–trace (0–30)	Neg	Neg	0 or Occ	0 or Occ	0 or Occ	Hyaline casts
Fever	↓	↑	Trace or 1+ (<30)	Neg	Neg	0	Occ	0 or Occ	Hyaline casts, tubular cells
Congestive heart failure	↓	↑ (varies)	1–2+ (30–100)	Neg	Neg	None or 1+	0	1+	Hyaline and granular casts
Eclampsia	↓	↑	3–4+ (30–2000)	Neg	Neg	None or 1+	0	3–4+	Hyaline casts
Diabetic coma	↑ or ↓	↑	1+ (30)	Neg	Neg	0	0	0 or 1+	Hyaline casts
Acute glomerulonephritis	↓	↑	2–4+ (100–2000)	Pos	Neg	1–4+	1–4+	2–4+	Blood; RBC, cellular, granular, and hyaline casts; renal tubular epithelium
Nephrotic syndrome	N or ↓	N or ↑	4+ (>2000)	Neg	Neg	1–2+	0	4+	Granular, waxy, hyaline, and fatty casts; fatty tubular cells
Chronic renal failure	↑ or ↓	Low; invariable	1–2+ (30–100)	Neg	Neg	Occ or 1+	0	1–3+	Granular, hyaline, fatty, and broad casts

TABLE 8–24 (CONTINUED).

Disease	Daily Volume	Specific Gravity	Protein[2] (mg/dL)	Esterase	Nitrite	RBC	WBC	Casts	Other Microscopic Findings
Collagen-vascular disease	N, ↑ or ↓	N or ↓	1–4+ (30–2000)	Neg	Neg	1–4+	0 or Occ	1–4+	Blood, cellular, granular, hyaline, waxy, fatty, and broad casts; fatty tubular cells; telescoped sediment
Pyelonephritis	N or ↓	N or ↓	1–2+ (30–100)	Pos	Pos	0 or 1+	4+	0 or 1+	WBC casts and hyaline casts; many pus cells; bacteria
Hypertension	N of ↑	N or ↓	None or 1+ (<30)	Neg	Neg	0 or Occ	0 or Occ	0 or 1+	Hyaline and granular casts

[1] Modified, with permission, from Krupp MA et al (editors): Physician's Handbook, 21st ed. Originally published by Appleton & Lange. Copyright © 1985 by The McGraw-Hill Companies, Inc.

[2] Protein concentration in mg/dL is listed in parentheses.

TABLE 8–25. VAGINAL DISCHARGE: LABORATORY EVALUATION.[1]

Diagnosis	pH	Odor With KOH (Positive "Whiff" Test)	Epithelial Cells	WBCs	Organisms	KOH Prep	Gram Stain	Comments
Normal	<4.5	No	N	Occ	Variable, large rods not adherent to epithelial cells	Neg	Gram-positive rods	
Trichomonas vaginalis vaginitis	>4.5	Yes	N	↑	Motile, flagellated organisms	Neg	Flagellated organisms	
Bacterial vaginosis (*Gardnerella vaginalis*)	>4.5	Yes	Clue cells[2]	Occ	Coccobacilli adherent to epithelial cells	Neg	Gram-negative coccobacilli	
Candida albicans vaginitis	<4.5	No	N	Occ slightly increased	Budding yeast or hyphae	Budding yeast or hyphae	Budding yeast or hyphae	Usually white "cottage cheese" curd
Mucopurulent cervicitis (*N gonorrhoeae*)	Variable, usually >4.5	No	N	↑	Variable	Neg	Intracellular gram-negative diplococci	

[1] Modified, with permission, from Kelly KG: Tests on vaginal discharge. In: Walker HK et al (editors): Clinical Methods: The History, Physical and Laboratory Examinations, 3rd ed. Butterworths, 1990.

[2] Epithelial cells covered with bacteria to the extent that cell nuclear borders are obscured.

TABLE 8–26. VALVULAR HEART DISEASE: DIAGNOSTIC EVALUATION OF CARDIAC VALVULAR DISEASE. [1]

Diagnosis	Chest X-ray	ECG	Echocardiography	Comments
MITRAL STENOSIS (MS) Rheumatic disease	Straight left heart border. Large LA sharply indenting esophagus. Elevation of left main bronchus. Calcification occ seen in MV.	Broad negative phase of biphasic P in V$_1$. Tall peaked P waves, right axis deviation, or RVH appear if pulmonary hypertension is present.	**M-Mode:** Thickened, immobile MV with anterior and posterior leaflets moving together. Slow early diastolic filling slope. Normal to small LV. **2D:** Maximum diastolic orifice size reduced. Reduced subvalvular apparatus. Foreshortened, variable thickening of other valves. **Doppler:** Prolonged pressure half-time across MV. Indirect evidence of pulmonary hypertension.	"Critical" MS is usually defined as a valve area <1.0 cm^2. Balloon valvuloplasty has high initial success rates and higher patency rates than for AS. Open commissurotomy can be effective. Valve replacement is indicated when severe regurgitation is present. Catheterization can confirm echo results.
MITRAL REGURGITATION (MR) Myxomatous degeneration (MV prolapse) Infective endocarditis Subvalvular dysfunction Rheumatic disease	Enlarged LV and LA.	Left axis deviation or frank LVH. P waves broad, tall, or notched, with broad negative phase in V$_1$.	**M-Mode and 2D:** Thickened MV in rheumatic disease. MV prolapse; flail leaflet or vegetations may be seen. Enlarged LV. **Doppler:** Regurgitant flow mapped into LA. Indirect evidence of pulmonary hypertension.	In nonrheumatic MR, valvuloplasty without valve replacement is increasingly successful. Acute MR (endocarditis, ruptured chordae) requires emergent valve replacement. Catheterization is the best assessment of regurgitation.
AORTIC STENOSIS (AS) Calcific (especially in congenitally bicuspid valve) Rheumatic disease	Concentric LVH. Prominent ascending aorta, small knob. Calcified valve common.	LVH.	**M-Mode:** Dense persistent echoes of the AoV with poor leaflet excursion. LVH with preserved contractile function. **2D:** Poststenotic dilatation of the aorta with restricted opening of the leaflets. Bicuspid AoV in about 30%.	"Critical" AS is usually defined as a valve area <0.7 cm^2 or a peak systolic gradient of >50 mm Hg. Catheterization is definitive diagnostic test.

			Doppler: Increased transvalvular flow velocity, yielding calculated gradient.	Prognosis without surgery is less than 50% survival at 3 yr when CHF, syncope, or angina occur. Balloon valvuloplasty has a high restenosis rate.
AORTIC REGURGITATION (AR) Bicuspid valves Infective endocarditis Hypertension Rheumatic disease Aorta/aortic root disease	Moderate to severe LV enlargement. Prominent aortic knob.	LVH.	**M-Mode:** Diastolic vibrations of the anterior leaflet of the MV and septum. Early closure of the valve when severe. Dilated LV with normal or decreased contractility. **2D:** May show vegetations in endocarditis, bicuspid valve, or root dilatation. **Doppler:** Demonstrates regurgitation. Estimates severity.	Aortography at catheterization can demonstrate AR. Acute incompetence leads to LV failure and requires AoV replacement.
TRICUSPID STENOSIS (TS) Rheumatic disease	Enlarged RA only.	Tall, peaked P waves. Normal axis.	**M-Mode and 2D:** TV thickening. Decreased early diastolic filling slope of the TV. MV also usually abnormal. **Doppler:** Prolonged pressure half-time across TV.	Right heart catheterization is diagnostic. Valvulotomy may lead to success, but TV replacement is usually needed.
TRICUSPID REGURGITATION (TR) RV overload (pulmonary hypertension) Inferior infarction Infective endocarditis	Enlarged RA and RV.	Right axis deviation usual.	**M-Mode and 2D:** Enlarged RV. MV often abnormal and may prolapse. **Doppler:** Regurgitant flow mapped into RA and venae cavae. RV systolic pressure estimated.	RA and jugular pressure tracings show a prominent V wave and rapid Y descent. Replacement of TV is rarely done. Valvuloplasty is often preferred.

[1] Modified, with permission, from Tierney LM Jr, McPhee SJ, Papadakis MA (editors): Current Medical Diagnosis & Treatment 2000. McGraw Hill, 2000.
RA = right atrium; **RV** = right ventricle; **LA** = left atrium; **LV** = left ventricle; **AoV** = aortic valve; **MV** = mitral valve; **TV** = tricuspid valve; **LVH** = left ventricular hypertrophy; **RVH** = right ventricular hypertrophy; **CHF** = congestive heart failure.

TABLE 8–27. WHITE BLOOD CELLS: WHITE BLOOD CELL COUNT AND DIFFERENTIAL.[1]

Cells	Range ($10^3/\mu L$)	Increased in	Decreased in
WBC count (total)	3.4–10.0	Infection, hematologic malignancy.	Decreased production (aplastic anemia, folate or B_{12} deficiency, drugs [eg, ethanol, chloramphenicol]); decreased survival (sepsis, hypersplenism, drugs).
Neutrophils	1.8–6.8	Infection (bacterial or early viral), acute stress, acute and chronic inflammation, tumors, drugs, diabetic ketoacidosis, leukemia (rare).	Aplastic anemia, drug-induced neutropenia (eg, chloramphenicol, phenothiazines, antithyroid drugs, sulfonamide), folate or B_{12} deficiency, Chédiak-Higashi syndrome, malignant lymphoproliferative disease, physiologic (in children up to age 4 years).
Lymphocytes	0.9–2.9	Viral infection (especially infectious mononucleosis, pertussis), thyrotoxicosis, adrenal insufficiency, ALL and CLL, chronic infection, drug and allergic reactions, autoimmune diseases.	Immune deficiency syndromes.
Monocytes	0.1–0.6	Inflammation, infection, malignancy, tuberculosis, myeloproliferative disorders.	Depleted in overwhelming bacterial infection.
Eosinophils	0–0.4	Allergic states, drug sensitivity reactions, skin disorders, tissue invasion by parasites, polyarteritis nodosa, hypersensitivity response to malignancy (eg, Hodgkin's disease), pulmonary infiltrative disease, disseminated eosinophilic hypersensitivity disease.	Acute and chronic inflammation, stress, drugs (corticosteroids).
Basophils	0–0.1	Hypersensitivity reactions, drugs, myeloproliferative disorders (eg, CML), myelofibrosis.	

[1] In the automated differential, 10,000 WBCs are classified on the basis of size and peroxidase staining as neutrophils, monocytes, or eosinophils (peroxidase-positive) and as lymphocytes or large unstained cells (LUC), which are peroxidase-negative. LUCs, larger than normal lymphocytes, may be atypical lymphocyte or peroxidase-negative blasts.
Basophils are identified using two-angle light scattering, based on their singular resistance to lysis.
The reproducibility of 100-cell manual differentials is notoriously poor. Review of blood smears is useful to visually identify rare abnormal cells, blasts, nucleated RBCs, morphologic abnormalities (eg, hypersegmentation, toxic granulation, sickle cells, target cells, spherocytes, basophilic stippling) and to look for rouleaux (stacking of red cells due to increased globulins) and clumped platelets.
WBC differential is unlikely to be abnormal with a normal WBC count or to be changed if the total WBC count is unchanged.
ALL = Acute lymphocytic leukemia; **CLL** = Chronic lymphocytic leukemia; **CML** = Chronic myelocytic leukemia.

TABLE 8-28. TRANSFUSION: SUMMARY CHART OF BLOOD COMPONENTS.[1]

Component	Major Indications	Action	Not Indicated For—	Special Precautions	Hazards[2]	Rate of Infusion
Whole blood	Symptomatic anemia with large volume deficit	Restoration of oxygen-carrying capacity, restoration of blood volume	Condition responsive to specific component	Must be ABO-identical Labile coagulation factors deteriorate within 24 hours after collection	Infectious diseases; septic/toxic, allergic, febrile reactions; circulatory overload; GVHD	For massive loss, as fast as patient can tolerate
Red blood cells; red blood cells with adenine-saline added[3]	Symptomatic anemia	Restoration of oxygen-carrying capacity	Pharmacologically treatable anemia Coagulation deficiency	Must be ABO-compatible	Infectious diseases; septic/toxic, allergic, febrile reactions; GVHD	As patient can tolerate, but less than 4 hours
Red blood cells, leukocyte-reduced	Symptomatic anemia, febrile reactions from leukocyte antibodies or cytokines, prevention of platelet refractoriness due to alloimmunization, decrease in infections and cancer recurrence (controversial)	Restoration of oxygen-carrying capacity	Pharmacologically treatable anemia Coagulation deficiency	Must be ABO-compatible	Infectious diseases; septic/toxic, allergic reactions (unless plasma also removed, eg, by washing); GVHD	As patient can tolerate, but less than 4 hours
Fresh-frozen plasma[3]	Deficit of labile and stable plasma coagulation factors and TTP	Source of labile and nonlabile plasma factors	Condition responsive to volume replacement	Must be ABO-compatible	Infectious diseases, allergic reactions, circulatory overload	Less than 4 hours

TABLE 8–28 (CONTINUED).

Component	Major Indications	Action	Not Indicated For–	Special Precautions	Hazards[2]	Rate of Infusion
Liquid plasma; plasma; and thawed plasma	Deficit of stable coagulation factors	Source of nonlabile plasma factors	Deficit of labile coagulation factors or volume replacement	Must be ABO-compatible	Infectious diseases; allergic reactions	Less than 4 hours
Cryoprecipitate AHF	Hemophilia A,[4] von Willebrand's disease,[4] hypofibrinogenemia, factor XIII deficiency	Provides factor VIII, fibrinogen, von Willebrand factor, factor XIII	Deficit of any plasma protein other than those enriched in cryoprecipitated AHF	Frequent repeat doses may be necessary for factor VIII	Infectious diseases; allergic reactions	Less than 4 hours
Platelets; platelets from pheresis[5]	Bleeding from thrombocytopenia or platelet function abnormality	Improves hemostasis	Plasma coagulation deficits and some conditions with rapid platelet destruction (eg, ITP)	Should not use some microaggregate filters (check manufacturer's instructions)	Infectious diseases; septic/toxic, allergic, febrile reactions; GVHD	Less than 4 hours
Granulocytes from pheresis	Neutropenia with infection	Provides granulocytes	Infection responsive to antibiotics	Must be ABO-compatible; do not use microaggregate filters or leuko-depletion filters	Infectious diseases; allergic, febrile reactions; GVHD	One unit over 2–4 hours. Observe closely for reactions.

[1] From: American Association of Blood Banks, American Red Cross, American Blood Centers. Circular of information for the use of human blood and blood components. Bethesda: American Association of Blood Banks 1999, 13th ed.

[2] For all cellular components, there is a risk the recipient may become alloimmunized.

[3] Solvent detergent pooled plasma is an alternative in which some viruses are inactivated, but clotting factor composition is changed.

[4] When virus-inactivated concentrates are not available.

[5] Red blood cells and platelets may be processed in a manner that yields leukocyte-reduced components. The main indications for leukocyte-reduced components are prevention of febrile, nonhemolytic transfusion reactions and prevention of leukocyte alloimmunization. Risks are the same as for standard components except for reduced risk of febrile reactions.

AHF = antihemophilic factor; **GVHD** = graft-versus-host disease; **ITP** = idiopathic thrombocytopenic purpura; **TTP** = thrombotic thrombocytopenic purpura.

Index

Page numbers followed by *t* denote tables. Those followed by *i* denote illustrations.

NOTES

NOTES

NOTES

NOTES

NOTES

NOTES

NOTES

NOTES